5 AND LESS PAIN

FIBROMYALGIA

NEW SCIENCE – REAL HOPE

A Guide to Prepare, Be Heard and Get Results

Dr. Robert J. Langone DC

ISBN: 1496033566
ISBN 13: 9781496033567
Library of Congress Control Number: 2014903713
CreateSpace Independent Publishing Platform
North Charleston, South Carolina

DISCLAIMER

Note to Readers

This book is written as educational material with no intention of diagnosing, treating, or consulting its readers.

The book is sold with the understanding that the author is not engaged in rendering medical or health advice of any kind, and, as such, this book does not constitute a doctor-patient relationship. Each reader should consult with his or her medical/health-care professional before adopting any of the suggestions in this book or drawing inferences from it.

The author and publisher specifically disclaim all responsibility or liability due to loss or risk (personal or otherwise) which may be incurred as a consequence, directly or indirectly, of the use or application of any of the contents of this book.

Vicki G.

FIBROMYALGIA:

NEW SCIENCE – REAL HOPE

INTRODUCTION

New Science–Real Hope

Why would, or should, a book such as this be concerned about hope? After all, you must already have hope or you wouldn't be reading this introduction. Why not just discuss diagnosis; the aches, pains, fatigue, and the sleeplessness of fibromyalgia; new medications and exercise, etc.? The answer is that if I did that, this book would be nothing more than a rehash of all the other books, blogs, and web information you have read in the past and can readily find with a click of your mouse. My job is to arm the reader so that he or she will be prepared to decipher and understand it all and be able to negotiate through the health-care community.

Over the past twenty years, I have found that in spite of evolving science, cutting-edge medical advances, and diverse interdisciplinary opportunities that exist, patients have little choice but to educate themselves. Patients must learn about the medical science of fibro and understand the multidisciplinary and diverse opportunities outside of their favorite doctor's office. The most successful patients are those who are willing to contribute to the knowledge base of the very doctors that they turn to for answers. Then, together, they can piece together a comprehensive diagnosis and treatment plan.

Fibromyalgia patients must do this in the midst of their personal battle with pain, fatigue, depression, and a myriad of other coexisting conditions, to say nothing of the physical and emotional stresses of everyday life—having to balance relationships and checkbooks, as well as jobs and home upkeep.

As you read, you may find the most meaningful and useful understandings are contrary to your present beliefs, and subsequently, find that your doctor is surprised or offended by your confident self-advocacy when you begin to question his or her thoughts with your newfound knowledge. Remember, this is about you and your family, not the doctor. There are things doctors don't know; first because not all doctors specialize in fibromyalgia; second, even if they do, they have tight/busy practice times and are overloaded with paperwork and managed-care constraints; hence they find it impossible to keep up with evolving science.

We will cover such things as the role that posture plays in fibromyalgia, nutritional nuances, what a person might have inherited from his or her mother, or how other conditions such as IBS, restless legs, or burning muscles relate to fatigue, the inability to sleep, headaches, and brain fog. You will learn where the pain comes from, why, and most importantly, what you can do about it.

This writing focuses primarily on women—not because they're more naïve or less capable than men when it comes to advocating for themselves, but simply because 80 to 90 percent of fibromyalgia sufferers are women. However, we have dedicated Chapter 6 to Fibro men, recognizing that there are some unique differences between genders.

We find that patients are often swept along diagnostic and treatment paths that neither they nor their doctors realize are limited by a medical paradigm that has passed its prime. My intention is to expose the unintentional lies, inconsistencies, and misunderstandings inherent in traditional Western medicine, to prepare fibromyalgia sufferers for confident self-advocacy, and to help them live a more energetic life with less pain. In turn, they can help protect their children from suffering in these same ways.

Let's backtrack for a minute. I am not offering hope as a vague concept, but rather, in concrete terms and with explanations that pivot from insights into:

- How to reduce pain without taking pills
- What causes chronic pain and fatigue
- Which medications work, and how
- Reducing confusion and frustration with doctors
- How to avoiding being overwhelmed physically and emotionally
- How MRI can confirm and help erase pain
- Knowing the limits of your doctor's education
- Mindfulness as an opportunity for recovery
- The science linking fibro to IBS, insomnia, CFS, muscle/joint pain
- The fibro-science behind burning, tingling, migraines, etc.
- Men and children who have fibro
- Knowing that fibromyalgia is real and is not the patient's fault

Does hope seem like too much to hope for sometimes? You may find that by completing a "Happiness/Optimism Quiz" your personal emotional roadblocks are revealed. To complete the quiz, go to www.fibro-doc.com and click on the Resources tab.

Score yourself and put the score on the inside front cover of this book. After you complete the book, go back and retake the quiz, calculate your score, and enter it on the back cover of the book. I believe that your results will be inspiring. In any case, I would love to hear from you to learn what happened to your score and what the book meant to you. I would love for you to share your thoughts, criticisms, suggestions, and questions. Share with me what it was like trying to put your doctoring team together and what kinds of attitudes and roadblocks came up in the process. And, of course, I'd love to hear your fibro story right from the beginning—you can do this on our website as well by clicking on "My Fibro Story."

Why do I want to hear your story? It is because this book and its mission are all about you. This is the ultimate point of all the information that I will share. Your journey is important, and every tool available should be offered for you to evaluate and implement or set aside, depending on your specific needs. You should have all the information--from the science behind how cells produce energy to the science of how the brain perceives pain—and not just from a "medication" standpoint, but from the ancient arts of Chinese energy medicine to the centuries-old practices of yoga and other meditative exercises, from MRIs to chiropractic, acupuncture, self-help and everything in between. This book is all about you, your life, your health, your success; it is about you as your own best advocate.

I am excited and honored to put this book into your hands. More than anything, I want to give the gift of hope to you. I invite you to turn the page and take the first step on a unique and candid road of discovery to empower understanding, and a life with more energy and less pain.

LETTER TO NORMALS

by Claudia Marek

Here is my letter written to explain to family and friends what it's like to have fibromyalgia. It won't work miracles: it's hard to understand our illness from the outside looking in. But it is a start and can open the door to important dialogues. You are all welcome to use it, either as-is, or as a basis for writing your own. Remember that you have a responsibility to tell those close to you what is wrong and to communicate as clearly as you can how you feel and what you need. The best time to do that is when you are not upset!

Fibromyalgia isn't all in my head and it isn't contagious. It doesn't turn into anything serious and nobody ever died from fibromyalgia (though on really awful days they might have wished they could!). If you want to read articles or books about fibromyalgia, I can show you some that I think are good. If you just want to learn as we go along, that's fine too. This is definitely going to be a process. The first step is for you to believe that there is an illness called fibromyalgia and that I have it. This may sound simple, but when you hear about my symptoms, I don't want you to think I'm making this all up.

Fibromyalgia is a high-maintenance condition with lots and lots of different kinds of symptoms. There's no way to just take a pill to make it go away, even for a little while. Sometimes a certain medication can make some of my symptoms more bearable. That's about the best I can hope for. Other times I may take a lot of medication but still won't feel any better. That's just the way it goes. I can't control how often I feel good or when I'm going to feel terrible. Lots of people have been cutting new drug advertisements out of magazines for me and I appreciate the thought, but I've seen them too. Look at the list of side effects and the few symptoms they help in return. Even in the best studies, those expensive compounds didn't help more than half the people who have tried them. No matter how happy the people in the pictures look, there's still no miracle drug available.

There's no cure for fibromyalgia, and it won't go away. If I am functioning normally, I am having a good day. This doesn't mean I'm getting better—I suffer from chronic pain and fatigue for which there is no cure. I can have good days, several good weeks or even months. But a good morning can suddenly turn into a terrible afternoon. I get a feeling like someone has pulled out a plug and all the energy has just run out of my body. I might get more irritable before these flares and suddenly be more sensitive to noise, or just collapse from deadening fatigue. Weather changes can have a big effect on how I feel. Other times there may be no warning; I may suddenly just feel awful. I can't warn you when this is likely to happen, because there isn't any way for me to know. Sometimes this is a real spoiler and I'm sorry. The sadness I feel for what my illness does to those around me is more than I can easily describe. You may remember me as a light-hearted, fun-loving person—and it hurts me that I am no longer what I was.

Fibromyalgics have a different kind of pain that is hard to treat. It is not caused by inflammation, like an injury. It is not a constant ache in one place, like a broken bone. It moves around my body daily and hourly and changes in severity and type. Sometimes it is dull and sometimes it is cramping or prickly. Sometimes it's jabbing and excruciating. If Eskimos have a hundred words for snow, fibromyalgics should have a hundred words for pain. Sometimes I just hurt all over like I've been beaten up or run over by a truck. Sometimes I feel too tired to lift up my arm.

Besides pain, I have muscle stiffness that is worse in the mornings and evenings. Sometimes when I get up out of a chair I feel like I am 90 years old. I may have to ask you to help me up. I'm creaky and I'm klutzy. I trip over things no one can see and I bump into the person I am walking with and I drop things and spill things because my fingers are stiff and my coordination is off. I just don't seem to connect the way I should. Hand-eye, foot-eye coordination—it's all off. I walk slowly up and down stairs because I'm stiff and I'm afraid I might fall. When there's no railing to hold on to, it's terrifying.

Because I feel bad most of the time, I am always pushing myself, and sometimes I just push myself too hard. When I do this, I pay the price. Sometimes I can summon the strength to do something special, but I will usually have to rest for a few days afterward because my body can make only so much energy. I pay a big price for overdoing it, but sometimes I have to. I know it's hard for you to understand why I can do one thing and not another. It's important for you to believe me, and trust me about this. My limitations—like my pain and my other symptoms—are invisible, but they are real.

Another symptom I have is problems with memory and concentration, which is called fibro-fog. Short-term memory is the worst! I am constantly *looking for things. I have no idea where I put down my purse, and I walk into rooms and have no idea why. Casualties are my keys, which are always lost, and my list of errands, which I write up and leave on the counter when I go out. Even if I put notes around to remind myself of important things, I'm still liable to forget them. Don't worry; this is normal for fibromyalgics. Most of us are frightened that we are getting Alzheimer's. New kinds of brain scans have actually documented differences in our brains.*

I mentioned my sensitivities earlier and I need to talk about them again. It's more like an intolerance for everything. Noise—especially certain noises like the television or shrill noises—can make me jittery and anxious. Smells like fish or some chemicals, or fragrances or perfume, can give me headaches and nausea. I also have a problem with heat and cold. It sounds like I'm never happy, but that isn't it. These things make me physically ill. They stress me out and make my pain worse, and I get exhausted. Sometimes I just need to get away from something—I just don't know how else to say it. I know sometimes this means I will have to go outside, or out to the car, or go home to sit alone, and that's really all right. I don't want or need you to give up doing what's important to you. That would only make me feel worse. Sometimes when I feel lousy I just want to be by myself. When I'm like this, there's nothing you can do to make me feel better, so it's better to just let me be.

I have problems sleeping. Sometimes I get really restless and wake up and can't get back to sleep. Other times I can fall into bed and sleep for fourteen hours and still be tired. Some nights I'll toss and turn and not be able to sleep at all. Every little thing will keep me awake. I'm sure that's confusing to be around, and I know there are times when my tossing and turning and getting up and down to go to the bathroom disturbs you. We can talk about solutions to this.

All these symptoms and the chemical changes in my brain from pain and fatigue can make me depressed, as you may imagine. I get angry and frustrated and I have mood swings. Sometimes I know I'm being unreasonable, but I can't admit it. Sometimes I just want to pull the covers over my head and stay in bed. These emotions are all very strong and powerful. I know this is a very hard thing about being with me. Every time you put up with me when I'm in one of my moods, secretly I'm grateful. I can't always admit it at the time, but I'm admitting it now. One thing I can tell you is that it won't help to tell me I'm irrational. I know I am, but I can't help it when it's happening.

I have other symptoms like irritable bowel, muscle spasms, and pelvic pain that will take their toll on our intimacies. Some of these symptoms are embarrassing and hard to talk about, but I promise to try. I hope that you will have the patience to see me through these things. It's very hard for me too, because I love you and I want to be with you, and it makes everything worse when you are upset and tired of dealing with all my problems. I have made a promise to myself, and now I am making it to you: I will set aside time for us to be close. During that time we will not talk about my illness. We both need time to get away from its demands. Though I may not always show it, I love you a million times more for standing by me. Having to slow down physically and having to get rid of unnecessary stresses will make our relationship stronger.

This letter was generously offered to the world by Claudia. She wrote it to share fibromyalgia and its struggles with family and friends with the hope that their understanding will help others to maintain a more normal life.

INSIGHT #1

IN PERSPECTIVE: FIBRO 101

The Longest Journey Is the Journey Inward.
—Dag Hammerskjöld

CHAPTER 1

In Perspective: Fibro 101

Understanding the Basics of Fibromyalgia

Putting Fibromyalgia into Real-Life Perspective

Six to nine million Americans suffer from fibromyalgia. This estimate does not include the many unreported and undiagnosed cases, particularly of men, adolescents, and the geriatric population. While much more is known today about the diagnosis and treatment of this chronic pain syndrome, some physicians still treat it as a "wastepaper diagnosis"—a term coined by Dr. Frederick Wolf. Some doctors won't even acknowledge the syndrome's existence, and treat patients who have fibromyalgia as nothing but "chronic complainers."

To those who truly suffer from fibromyalgia, however, the syndrome is very real, and it can wreak havoc on their health, their lives, and their families. What follows are the basics to begin putting fibromyalgia into real-life perspective.

Fibromyalgia, to many sufferers, has been termed the "I hurt everywhere syndrome." This definition seems most easily relatable to sufferers and helps to establish common ground for discussion.

A more technical definition of fibromyalgia, however, involves breaking down the word into three pieces: "fibro" describes the soft tissues of the body; "my/myo" means muscles; and "algia" describes pain. Together, these three pieces lead to the technical definition of fibromyalgia as "pain in the muscles and soft tissues of the body."

Simply knowing what the word means, however, doesn't mean that we fully understand fibromyalgia. To do this, we need to gain a more specific understanding of how and why it comes about in the first place and what it means to the sufferer.

Most recently, fibromyalgia has been termed a *Central Sensitivities Syndrome* (CSS). CSS simply means that something has caused the central nervous system to become overly sensitive. This oversensitivity has the potential to cause various symptoms. When multiple symptoms exist concurrently, the malady is then called a *syndrome*. Although there are many symptoms, the majority of patients, 98 percent, report widespread pain as their major concern.

Putting pain and suffering into perspective is a crucial part of understanding fibromyalgia.[75] Pain is subjective; what one person considers painful may not even affect another. In the past, the perception of pain was thought to exist only in one's mind and feelings, as there didn't seem to be any way to document evidence of pain, and nothing to measure objectivity. We are gaining ground, however. We know that a very real neurological and chemical mechanism exists within the brain that actually accounts for a patient's personal experience/interpretation of pain.

There are endless possibilities for how the nerves and chemicals in the brain can interact to form an interpretation, opinion, and reaction to any given situation. Understanding of these mechanisms is evolving; however, as pain is subjective, it is doubtful that we will ever be able to truly understand each other's experiences and pain tolerances. You can feel pain, and you can describe how you feel, but another person will not experience your pain as you do.

The medical world has and continues to deal with the concept of pain as if it were purely abstract in nature. In a court of law, pain would be considered hearsay and not be admissible, as it's impossible to document objectively and hence would not be used as evidence. In a doctor's office, however, your doctor will be the judge of whether the pain *you say* you feel is "admissible." Where there is evidence that your pain exists, your doctor may accept it as real. Where there isn't, your doctor may not believe that you are actually in pain. Unfortunately, some people who are in pain may already have experienced this rejection.

At first glance, we may assume that where there is pain, there is suffering. However, we find that this is not always the case.

Suffering, when noted, is a frustration and embarrassment to the medical community. Suffering inherently suggests an emotional component. A woman in childbirth may be in great pain but not feel as though she is suffering.[75]

In *The Nature of Suffering*, author E.J. Cassell defined suffering as "...the state of severe distress, associated with evidence that threatens the intactness of a person." We find that if a person realizes purpose in their pain and has understanding, there is hope. He or she can then rationalize that the pain they feel holds no threat to their intactness. It is easy for a patient to rationalize pain when she feels a sense of control, hence minimizing suffering.

Fibromyalgia, however, is difficult for patients to rationalize, as it brings both pain and suffering. Patients feel pain due to the transmission of nerve signals within their brains; patients suffer because the pain is ongoing, seems out of control, and seems to have no rhyme, reason, or purpose.

Why is it that some sufferers seem to cope with fibromyalgia better than others? A reasonable explanation may lie in interpretation. Patients with a positive attitude, who have learned mental and physical exercises to help them literally train their brains to interpret pain signals differently (it can be done), seem to endure the pain and cope with fibromyalgia rather well. Others may have expectations that cause them to interpret pain in a way that reduces their ability to cope.

For example, I had confirmed the diagnosis of FM in a 46-year-old patient in 1999. She had suffered for seven years. She expressed a feeling of hopelessness because she couldn't feel the way she did when she was 24 years old: young, full of energy, healthy, and happy. She felt as if there was no reason to go on living. Her expectations and attitude sabotaged her every effort to feel better. Her brain corroborated with an appropriate level of suffering based on her expectations and attitude. Similarly, each of us may play a large and controllable role in how much we suffer.

This brief explanation of the major emotional components of fibromyalgia is just one piece of the puzzle that leads to a full understanding of fibromyalgia and fibromyalgia-like conditions. However, we find that recognizing the basic emotional issues surrounding the syndrome can help confused sufferers understand their complaints rather than seeming to be just complaining. With new understanding, communication improves, allowing doctors and patients alike to realize the pain is *very real*. This validation brings hope.[75]

CHAPTER 2
100 Years of Pain and Fatigue

History

I imagine that since the beginning of time people have had complaints, aches, pains, headaches, and episodes of sometimes not sleeping well. Back in 1978, patients who are now known to be fibromyalgia patients were commonly described as having fibrosis, fibro-myositis, and rheumatism. Previous to that, there is more than a hundred years of history, different terms, and different perspectives on the ailment. Our history writing will be a bit atypical. If you feel you would like a historian's version of fibro history, I will refer you to *Fibromyalgia Syndrome* by Leon Chaitow. He does a great job with a family-tree version. In the meantime, I will begin circa1990 when The American College of Rheumatology (ACR) set forth a formal classification. As you'll see, it has lost the majority of its validity, yet it helps to put in perspective where we've come from.

First, from Arthritis and Rheumatism, Vol. 33, No. 2 (February 1990)

The percentage of patients reporting specific symptoms breaks down as follows:

Condition	% of FMS Symptoms
Muscular Pain	100
Fatigue	96
Insomnia	86
Joint Pains	72
Headaches	60
Restless Legs	56
Numbness and Tingling	52
Impaired Memory	46
Leg Cramps	42
Impaired Concentration	42
Nervousness	32
Depression	22

The American College of Rheumatology (ACR) Classification of Fibromyalgia

Fibromyalgia is a distinctive syndrome that can be diagnosed with clinical precision. It may occur in the absence (primary fibromyalgia) or presence (concomitant fibromyalgia) of other conditions such as rheumatoid arthritis or systemic lupus erythematosus. It is rarely secondary to another disease; alleviation of the associated disease does not cure the fibromyalgia. It may be confidently diagnosed in patients with widespread musculo-skeletal pain and multiple-tender points.

History of widespread pain that has been present for at least three months

Definition: Pain is considered widespread when all of the following are present:

- Pain in both sides of the body
- Pain above and below the waist. In addition, axial skeletal pain (cervical spine, anterior chest, thoracic spine, or low back pain) must be present. Low back pain is considered lower segment pain.

Pain in 11 of 18 tender-point sites on digital palpation

Definition: Pain, upon digital palpation, must be present in at least 11 of the following 18 tender point sites as pictured below:

Digital palpation should be performed with an approximate force of 4 kg (8 pounds). A tender point has to be painful on palpation, not just "tender."

Illustration of Tender Points

Tender Points of Fibromyalgia

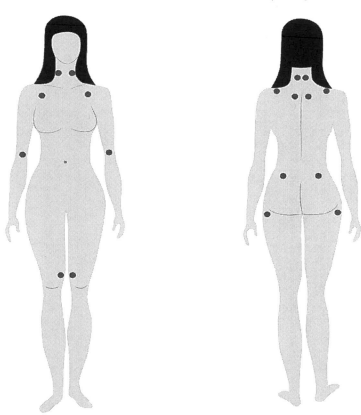

The above notes the common 18 fibromyalgia tender points frequently referred to. They are the points that most practitioners subscribe to as being definitive of fibromyalgia, however subjective and invalid they may be diagnostically. As we go on, we'll see that these diagrams serve little to no purpose in actually understanding a particular patient's condition. All definitions and all perspectives about fibromyalgia to date should be considered evolving, and each of them individually could be labeled only a hypothesis.

Some of the major flaws and inconsistencies relating to the ACR definition of 1990 are:

1. The evaluation of the 18 tender points was at best a working effort to identify fibromyalgia but had very little scientific basis and, in retrospect, would be considered arbitrary.
2. The evaluation was dependent on the skill of the examiner and the subjective interpretation of the amount of pressure used. It's almost impossible to standardize arbitrary pressure.
3. The patient's physical and emotional condition at the time of examination were not evaluated. We'll see that the physical, emotional, and chemical state of the patient at the time could vary the intensity of the tender points, and hence the patient's feedback to the doctor. This means that a person who has fibromyalgia may not be diagnosed because she happens to be having a good day; or a person who doesn't have fibromyalgia may be diagnosed as having fibromyalgia because he is having a bad day.

Fast-Forward to 2010

Let's fast-forward and look at the most contemporary definition of fibromyalgia.

- The American College of Rheumatology (ACR) 2010 criteria is used for clinical diagnosis and severity classification. Diagnosis is based on:
- Widespread Pain Index (WPI) >7 and a symptom severity scale (SS) >5 or WPI 3-6 and SS >9.
- Symptoms have been present at a similar level for at least three months.
- The patient does not have a disorder that would otherwise explain the pain.

You'll notice that this definition is simpler than the one put forward by the American College of Rheumatology in 1990. The 2010 definition is far more useful and allows physicians the flexibility to ignore previously set criteria that have not stood the test of time and clinical significance.

There is no shortage of confusing history, opinions, and hypotheses attempting to explain the path from which we have come; attempting to connect the dots between classic/true fibromyalgia and the multitude of symptoms and conditions raises the question as to whether the symptoms are simply coexisting due to other conditions, or whether they have a common causal relationship. The hypothesis that seems to surface most strongly, and is the most feasible explanation, is that fibromyalgia is an aberration and/or adaptive mechanism of the central nervous system's pain pathways and their relationship to the corruption of other nerve pathways and bodily systems. The term for this explanation is central sensitivity syndrome. In central sensitivity syndrome, the body triggers pain signals and/or amplifies normal pain signals and proceeds to interpret them inappropriately. This represents a malfunction or a primitive protective mechanism within the brain and central nervous system, accounting for the many coexisting conditions—the neurological equivalent of friendly fire. A few of the feasible explanations follow.

Causes and Management

Rheumatology or Neurology?

The concept of central sensitivity syndrome brings us to the realization that fibromyalgia may be reclassified as a neurological disorder, and accordingly should be under the auspices of the study and practice of neurology. In the early days, as you can see from the 1990 definition of fibromyalgia, it was assumed to be some type of soft tissue, joint, or autoimmune disease, and was therefore adopted by the rheumatologic community. While this interpretation appeared valid and appropriate at the time, it may have served to stall and confound advancements in fibromyalgia diagnosis and treatment.

Now, research is uncovering abnormalities within muscle tissues. Could this be the actual cause of fibro? Studies show abnormalities in muscle cells and circulation, damage to fibers due to prolonged contractions, and fragmented DNA, all of which can cause muscle fatigue and general stamina depletion. These signs/symptoms resemble premature aging. Dr. Alex Vasquez feels these finding establish fibromyalgia as a disease of metabolic dysfunction vs a syndrome, and therefore rejects other possible causes such as central sensitivity syndrome. So the plot thickens. We will contrast the theories in later chapters. My research shows that metabolic dysfunction may be one of the causes, or may represent the results of a disrupted nervous system. That still leaves the question: What type of doctor should manage your fibro?

As of this writing, it's hard to say whether a fibro sufferer would be better off primarily managed by a rheumatologist or neurologist. My opinion is that the initial diagnosis would best be made by a rheumatologist, subsequently to be co-managed by a neurologist, at least for the prescriptions that may be appropriate—with the criteria that each of them must have an abiding interest in the study of fibromyalgia. In later chapters we will discuss the necessity of what I might call triaging and co-managing with Non-medical physicians whose disciplines take a broader health and healing approach.

Relationship to Other Symptoms

The central sensitivity syndrome theory looks at the corruption of brain circuits and helps explain fibromyalgia's connection to commonly found coexisting conditions with fibromyalgia, such as fatigue, stiffness, insomnia, non-refreshing sleep, headaches, irritable bowel and/or irritable bladder, dysmenorrhea, candidiasis, sensitivity to cold, tingling, numbness, intolerance to physical activity/exercise, and anxiety and/or depression.

Many physicians feel that anxiety and depression are more commonly a result rather than a cause of the pain and disability of fibromyalgia. Let's accept that if anxiety and depression did not help to cause fibromyalgia, they will definitely be part of the clinical picture and subsequently help to confound/perpetuate the clinical picture.

When emotional factors are causative, they may be termed psychosomatic; however, as of late, in respect to the aforementioned central sensitivity syndrome, Dr. Jay Goldstein uses the term "neurosomatic." Neurosomatic is a much more appropriate term, helping to look at the condition through its true neurology as opposed to the term "psycho" somatic, which stigmatizes a suffer as a nut-job. When physicians understand patients' conditions to be psychosomatic, they are likely to attenuate the diagnostic process, quickly prescribe antidepressants, and refer the patient for counseling. We are a society sensitive to terms—giving up the term psychosomatic will help prevent regressing to the '60s and '70s, when the validity of the fibromyalgia diagnosis was questioned.

Is This My Fault? What Happened to Me?

The short answer is no, it's not your fault. As far as what has happened to you, while the scientific community is still at odds as to the exact underlying cause or causes, one thing is for sure: your body's homeostasis has been upset, demonstrated by an upset in physical, emotional and chemical balance, as well as in its ability to unlearn neurological patterns once established. It has always amazed me how quickly we can learn a new behavior or response, whether automatic or intentional, and then how difficult it is to unlearn or change our original adaptation. I remember setting up the kitchen in my first house. There was a cutting board and set of knives on the counter to the right of the sink and work area. Thoughtlessly, and with ease, I adapted to my new kitchen set-up. Several years later we remodeled the kitchen and when we did so, the knives were relocated to the left of the work area. To this day, some 16 years later, I'll catch myself reaching to the right for the knives. This is an example of the brain's easily adapting and learning a task or response, yet never completely letting go of an original pattern established. This is an important lesson that we will revisit in many chapters ahead.

So how did this fibromyalgia/neurological pain pattern happen to you? What has challenged your adaptive responses, upset your homeostasis, and caused what seems to be a permanent pattern/condition? Some of the possibilities are as follows:

1. Genetic predisposition
2. Nutritional deficiencies
3. Toxicity
4. Spinal subluxation
5. Trauma
6. Immune failure
7. Infections (viral, bacterial/fungal)
8. Chemical sensitivities
9. Emotional factors
10. Metabolic disease

You might say to yourself that this same list is true for many different illnesses: cancer, heart disease, chronic fatigue, fibromyalgia, etc. And that's true. Additionally, research has not definitively labeled any one of these particular possibilities as a causative, aggravating, perpetuating, or coexisting factor. Yet they are all very possible. In 2007, researchers Chmidte-Wilke as well as Sundgren studied brain MRIs. They found that there were physical differences between a fibromyalgia patient and a controlled group of patients in areas of the brain that interpret emotions, as well as in the thalamus. The thalamus receives and helps to interpret and distribute information that comes from the body in reference to our senses. The thalamus is also the center for appreciation of the sensation of pain, crude touch, and temperature. What's unclear is whether or not the changes demonstrated on an MRI were the cause of fibromyalgia symptoms, or the result of chronic pain—the chicken and egg dilemma, nevertheless shedding light on areas to be studied to understand neurological resistant to change.

Blood Type

In 2002 D'Adamo found that a person's blood type could play a significant role in fibromyalgia symptoms and patients with blood type O responded well to a wheat-free diet. The theory is that wheat challenges the immune system. By restricting wheat for a long enough period of time, inflammation will be reduced and the immune system will regain strength. In our clinic we find that restricting wheat is very resourceful in almost all pain syndromes, especially those with an inflammatory component. If you've ever tried restricting wheat for weight-loss purposes you know that it's a challenge. Wheat products are tasty, convenient, cheap, and everywhere. Most patients find it difficult to restrict wheat for a long enough period of time to get results. However, once restricted, energy improves, cravings are reduced, pain reduces, and weight is controlled better.

To me the flaw in the theory is that we're not convinced that fibromyalgia is an inflammatory disease. Therefore, the restriction of wheat is likely to be a pain-management method of coexisting conditions. But that's okay. With a little coaching and reorganization of our cupboards, it's easy to test out how we respond to reduced wheat.

Trauma

Trauma, such as a whiplash injury, has been noted as a frequent prelude to fibromyalgia. The whiplash injury does not have to be severe; minimal or undetectable damage can trigger hypersensitivity, subluxation, and chronic pain anywhere in the body.[10] One of the dilemmas for sufferers is to find a neurologist, orthopedist, or primary care physician (PCP) who is well-versed in the traumatic aspects of neuromuscular skeletal injury and how it relates to the long-term impact on a person's brain and central nervous system. Insurance companies often dismiss low-impact whiplash injuries as being inconsequential, in spite of a person's pain. In the meantime, the neurological damage can take its toll for a lifetime, generating what's frequently termed "invisible disabilities," including conditions such as fibromyalgia syndrome (FMS), reflex sympathetic dystrophy (RSD), idiopathic pain, and chronic subluxation complex.

Spinal Subluxation

Spinal subluxation connotes a hybrid of clinical concerns involving both the spine and the nervous system. Subluxation has a profound relationship to central sensitivity syndrome, as mentioned above.

Life's stressors will affect the central nervous system (CNS) and may cause it to generate distorted or exaggerated signals to the rest of the body, causing a multitude of functional aberrations involving muscles, ligaments, regional tissue, circulation, discs, organs, and systems of the body. However, the ways that stress affects spinal bones, joints, and the nerves entering and exiting the spine have the most impact on fibromyalgia. Spinal joints once disturbed may lose proper alignment and motion, which will corrupt nerves and account for distorted/exaggerated signals to and from the brain. This may cause and or perpetuate fibro pain.

On a case-by-case basis, there is some question as to what came first: compromised neurology due to stress, or physical stress directly disturbing spinal bones and joints. One way or another, they will both exist at the same time, constituting a subluxated condition or subluxation complex. The word "complex" is used due to the consequences that insult the complex of muscles, tendons, and ligaments as well as circulation and contiguous nerves, joints, and general physiology in the area. Uncorrected, subluxation can lead to a host of problems including spinal arthritis, degeneration, and a cascade of adaptive changes in body chemistry and general function. Ultimately, subluxation is of primary concern in all fibromyalgia cases. Let's take a look at how this might happen.

The initial stress on the CNS could come from physical, chemical, or emotional stress. Physical stress, such as a strain/sprain, or some type of injury like a whiplash or sports injury, frequently will directly damage spinal joints and nerves. Chemical stress, such as alcohol, smoking, or toxic diet/lifestyle, takes its toll over time. Emotional stress, such as job stress, financial stress, and relationship stress is unavoidable for most.[12] Regardless of the initial stress, a feedback loop—spine to brain/brain to spine—will ultimately lead to the scenario described above.

Subluxation is primarily diagnosed by physical exam, possibly with the help of electromyography (EMG). Subsequently, X-rays of the spine may be used to further understand and demonstrate adaptive changes that bones, joints, and discs have suffered as well as ruling out other conditions; subsequently helping to guide treatment. This was first reported in the early 1900s through the research of Dr. D.D. Palmer.

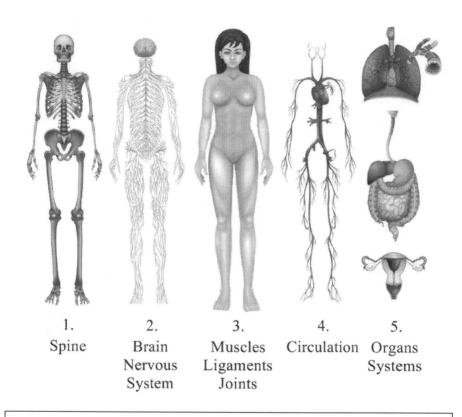

1.	2.	3.	4.	5.
Spine	Brain Nervous System	Muscles Ligaments Joints	Circulation	Organs Systems

1. Abnormal positioning or motion of spinal bones will **2.** corrupt the nervous system including the brain (subluxation). Left untreated, this will lead to **3.** muscle, ligament, and joint problems (PAIN), and **4.** abnormal circulation as well as **5.** organ/systems malfunctions, such as respiratory problems (examples: asthma/allergies) and digestive issues (examples: indigestion, IBS). Additionally, hormonal disturbances encouraging PMS, mood swings, adaptive response to stress, and sleep deprivation are likely to advance.

Subluxation is of epidemic proportions. It is likely to take its toll silently and painlessly, more like cancer or diabetes in the early stages, and to progress without being noticed. Over time it will cause imbalance within the brain, as in central sensitivity syndrome. Left uncorrected, it can lead to chronic degenerative diseases such as IBS/Crohn's, arthritis, fibromyalgia, diabetes, etc. If it's disturbing the central nervous system and the body's ability to communicate with itself, there is potential to upset any and all bodily functions, as well as to retard if not prevent recovery from illness.

The effect of a subluxation is of great importance to Fibros (in this book, I will use the term "Fibro" to refer to someone suffering from fibromyalgia). Subluxation causes a state of hyper- or hypo-excitability in and around the joints of the spine, distorting and generating in-valid /error messages to and from the brain (feedback loop) as well as to other tissues surrounding the area. Over-excited or under-excited muscles eventually lead to pain and/or develop trigger points, aka myofascial trigger points. If someone has fibromyalgia and has myo-fascial trigger points (most do), they usually will hate to have those areas touched in spite of the fact that treatment may bring relief. The dilemma is that without directly treating the subluxated segments of the spine, trigger points will continue to appear and reappear, regard-less of how effective a trigger point therapy or physical therapy session appears to be. We'll discuss the finer points of subluxation, posture, the spine, and trigger points later.

By the same token, headaches, joint pain and stiffness, digestive problems, tingling, fatigue, and a host of other symptoms may con-tinue to appear and reappear regardless of how effective medication, diet, or lifestyle changes seems to be in the short run.

Treat the Body, Not the Disease
There is an evolving hypothesis gaining recognition by naturo-pathic physicians, functional medicine specialists, and chiropractors. They are starting to see chronic pain, at least in part, as a result of chronic dysfunction of organ systems and metabolism over time, which creates disease and challenges a person's genetic makeup. Functional medicine isn't new. It represents a return to the roots of medicine before pharmaceutical companies became so powerful and influen-tial. One of the first professors at Johns Hopkins University School of Medicine and later its Physician-in-Chief was Sir William Osler. He was quoted as saying: "The good physician treats the disease; the great physician treats the patient who has the disease." Functional medicine is patient-centered care at its best. Instead of looking at and treating health problems as isolated diseases, it treats individuals who may have bodily symptoms, imbalances, and dysfunctions.

In this vein, diagnostic and treatment emphasis is on nutrition, or-gans and systems function, along with physical, emotional, and chemi-cal toxicity issues. The health of a person's gut is often the first pivotal consideration. The gut (digestive system) in large part will dictate the general health of a person, influencing toxicity levels, chemical balance, and synergy of non-human organisms that we share with our bodies. Ninety percent of all cells and organisms in the human body are not human cells. When you read or hear information about acidophilus, bacterial overgrowth, yeast, Candida, fungus, mucus in the gut, etc., it's relating to the chronic chemical imbalances that challenge all systems of the body. Some functional-medicine doctors look at this as possibly the definitive cause of fibromyalgia. It is at the very least coexisting and a major complicating/perpetuating factor. Therefore it must be dealt with on some level for a person to reach maximum improvement. I believe it's naïve to adopt any single protocol as the only answer, but these general body-chemistry considerations must be included in a comprehensive clinical effort.

CHAPTER 3

Is There a Cure?

Chapter Topics:
Is Fibro Real?
Am I Crazy?
What It Feels Like
How Could This Happen To Me?
Help vs. Hope

Is There a Cure?

If by "cure" we mean that the patient will never have another ache or pain, then the short answer is no, there is no cure as of this writing. But that doesn't mean you can't feel better, have more energy and less pain, and live the life that you choose for yourself and your family.

The first step is to come up with a procedure to make a definitive diagnosis. The scientific community is working frantically to do just that. In our chapter on New Science, Real Hope, you'll learn about some of the truly hopeful methods. In the meantime, the best you can do is to continue to improve your understanding and your perspective, and to gain a vocabulary that will help you ask better questions of yourself and of your health team.

Follow as many of the principles and recommendations in this book as you can. The best thing you can do for yourself is to be willing to grow and to change. The first thing you can do to empower yourself is to take control, follow the steps, and put it right at the top of your list that your number-one job and priority is to improve your health.

Once a definitive fibromyalgia diagnosis has been made, a patient will feel great therapeutic relief. A diagnosis is like a label on your suffering that identifies and validates it. You have a disease or a problem; you're not crazy, you're in the company of over 15 million other people with fibromyalgia. A diagnosis helps to put things into perspective. It makes it easier for your heart and your head to tolerate the discomforts. It helps with communication and relationships.

And yet, we find that approximately 12-15 percent of people who have been diagnosed with fibromyalgia do not actually have it. They've either been misdiagnosed or simply misled by their own research and are now convinced that they have fibromyalgia. However, it's very upsetting if you tell a person who believes she has fibromyalgia that she may not. It breaks down a component of stability and confidence in herself and her life if a doctor takes away the label. The label is also a way of giving a person direction to feel like she has some power, because now she has something definitive to research, to read about, and to talk about. So a person may feel disempowered, confused, and often overwhelmed if the label is removed.

Why am I telling you that some people diagnosed with fibromyalgia don't actually have it? I am telling you because the major part of this book puts into perspective and into motion principles that will serve you whether you have fibromyalgia or some type of fibromyalgia look-alike. Simply by following the principles, you'll find that individual symptoms often can be cleared up or improved. When one area of your body or condition improves, other areas feel better as well. So the worst thing that can happen by following through using this book as your guide is that you'll feel more in control and more confident to control your life. You'll start feeling better both emotionally and physically, and at the end of the day you'll either be a fibromyalgia patient who feels better, or you'll be someone who feels better but never has had fibromyalgia. In the meantime, science will continue to evolve, working toward a definitive diagnosis and cure.

Throughout this book you may feel that there are contradictory concepts, anecdotes, and treatment protocols offered. Don't be worried by those seeming contradictions. Remember that the study of fibromyalgia is an evolving science, and with technology moving forward exponentially from year to year, specialized scans are able to observe in real time neurological functions within the brain, helping us to understand inflammation, cell communication, and the quirky primitive wiring that our brains don't seem to want to give up from caveman days. As technology, protocols, and philosophies evolve, so do ideas and treatments. My original comment that there is *no cure* means right this minute there is no permanent cure. Waking every morning and asking the question, "Will I have pain today?" is analogous to watching a pot boil (as my grandmother would say). This is a bad way to start the day. The truth is you probably will have some pain, but the pot will boil and most people reading this text will be better able to manage their pain soon without problematic reliance on drugs.

Until the late 1800s, infections could cause uncontrollable fevers, a normal defense mechanism. It was possible for the fever to go rogue and reach temperatures that could damage brain cells. When aspirin came on the scene, it was considered a wonder drug.

Medications are being developed now to control and mitigate chronic neuropathic pain and its central sensitivity component. Additionally, there is physical medicine; in physical medicine we include chiropractic, osteopathy, and nutrition as well as physical therapy, all of which are refining the understanding of peripheral neurology and the effects of trauma and repetitive insults, movement, and coordination. And let's not forget working with a doctor who believes in you, believes in fibromyalgia, and has an abiding interest in evolving science and the management of chronic pain. The patients who do the best are those who work at avoiding being overwhelmed (Chapter 19). This will get your head and heart straight each day and help to sidestep the brain static, fear, and confusion from the overload of information, suggestions, and advice you will be bombarded with. All patients will have their own demons and baggage kicking around in their heads to deal with, just like the rest of us. Things that you and only you can implement for yourself will help reduce and control many of the signals that trigger pain in the first place. For more technical perspectives, reference Chapter 20.

Many efforts can be undertaken right now and for the most part can be self-managed. They are effective and active efforts that support body, mind, and spirit. Many people with fibromyalgia have been able to minimize and control their symptoms, toning them down to not much more than episodes of annoyance, and getting on with living their life.

The Big Question

"Is Fibromyalgia Real?"

Anyone who doesn't believe that fibromyalgia is a real clinical entity to be reckoned with must have been living under a rock for the last 20 years. Although the number of disbelievers in the medical community has dwindled markedly, there are still those who will not accept fibromyalgia as a legitimate diagnosis. There is, however, no question as to whether or not the symptoms of fibromyalgia exist and in fact have real connection to each other. At the very least, all should be willing to accept the term "fibromyalgia" as an opportunity to understand the suffering, the causes, and the possible solutions of this often invisibly disabling condition. The rheumatologic community has worked for decades to understand fibromyalgia. However, neurobiologists are weighing in with research that places fibro as a neurological problem—a hopeful evolution.

Am I Crazy/Am I The Only One?

While it may feel like you are alone or crazy, you're definitely not.

The following are some brief data on the number of diagnosed fibromyalgia cases:

USA: upwards of 5 million *(CDC 2012 statistics)*

Canada approximately 400,000 (Ontario, Canada, action network)

(Numbers of cases have been extrapolated from prevalence statistics and the assistance of right diagnosis by health grades) [15]

France: 822,000

Germany: 1,121,000

Spain: 548,000

Mexico: 1,428,000

United Kingdom: 820,000

Italy: 790,000

India: 15,000,000

Israel: 84,000

Before someone is diagnosed with fibromyalgia, there are many symptoms that in retrospect signal systemic neurological breakdown. When you think back, you may have had isolated symptoms that we all tend to slough off as "stuff we go through"—things like growing pains; diarrhea, gas, or bloating and other digestive or bowel conditions; depression; sleeping problems. There may be a recurrence of infections—sinus or bronchial or bladder. Frequently, women will have a history of severe PMS. You weren't alone before fibromyalgia, and you're not alone or crazy now.

What Does It Feel Like?

We're not going to labor over the symptoms in this section. They've been well- documented and you can pick up any text or any reference on the web to find the list and the details of the symptoms. However, I will offer a short list that is typical. The most commonly reported is diffuse pain and tenderness of muscles, or what may be described as a lame feeling, as if a person is fighting the flu. Restorative sleep is difficult if not impossible. Certainly there are many areas of tenderness when touched. Stiffness and joint pain are frequently reported, as well as emotional swings and depression. Some physicians will suggest that depression and your mental state is the cause of fibromyalgia. We're not convinced that it is the cause by any means; however, there will be emotional considerations and depression; if not causative, at least as a result of the pain and the fatigue endured. In later chapters we will discuss an interesting neurological relationship between emotions at the time of a physically traumatic event, and the establishment of chronic pain patterns. Brain-fog, aka fibro-fog, may cloud judgment and memory. Frequently patients will have a history of arthritis, depression, TMJ disorders, carpal tunnel syndrome, and possibly a history of thyroid and/or adrenal fatigue.

How Could This Happen to Me?

Unfortunately, the understanding and the science of fibromyalgia is incomplete. In a Fibromyalgia Network newsletter, 1999, it was reported that many sufferers were physically and emotionally traumatized immediately before the onset of fibromyalgia symptoms. Others reported a reaction to taking medication or receiving some kind of immunological shot. There have also been reports of symptoms beginning right after a bacterial or viral infection—possibly after a high fever. Toxins and allergies have been implicated by some physicians. Some people have had a history of mononucleosis, herpes, hepatitis, Lyme disease, or fibro onset after major surgery.

What seems to be clear is that fibromyalgia is preceded by emotional, physical, or chemical events that tip the scales of the body's homeostasis and cause the nervous system, immune system, and chemical modulators to be disturbed.

Leon Chaitow, in his book *Fibromyalgia Syndrome,* reports that a basic survey, which was conducted on behalf of the Forest General Hospital in Mississippi and subsequently reported results in the Fibromyalgia Network Newsletter, notes that the co-existing and pre-existing conditions that may give us direction and understanding for how a person develops fibromyalgia are as follows:

65% arthritis
62% depression
52% irritable bowel syndrome
41% TMJ problems
30% carpal tunnel

24% hypothyroid
23% panic attacks
19% blood sugar imbalance

Is There Any Help or Hope?

Yes, there is help and hope. However, even the most accurate diagnosis and effective treatment will require patients to play an active, educated role in their recovery. Just getting this far in the book means you are on your way. The key is empowerment: empowering yourself first as a student, and secondly as a trainer/educator of people around you. This may include helping your doctor to understand. I know this sounds like the tail wagging the dog, but with your efforts, you are very likely to end up knowing more than the doctors you're working with. You must ask better questions of them, and subsequently hold them responsible for the answers—which, by the way, you would be wise to confirm.

You'll find that rest, cognitive therapies, nutrition, body mechanics, and exercise will surface as common denominators in any clinical effort. The degree to which they will be effective will in large part be related to coexisting or fibromyalgia look-alike symptoms/conditions. For instance, in our clinic when we work with a fibromyalgia patient, one of their major complaints is likely to be low back pain. When addressing low back pain with chiropractic, we must employ the most contemporary subtleties of neuromuscular and neurochemical understandings as we strive to minimize the use of drugs. The patient usually reports relief quickly. However, that doesn't mean that fibromyalgia has been treated successfully—at least not yet. Rather, the relief is a signal that there is a reduction in central nervous system excitability, hence confirming that chiropractic must be at least part of a comprehensive fibro recovery plan.

There is a long list of possibilities for patients. The results certainly vary from patient to patient. There is everything from over-the-counter-drugs to prayer, stretching, physical therapy, Tens Unit, and acupuncture, to name a few. However, as mentioned, almost all of these efforts are directed at symptoms and not the cause. The most promising research to get at the underlying cause of fibromyalgia is the science of neurological and chemical dysregulation in the body—that is to say, the miscommunication and imbalance between chemical and neurological factors that take their toll primarily within the central nervous system and the brain. I intentionally accept redundancy in this section with the intent of establishing familiarity with new vocabulary and concepts that will make subsequent chapters more comfortable and understandable.

There are other things that can help and offer hope, such as specialized computers, scans and microscopes, Bio-Nano Robotics (internal body drones investigating and reporting back data on every aspect of what and who we are from the inside out). Luckily, research has become big business; big business drives discovery. Additionally, we find hope in realizing that more physicians are becoming aware of the need for natural and multidisciplinary approaches to health care. Admittedly, this sounds negative and challenging for doctors and patients alike. However, all told, awareness, education, desire, and need offer more hope for fibro sufferers than ever before. For now, let's continue to understand fibromyalgia, put it in perspective, and manage our lives.

It only feels like you are crazy sometimes—you're not! Fibromyalgia is real, but it doesn't mean you can't feel better and have more energy and less pain, and live the life that you choose for yourself and your family.

CHAPTER 4

Medication Rx and Diet

Chapter Topics:
   Medications
   Guaifenesin
   Carbohydrates

Medication

Medicines that are approved for the treatment of fibromyalgia and prescribed frequently by MDs are:

- Antidepressants generally, and specifically Savella, which helps with mood and brain fog. Many of them are serotonin or norepinephrine reuptake inhibitors. Antidepressants can have a stronger effect on neurotransmitters, helping to inhibit pain signals. Cymbalta falls into this category; however, it is not approved to treat fibromyalgia specifically. As with all medication, antidepressants come with side effects.
- Non-steroidal anti-inflammatories that decrease inflammation. These drugs have been used frequently in spite of the fact that we are unable to document inflammation as a clinical component of fibromyalgia. They nevertheless seem to have at least a marginal effect, if for no other reason than that they afford a decrease in the discomfort of inflammation due to coexisting conditions, such as arthritis, subluxation, strains and sprains, etc.
- Lyrica has been approved by the FDA. It decreases the hypersensitivity/excitability of nerves by controlling calcium's effect on nerves in the central nervous system.
- Sleep aids. While sleep aids have not been approved specifically for the treatment of fibromyalgia, they are frequently used effectively to improve sleep patterns, in turn helping to modulate pain, fatigue, and various other symptoms.

The clinical trials with these drugs have been shown to be effective with acceptable side effects, but not for everyone. We won't get into the details of each medication and their side effects; suffice it to say that side effects could include dizziness, dry mouth, swelling, blurred vision, and weight gain, as well as abnormal thinking, and possibly nausea and constipation. We will cover medication in more detail shortly.

Guaifenesin

Guaifenesin protocol in the treatment of fibromyalgia is arguably substantiated by research. However, the developer, Dr. Paul St. Amand MD (endocrinologist), would disagree. All in all, this protocol deserves serious consideration as a possible solution for some sufferers with no more or less validity than any other theory, and may actually net better and longer-lasting results if applied *exactly* as Dr. Amand recommends.

The FDA has not approved guaifenesin for the treatment of fibromyalgia. But then again, the few treatments that have been approved are marginally effective, with many side effects.

Dr. Paul St. Amand's Protocol

Dr. St. Amand has developed his guaifenesin protocol over the last 40-plus years. He sees fibromyalgia as a lack of cellular energy. As a side note, most doctors and researchers agree up to this point, that in fact fibro sufferers have a generalized deficit of cellular energy. Dr. St. Amand sees the ubiquitous lack of cellular energy accounting for the plethora of symptoms. His theory basically dictates that the lack of cellular energy (adenosine triphosphate, or ATP) is due to excess phosphate inside cells, specifically in the part of the cell called the mitochondria. The short story is that guaifenesin takes its effect on the kidneys, helping to pull excess phosphate out of cells and, over time, with the assistance of other aspects of his protocol, the treatment will net a relatively consistent increase in energy and abatement of most or all symptoms.

Guaifenesin is famous as an expectorant that loosens mucus and phlegm. It is the active ingredient in Mucinex and other decongestants. Side effects have been reported, but within a protocol and considering the mild or nonexistent side effects, it would be very difficult to decipher side effects from a symptom that was part and parcel of fibromyalgia. The bottom line is that it's generally considered safe. However, as with all information in this book or any other book you read, theories, recommendations, and anecdotes should be approved by your doctor and not be undertaken on your own.

Carbohydrates

The guaifenesin theory seems to correlate nicely with the understanding of hypophosphatemia, an electrolyte disturbance in which there is an abnormally low level of phosphate in the blood. This condition is most commonly seen in malnourished individuals with an overconsumption of carbohydrates. Particularly for those of us who are carbohydrate- sensitive, the greater the consumption of carbohydrates, the greater chance we have of creating high demand within the cells for phosphorous. When this demand exists, phosphorous is pulled from the blood and driven into the cells, eventually causing intercellular excess and extracellular depletion. Another cause of low blood phosphorous is malabsorption syndrome, seen in gastrointestinal problems such as irritable bowel syndrome, lack of vitamin D, or chronic use of NSAIDs (the chronic use of NSAIDs is of epidemic proportion due to over-the-counter availability and quick symptom relief, regardless of the side effects).

Symptoms of malabsorption syndrome include:

*altered muscle physiology
*cognitive alteration such as confusion and brain fog
*rickets
*alteration of nerve physiology

Proper levels of phosphorus are so crucial that rickets could develop even if a person has an adequate supply of vitamin D and calcium. Low phosphate levels can be seen in other conditions as well, such as Falconi syndrome caused by Dent's disease.

My experiences with chronic pain patients is that restricting carbohydrates, particularly grains, will help to manage blood sugar and subsequently pain, as well as energy, at least to some degree, in just about everyone. It's possible that much of the success that Dr. St. Amand reports is more directly related to carbohydrate restriction and blood-sugar management than the therapeutic effect of guaifenesin.

Evaluation

The evaluation used within a guaifenesin protocol is interesting and controversial. St. Amand does not palpate for "tender points" as defined and recognized as pathognomonic of fibromyalgia by the

American Board of Rheumatology (ABR), but rather he palpates to map out areas of the body that demonstrate swollen areas. The result can be many more than the typical 18 tender points which are referred to in every text ever written about fibromyalgia. He notes that these swollen areas may be nodulated, rigid, or tender—but not necessarily. They can be found in muscles, tendons, ligaments, either superficially and/or around joints. They are mapped out on a diagram of the patient. After a period of time on his protocol, a re-evaluation with remapping would take place, looking for the lumps and bumps to become smaller, softer, and more mobile. I have to admit that I like the objectivity of his evaluation, a quality that is lacking in the more common "18 tender points" assessment, which is primarily subjective and nearly worthless in its diagnostic validity.

Protocol

The protocol must be managed precisely. Proper dosing and timing of guaifenesin is crucial, requiring an experienced practitioner to guide the patient through the process. In addition to dosing and timing, there are strict dietary parameters. Carbohydrates must be limited to a strict diabetic-type diet for obvious reasons, as stated above. In addition, there are some crucial restrictions that, if not adhered to, will block the effect that guaifenesin will have on phosphate.

The following should be strictly eliminated in the protocol:

*aspirin or any other medication that contains salicylates
*topical creams, lotions and cosmetics that may have natural salicylates
*plant oil gels or extracts
*mint flavors, mint oil, menthol
*plant compounds such as camphor
*all herbal medications/nutritional supports

Perspective

Dr. St. Amand, in fact, suffers from fibromyalgia himself, and that is one of the reasons that he's so passionate and committed as a physician and researcher to helping other fibromyalgia patients. In speaking with him, I've found him to be charming, articulate, and very clear on the necessity for guaifenesin. His book has sold over 200,000 copies. The statistics that he presents are impressive. However, I've been able to find very little corroborating science or research to support his assertions. I have no doubt that he has been able to help many people, but his protocol does not seem to have been able to be duplicated by many other physicians. My staff and I called 90 percent of the doctors and clinics listed in 2013 on his website as being trained and implementing his protocols. The doctors we spoke with, who have worked with the protocol, reported their results to be disappointing and they no longer use the protocol. When pressing them for details of the protocol, it became obvious that the protocol is so specialized and detailed that doctors, their staff, and their patients were unable or unwilling to follow through precisely as St. Amand has designed. Consequently, it seems reasonable to believe that's why he's one of very few who are getting results with the protocol.

The challenge, as I've alluded to above, would be to find a clinic or doctor who could actually implement the protocol effectively. I'm in hopes that someone will come forward substantiating/duplicating the guaifenesin protocol successfully. Regardless of the controversy, St. Amand's protocol does not appear to have any less validity than any other theory to date.

> Medications, protocols, and special diets come in and out of favor. That doesn't mean that with a little trial and error you couldn't find relief with acceptable side effects. This effort should be undertaken as a tool to improve the quality of your life while working toward more organic/natural methods to balance the nervous system, reduce pain, and increase energy.

CHAPTER 5

The Great Imposters

Chapter Topics:

Chronic Fatigue Syndrome	Lyme Disease
Myofascial Pain Syndrome	Lupus
Trigger Points	Connective Tissue Disease
Comparative Chart	Reflex Sympathetic Dystrophy

There are many conditions that share symptoms with fibromyalgia, which frustrate and complicate the diagnosis and understanding. Among them are:

*Autoimmune diseases such as lupus, rheumatoid arthritis, and Sjogren's syndrome
*Neurological disorders such as subluxation, myasthenia gravis and multiple sclerosis
*Connective tissue disease
*Chronic fatigue syndrome
*Temporal mandibular joint dysfunction (TMJ)
*Osteoarthritis
*Hypothyroidism
*Adrenal exhaustion
*Depression
*Magnesium deficiency
*Gluten / Carbohydrate sensitivity

Many of these will be discussed throughout the book. However, for this chapter we're going to cover chronic fatigue syndrome, myofascial pain syndrome, trigger points, and Lyme disease.

Physicians with many contact hours working with fibro patients will differ on the causative factors and whether or not chronic fatigue syndrome (CFS) and/or myofascial pain syndrome (MPS) are just a variance of fibromyalgia syndrome. It is my opinion that they are distinctly different.

We're going to discuss findings and factors that help put these syndromes in perspective. The disagreement as to causative factors revolves around simple questions: do the signs and symptoms simply coexist? Are any of them causative—possibly a consequence of each other—or altogether disconnected and simply guilty by association?

Definition of Fibromyalgia

I have included the definition of fibromyalgia from the American College of Rheumatology to clarify and refresh your perspective from our chapter on history:

The American College of Rheumatology (ACR) 2010 criteria is used for clinical diagnosis and severity classification. Diagnosis is based on:

- Widespread Pain Index (WPI) >7 and a symptom severity scale (SS) >5 or WPI 3-6 and SS >9.
- Symptoms have been present at a similar level for at least three months.
- The patient does not have a disorder that would otherwise explain the pain.

Chronic Fatigue Syndrome/CFS

The search for the cause of chronic fatigue syndrome is convoluted. There are many different opinions and seemingly valid data to back up each opinion. Currently there are no objective tests to diagnosis CFS. Some researchers feel that fibromyalgia and chronic fatigue are two different sides of the same coin. When comparing patients' history and physiology, we find that there are emotional, physical, and/or chemical factors that have simply overwhelmed the body in each case. The tipping point or trigger with chronic fatigue seems to be that a person's body is being overwhelmed more in a chemically toxic way, which in turn affects the immune system. In concert with each other, these factors influence the nervous system and produce a typical chronic fatigue syndrome. In contrast, fibromyalgia reaches a tipping point when physical and/or emotional stress overwhelms a person's brain and central nervous system.

Sufferers will frequently have a history of infection from bacterial or viral origin. Mononucleosis, Lyme disease, and microbial infections, among others, have been cited. That's not to say that a challenge to the immune system cannot trigger fibromyalgia or complicate it, but it is clear that chronic fatigue is more obviously and consistently involved in a person's immune system being challenged.

Let's begin with an overview as taken from the Centers for Disease Control and Prevention, 1994 definition:

Chronic Fatigue Syndrome (CFS) is a debilitating and complex disorder characterized by intense fatigue. It does not improve with bed rest and symptoms may worsen physical or mental activity. People with CFS most often function at a substantially lower level of activity than they were capable of before the onset of the illness. The causes of CFS have not been identified and no specific diagnostic test is available. Therefore, in order to be diagnosed with chronic fatigue syndrome, a patient must satisfy the following criteria:

1. Having the onset of relentless or relapsing fatigue to a degree sufficient enough to reduce daily activities by 50 percent or more and last at least six months. Additionally the fatigue cannot be explained by any other medical condition.
2. Concurrently have four or more of the following symptoms:
    *   Impaired memory or concentration
    *   Un-refreshing sleep
    *   Muscle pain
    *   Multi-joint pain without redness or swelling
    *   Tender cervical or axillaries' lymph nodes
    *   Sore throat
    *   Headache
    *   Post-exertion malaise
3. The symptoms must have persisted or reoccurred during six or more consecutive months of illness and must not have predated the fatigue. Other commonly observed symptoms of chronic fatigue syndrome are:
    *   Abdominal pain
    *   Alcohol intolerance
    *   Bloating
    *   Chest pain
    *   Chronic cough
    *   Diarrhea
    *   Dizziness
    *   Dry eyes or mouth
    *   Earaches

- Irregular heartbeat
- Jaw pain
- Morning stiffness
- Nausea
- Night sweats
- Psychological problems (depression, irritability, anxiety, panic attacks)
- Shortness of breath
- Skin sensations such as tingling
- Weight loss

Physical Signs

Physical signs should have been documented by a physician on at least two occasions: in particular, low-grade fever, inflammation of the throat, and tenderness on palpation of the cervical and axillary lymph nodes.

Toxicity and CFS

While toxicity levels play a role in both chronic fatigue and fibromyalgia, there is an interesting distinction between the two when it comes to exercise. Fibromyalgia patients seem to benefit from exercise, at least temporarily, while chronic fatigue patients will not be able to tolerate exercise at all and tend not to have even temporary benefits.

We're all familiar with the fact that just being alive and having normal physiology will create free radicals/toxins every second of every day. During exercise, physiology speeds up and there are more free radicals and more toxic byproducts produced. Our bodies obviously have to deal with them. With our patients we find that in the early stages of a therapeutic program, neither fibromyalgia nor chronic fatigue patients benefit from exercise in spite of the initial impression (at least in the case of fibro) that it is helping. This initial impression is due to stimulation of endorphins, increased respiration, and improved oxygenation along with increased circulation and improved lymphatic flow—all of which sounds like a great idea, right?

However, the initial feeling of "This is a good thing" is short-lived, especially with chronic fatigue sufferers. The immune system is unable to deal with the increase in toxins, counteracting the benefits. Consequently, an exercise effort will end with another day lying on the couch.

Magnesium and CFS

Magnesium deficiency plays a role in fibromyalgia as well as in chronic fatigue. Particularly when it comes to exercise, magnesium deficiency encourages inflammation, with excessive production of oxygen-deprived free radicals. Magnesium is also a key nutrient in the process of glycolysis and the aerobic pathway, which helps mitochondria within each of our cells create energy[24]. Mitochondria create energy by generating ATP (adenosine triphosphate), and use this energy as you would suspect: for power and endurance, conducting everyday bodily functions, including thought and mental clarity. Additionally, cellular energy is required to repair injury and help our muscles recover from everyday activities. When mitochondria fail to keep up with the demand for ATP/energy, bodily fatigue sets in. Chronic fatigue sufferers are very familiar with what a decrease in ATP feels like. You'll hear them say, "I have to sit down and get off my feet," or "I just want to lie down." You may get tired of reading about ATP in so many different sections of this book. However, ATP/cellular energy is a common thread connecting all physiology and hypotheses.

Stress increases the need for ATP building blocks dramatically if a person is already suffering from chronic fatigue. It challenges nerve and muscle physiology, which will in turn increase the chances of developing myofascial trigger points, heaviness, and soreness and myofascial pain in the muscles. We will discuss this more in the next section; however, when we add myofascial symptoms to chronic fatigue, it is easy to see how someone could think that they have fibromyalgia. This judgment is no different in the clinical setting; doctors misjudge/misdiagnose the two regularly.

Assuming that myofascial trigger points have not developed, a chronic fatigue sufferer can at least expect that exercise will produce lactic acid. Lactic acid promotes tissue hypoxia (decreased oxygen), causing more toxins and inflammation, adding to the immune system's burden. This condition can cause muscles to become sore and tired. Although this happens to all of us to some degree after exercising, chronic fatigue sufferers are the least likely to tolerate it. Supplementing the diet with magnesium may help a person to participate in modest exercise, assuming they have their doctor's blessing.

There is no shortage of people who have chronic fatigue; lifestyle and eating habits alone could account for much of it, to say nothing of fatigue's relationship to other conditions—everything from diabetes to arthritis, heart disease to digestive problems. Kimberly Burnham

PhD, in the *Burnham Review* 2009 issues 9 to 13, reports that "Recent reviews of pharmacological therapies for fatigue remains inconclusive." Dr. Burnham reports that a literature search found non-pharmaceutical experimental studies about fatigue that concluded that exercise, and behavioral, nutritional and psychological interventions, were associated with statistically significant reduction in fatigue.

As with fibromyalgia, other diagnostic and treatment considerations would include further nutritional intervention, lifestyle choices, addressing food and environmental sensitivities, reaction to vaccines and medication, thyroid and adrenal imbalances, genetic factors, and carbohydrate metabolism, as well as spinal nerve conditions (subluxations). As a side note, I've never seen a patient with fibromyalgia, chronic fatigue, or myofascial pain syndrome who was not sensitive to carbohydrates.

In all considerations, the peripheral and central nervous systems' roles should be considered. In Chapter 11 we will discuss further details of the adaptive changes the nervous system goes through and how this understanding can benefit you with creative lifestyle and therapeutic decisions/solutions.

Myofascial Pain Syndrome
First, let's break down the term myofascial.

"Myo" means muscle. Muscle is a type of soft tissue (soft tissue is anything other than bone). Muscle cells contain protein filaments that slide past one another, producing a contraction that changes both the length and the shape of the cell, producing force and causing motion. They are primarily responsible for maintaining changes in posture and locomotion, as well as movement of internal organs, such as the contraction of the heart and movement of food through the digestive system. Muscles are controlled and take their cues from the nervous system and are influenced by hormones.

"Fascial" comes from the word fascia, which is a layer of fibrous soft tissue. The fibers of fascia form wavy ubiquitous sheets of tissue around muscles, groups of muscles, blood vessels, bones, and nerves. They also have intimate attachments to bones, joints, cartilage, and even the brain. They hold structures together in supportive bundles while allowing other structures and muscles to slide smoothly over each other. Fascia is extremely strong, with an ability to flex and stretch. Due to the waviness of their fibers, there is an ability to recoil back to their original shape and responsibility. They are made of the same collagen material that ligaments and tendons are made of.

Definition of Myofascial Pain Syndrome
The following was taken from the Mayo Clinic website,= (accessed July 1, 2014).

Myofascial Pain Syndrome (MFPS) is a chronic form of muscle pain. The pain of myofascial pain syndrome centers around sensitive points in your muscles called trigger points. The trigger points can be painful when touched, and the pain can spread throughout the affected muscle sometimes seemingly to refer pain to other areas. Some of the theories relating to the spread or referral of pain and sensory disturbance are that it is through disturbance of the skin (dermatomal), through muscles (myotomal), or through embryological factors (sclerodomal). Nearly everyone experiences muscle pain from time to time that generally resolves within a few days. But people with myofascial pain syndrome have muscle pain that persists or worsens. Myofascial pain has been linked to many types of pain including headaches, dizziness, jaw pain, neck pain, low back pain, pelvic pain, and arm and leg pain. Additionally there is some relationship to brain fog.

Other signs and symptoms of myofascial pain syndrome include:

- Deep aching pain in a muscle
- Pain that persists or worsens
- Muscle stiffness
- Joint stiffness near the affected muscle
- Areas of tension which feel knotted and may be sensitive to touch
- Difficulty sleeping due to pain
- Numbness
- TMJ issues
- Dizziness and brain fog
- Tingling

Risk Factors

- Muscle stress or injury. Examples are: A whiplash injury, repetitive motion as in painting a ceiling or UPS/FedEX delivering boxes all day. Another is chronic muscle tension when spending all day at a computer.
- Inactivity. This could be due simply to a sedentary lifestyle/job, recovering from an illness, disease, or surgery.

- Stress and anxiety. Chronic stress and anxiety are likely to encourage develop of trigger points, and their relationship to clenched teeth TMJ problems.
- Age. Myofascial pain syndrome is more likely in middle-aged adults. It seems to come with the territory of cumulative lifestyle factors particularly in the area of stress/ responsibility.

In our clinic, Enfield Integrative Health, located in Enfield, CT, we find that myofascial pain syndrome, including trigger points, is most commonly a regional finding, meaning it's confined to a particular muscle or group of muscles related to specific movements or responsibility. The distinguishing clinical feature is usually a tight, ropy, nodulated thickening with a loss of viscosity within a muscle, always attended by tenderness. When a trigger point is contacted the patient will flinch, tighten up, and either pull away or say, "Yeah, Doc—right there; you got it."

Myofascial pain syndrome (MPS) has equal occurrence between men and women. You'll notice in the literature that this is in obvious contrast to fibromyalgia and chronic fatigue syndrome, which tend to be found primarily in female patients.

The regions most likely to develop myofascial trigger points are neck, shoulder/between shoulders, and low back. We also find them about the hips and buttocks and thighs. Fibromyalgia, in contrast, is painful above and below the centerline of the body at the same time, and also to the right and to the left of a vertical centerline of the body.

Additionally, a distinguishing factor is that MPS usually is not accompanied with other problems such as digestion, emotional problems, energy problems, or brain fog. That's not to say that people can't have other problems; it's just that MPS tends to be more clearly a muscle issue. When chronic, the stressed fibers might develop scar tissue, causing a decrease in range of motion and weakness, leading to a relatively permanent condition and never be available for use again[69]. This will decrease enthusiasm to remain active and, over time, lead to emotional mood swings, interrupted sleep and fatigue. We caution patients not to cover up their discomfort with medication. The cover-up allows the real cause to continue and spread to surrounding tissues, hence developing more trigger points.

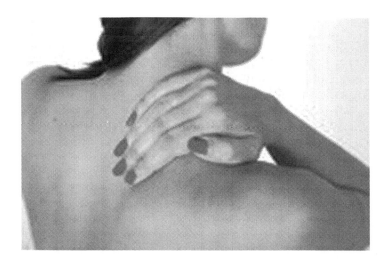

What Causes Trigger Points?

Trigger points can develop from local muscle damage such as some type of injury/trauma, infection, or simply overuse. But why do so many people develop them without having had an injury or obvious overuse of the affected area? Can they develop due to other types of stress, such as poor diet or emotional stress?

Poor diet and emotional stress can affect muscles just as negatively as overuse or direct damage. But if that's the case, why aren't trigger points more commonly developed all over the body? After all, there are around 600 muscles in the body. Why are they predominantly regionalized to the neck, shoulders/between shoulders, and low back?

The answer lies in the understanding that the muscles most susceptible to developing trigger points (and subsequently spreading to myofascial pain) are those already vulnerable or weakened for some reason.

A great example is a mild whiplash injury, which can occur from an auto mishap, sports injury, or a million other seemingly innocuous events which an adult may have experienced earlier in life. There may be no neck pain, but just enough disruption to dis-regulate joint neurology and movement, causing nerve irritation to affect muscles of the neck and shoulder region, rendering them vulnerable and weakened. This scenario so far is termed "subluxation complex." The word "complex" connotes the involvement of physical/dynamic alteration with neurological consequence. Let's add "subclinical subluxation complex" to be precise, simply because there may not be obvious pain...yet. The result is that everyday physical, emotional, and dietary stressors will take their toll on the most susceptible muscles first--in our case, the neck and shoulder muscles. This sets the stage to easily develop trigger points and myofascial pain.

So the answer to the question "Why are TP/MFP predominant-ly regionalized to the neck, shoulders/between shoulders and lower back?" is that they are the most neurologically rich and mechanically demanding, hence they are susceptible regions to develop sublux-ations, whether due to direct trauma or, as aforementioned, from life taking its toll on sub-clinically worn-down and vulnerable regions.

Solution

We're not going to spend a lot of time discussing the many indi-vidual techniques that attempt to resolve myofascial trigger points. We will, however, touch on the fundamentals that must be implemented regardless of the technique if MFT are to be radically decreased, if not resolved.

A variety of techniques can be employed to ease and attempt to resolve the trigger points directly where they occur in the muscle. Depending on the doctor you work with, acupuncture, acupressure, myofascial release, saline injections, Botox, ultrasound, laser therapy, etc., could be considered.

The treatment of choice will vary from doctor to doctor. Generally, all treatment of trigger points directly where they occur in the mus-cle has to do with stimulating specialized sensory nerves. Stimulating them is assumed to assist in reregulating the area in which the trig-ger points exist. By the way, the specialized sensory nerves are called mechanoreceptors. They directly influence the local fluid dynamics of arterioles, capillaries, and interstitial fluid. An acupuncturist would explain "the flow of meridian energy." When the treatment is effec-tive, tissues become more viscous, allowing muscles and fascia to flow and move over each other more smoothly and efficiently.[55]

There are fundamentals that must be implemented regardless of the technique if you hope to succeed and reduce the chances of the painful points returning. Specifically, the everyday stress on the muscles, posture, and the joints of the neck and low back must be dealt with. Also, regional subluxation complex must be suspected, di-agnosed, and corrected physically. Have you noticed that medication does little to nothing for trigger points? The reason is that you can only rarely take a chemical to fix the mechanical component of a problem. If you recall, subluxation complex, along with nerve irritation, has a mechanical component to it. If you suffer from myofascial pain and trigger points, they are likely to continue to recur unless the subluxation component is addressed. A chiropractor is likely to be the only doctor who can resolve this for you. However, if you are already working with a physical therapist who has an advanced degree in Integrative Manual Therapy IMT, or an osteopath, discuss it with them first.

Nutrition

Functional medicine/nutrition is also a fundamental necessity that has come to the foreground of almost any malady we could discuss. It is as important as subluxation correction. With improved nutrition, and by dealing with digestive and hormonal issues, we can greatly enhance patient recovery from MPS and reduce the chances of recurrences. Obviously, this addresses the dietary stress component we spoke of above. Generally, make sure to include a good source of minerals, amino acids, essential fatty acids, B vitamins, and vitamin D. Evaluation by a doctor (medical, naturopathic, chiropractic, or osteopathic) who specializes in functional medicine would be wise in an effort to pin down specific therapeutic nutrition for your case. Also tending to emotional issues is a type of nutrition that directly influences the nervous system and hormonal balance.

Note: The best approach would be to adopt an eclectic effort directed at the stressors of life, specific muscles involved, and the neurological component (subluxation). Without this combination, the likelihood of resolving trigger points and maintaining the improvement is remote. As part of our webinar series, we cover details and specific treatments related to trigger points that you can do for yourself at home—or discuss with your doctor. You can watch for our webinar schedule at www.Fibro-Doc.com.

Comparison Chart of Symptoms

Symptom Finding	Fibromyalgia	Chronic fatigue	Myofascial Pain
Pain	Primary Symptoms	Secondary Symptom	
Fatigue	Secondary Symptoms	Primary Symptom	
Sleep Problem			
High Spinal fluid levels of substance P	Yes	No	
Abnormal growth hormone levels	Yes, in some patients	No	
Problem with	Yes	Yes	
Poor concentration	Yes	Yes	
Chronic or frequent Sore throat	No	Yes	
Problems with short term memory	Yes	Yes	
Tender lymph nodes	No	Yes	
Chronic low grade fever	No	Yes	
Brain Fog	Yes	Yes	
Anxiety	Yes	Yes	
Depression	Yes	Yes	
Woman	Yes	Yes	
Man	Yes	Yes	Yes
Pain; head, shoulders,	Yes		Yes
Dr feels muscle	No		Yes
abnormality			Yes
Muscle abnormality	Yes		Yes
Wide spread pain	Yes		Yes
Regional Pain	Yes		Yes
Pinpoint Pain	Yes		Yes
Benefits from massage	Yes		Yes
Chiropractic Helps	Yes		Yes
Respond to medication	Yes	Yes	Yes
Fatigue improves with rest	No	Yes	
Headaches	Yes	Yes	If Neck
Joint pain	Yes	Yes	
Sensitivity	Yes	Yes	
Feel overwhelmed	Yes	Yes	
Digestive issues	Yes	Yes	

The questions still remain. Do the signs and symptoms simply co-exist? Are any of them causative, possibly a consequence of each other, or altogether disconnected and simply guilty by association? The answer is that all of these possible scenarios are possible, in any or all combinations depending on the specific case. Usually, over time, clarity comes in retrospect through the relationship you have with your doctors.

Lyme Disease—5,000 Years Old

In the year 2000, *National Geographic* reported that a mummified human 5300 years old (the Iceman) was found. A frenzy of analysis and testing took place. Of interesting note is that researchers found the genetic footprint of bacteria known as *Borrelia burgdorferi* in the Iceman's DNA—making the Iceman the earliest known human infected by the organism that causes Lyme disease

Is Lyme Disease Related to Fibromyalgia?

Lyme disease—along with the hepatitis C virus, HIV, and vaccinations—has been suspected of causing fibromyalgia. While all of them have the potential to cause symptoms that are suggestive of fibromyalgia, there is little to no science that confirms a causal relationship.

Considering Widespread Pain

Many conditions feature widespread pain, such as rheumatoid arthritis, ankylosing spondylitis, Lyme disease, polymyalgia rheumatica, lupus and fibromyalgia. Lyme is an infectious disease by inoculation of the spirochete Lyme bacterium due to a tick bite. Both researchers and doctors agree that early detection and treatment offers a very high cure rate. By the same token, there is agreement that, if not treated diligently, the illness can cause serious consequences for a lifetime, commonly affecting the brain, nerves, eyes, joints, and heart. Some cases have been reported to cause paraplegia due to directly affecting the brain.[68]

Dr. Sam Donta of Boston University notes that most people don't know that they've been bitten by a tick. Obviously this can lead to failure in seeking timely treatment. Additionally, even if treatment is sought, the illness is often misdiagnosed as some other condition with similar symptoms. The first six to eight weeks after infection are the most crucial for successfully diagnosing and treating the condition. Statistically, however, as reported by Lyme Disease Foundation cofounder Tom Forschner, it takes the average person twenty-two months and seven doctors to come to a final diagnosis. Further, it's estimated that 5 to 20 percent of all cases will end up with the patient suffering severe chronic symptoms.

There is some controversy as to whether or not chronic and lifetime consequences are due to the persisting infection itself, or the resolution of the infection leaving persistent symptoms due to its lingering effects on the autoimmune system response that was originally triggered. The Centers for Disease Control (CDC) estimates that over two million people have been infected. It's the most common tick-borne disease reported in North America and Europe. In the United States, we see most cases reported in New England, the Mid-Atlantic states, the east-north central United States, the south Atlantic and west-north central. It's found in Africa, Asia, Australia, Canada, Europe and the United Kingdom. Reported cases in South America are on the rise as well.

Signs and Symptoms

Symptoms will usually appear within one or two weeks of being bitten. May through September are the most dangerous months. There are cases of the infection that do not have symptoms at all; they are reported most often in Europe. In about 50 to 80 percent of the cases, a bull's-eye rash is described, with feverish qualities of redness and warmth. Flu-like symptoms, including headaches, muscle soreness, fever, and general malaise, are some of the early symptoms. It's easy to see how this condition would challenge a person's body, lower his resistance, and exacerbate if not trigger symptoms of fibromyalgia, rheumatic types of diseases, or other subclinical neuromuscular skeletal conditions resembling FMs, CFS, and MFPS.

Let's clarify the concept of one condition's triggering another. When a condition is triggered, we mean that condition A brings condition B to the surface. Maybe a person is genetically predisposed to, if not already suffering from, fibromyalgia, even if that person is unaware of it; condition A upsets their entire physiology and neuromusculoskeletal system, causing fibromyalgia to surface. But, as aforementioned, there's no science to document that Lyme disease actually causes fibromyalgia.

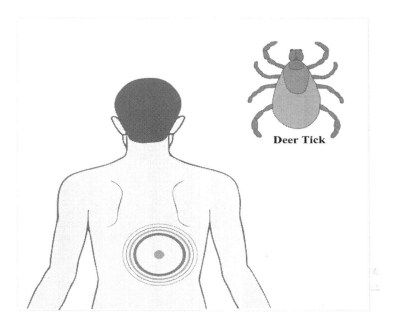

Deer Tick

The initial infection will be localized and then begin to spread through the bloodstream. Some cases have progressed and reported skin changes far removed from the site of the initial bite, as well as migrating pains in muscles, joints, and tendons, and heart palpitations and dizziness.

The organism itself (the spirochete bacterium) is an extremely resourceful and evasive organism with the ability to hide in and infect all body tissues and cells if not eradicated early on with antibiotics. In fact, the bacterium can spread to the brain even before the "bull's-eye" rash appears; this assumes that the rash appears at all. Once spread to the brain, the bacterium can cause facial paralysis, numbness and tingling, and cognitive problems such as memory loss, confusion, and difficulty in concentration (brain fog). Additionally, mood swings, changes in behavior and sensitivity to touch, noise, light, and smell may be noted.[29]

Diagnosis

Besides symptoms and history, objective data can be achieved by blood tests to evaluate antibodies; however, there is controversy on the reliability of these tests. Considering the severity and threat that untreated systemic infection poses, physicians frequently give the benefit of the doubt based on history and symptoms and choose to err on the side of treating a disease that doesn't exist rather than have it progress sub-clinically to a more destructive and complicated state.

Persons whose treatment has failed, or the victim who has been misdiagnosed or undiagnosed and consequently not treated, may progress into what some people call chronic Lyme disease or post-Lyme disease syndrome. This allows the infection to lurk sub-clinically and then express itself from time to time, mimicking fibromyalgia. It's the exacerbation and remission of the symptoms that most mimic fibromyalgia. Frequently it is impossible to judge with anything more than an opinion whether a patient has good old-fashioned arthritis, peripheral neuropathies, fibromyalgia, chronic fatigue, or a variety of other conditions that express themselves with widespread pain, fatigue and autonomic nervous system abnormalities—in general, flu-like symptoms.

The Gut

Gut health should not be over looked. Just about all inoculations by abnormal organism populations have the potential to express exactly the way we've discussed with Lyme disease. Of particular concern are abnormalities within the gut that are frequently overlooked by allopathic medicine and are potentially as harmful as Lyme disease. In this regard we're talking about overpopulation of fungus, yeast, or various other bacteria or viruses—all of which, like Lyme disease, may require intervention, first to kill the bad guys and subsequently to repopulate the gut with good guys (probiotics). Gut health is a recommended consideration in all fibro cases. This is the basis of the theory that some hold that fibromyalgia is primarily a metabolic disorder.

Treatment

Treatment for Lyme disease will frequently be dictated by the stage of the condition. However, antibiotic therapy is the treatment of choice, with very severe and prolonged cases possibly leading to IV antibiotic therapy. However, regardless of the apparent success of antibiotics, a holistic, whole-body program—to include supporting the immune system, nutritional considerations, detoxification, and tending to the gut and digestive issues, as well as behavior and lifestyle modifications—is necessary to make the maximum degree of restoration and reduce the chances of a subclinical deterioration/re-inoculation by dormant organisms leading to flare-ups. Therefore, even after antibiotic therapy, without proper follow-up a person who might be biologically or genetically susceptible to fibromyalgia is at risk.

Most patients with a history of Lyme disease, even when considered to have been fully cured, will still experience an inordinate amount of muscle and joint aching as well as issues with brain fog, chemical sensitivity, and low energy. Needless to say, this confuses the clinical picture. The bottom line is that in all cases of suspected fibromyalgia there should be a high suspicion of Lyme disease, and proper diagnostic tests and treatment should be done accordingly.

Lupus

Lupus is a chronic autoimmune disease that can damage skin, joints, muscles, ligaments, organs, and systems of the body including the spine, nervous system, and brain. Frequently symptoms come and go as they develop gradually over time and show fluctuating patterns throughout the disease.

When multiple symptoms are present, diagnosis can be challenging. A referral to a rheumatologist may be appropriate sooner rather than later. Your family doctor or a chiropractor could order tests to determine the level of inflammation or the presence of antibodies that might help point a finger toward/away from lupus, but there are a number of other possibilities that could account for the same symptoms that are best sorted out by a rheumatologist.

Lupus has many of the same symptoms that are found with rheumatoid arthritis, blood disorders, fibromyalgia, diabetes, thyroid problems, Lyme disease, and a number of heart, lung, muscle, connective-tissue disorders and bone disease.

The most common symptoms are:

- Fatigue
- Headaches
- Painful or swollen joints
- Fever
- Anemia
- Swelling in feet, legs, hands, and/or around eyes
- Pain in chest on deep breathing (pleurisy)
- Butterfly-shaped rash across cheeks and nose
- Sun or light sensitivity
- Hair loss
- Abnormal blood clotting
- Fingers turning white and/or blue when cold
- Mouth or nose ulcers

- Muscle pain
- Kidney problems

When lupus affects the central nervous system, additional symptoms may occur including:

- Headaches
- Confusion
- Depression
- Lupus fog/brain fog
- Seizures
- Strokes
- Vision problems
- Mood swings
- Difficulty concentrating

As with fibro, no single laboratory test can determine specifically whether or not a person has lupus. Test results can point to many other illnesses, and as with all laboratory tests, findings can vary from laboratory to laboratory, further confusing differential diagnosis. If there is any one distinction between fibro and lupus, it would be similar to rheumatoid arthritis in that there is an inflammatory component that by definition is not present with fibromyalgia.

Ninety-seven percent of those with lupus will have a positive "antinuclear antibody test" signaling that the body has begun attacking itself which can lead to autoimmune diseases diagnosis such as lupus, scleroderma, Sjögren's syndrome, polymyositis, dermatomyositis, mixed connective tissue disease, drug-induced lupus, autoimmune hepatitis, and juvenile arthritis. So you can see that even a positive ANA has poor specificity to lupus. Tests with greater specificity that are likely to support the diagnosis of Systemic Lupus Erythematosus SLE include the anti-dsDNA-antibody and anti-smooth-muscle (Sm) antigen tests. I won't get into specifics on these tests but mention them just so you're aware that they exist.

Two other tests will be commonly used to determine the body's state of inflammation but admittedly, once again, not specific to lupus. They are C-reactive protein (CRP) and erythrocyte sedimentation rate (ESR). ESR has lost its favor to CRP; however, ESR is useful to help decipher more acute/active lupus or an infection. Lupus can attack the kidneys without any warning signs, so urine tests are routinely suggested. I certainly haven't covered all diagnostic possibilities;

your rheumatologist will be managing your case. Keep in mind that many of these diseases have overlapping signs and symptoms. There are liable to be several diagnostic conclusions that could fit an individual's case.

Connective Tissue Disease

Connective tissue disease is a category of disease. A connective tissue disease is any disease that involves the connective tissues supporting organs and other parts of the body. Examples of connective tissue are fat, bone, muscle, and cartilage. These disorders often involve the joints, muscles, and skin, but they can also involve other organs and organ systems, including the eyes, heart, lungs, kidneys, gastrointestinal tract, and blood vessels. Connective tissues are made up of collagen and elastin, which are meant to hold/glue things together as well as maintain and recover shape due to their elastic qualities.

Many connective tissue diseases feature abnormal immune system activity with inflammation as a result of a compromised immune system, whereby the body attacks its own tissues. The specific causes of most connective tissue diseases are not known. However, it's likely that a combination of genetic risks and environmental factors are necessary for connective tissue disease to develop.

You may read/hear the term "undifferentiated connective tissue disease" (UCTD). This is used to describe symptoms and lab test results that indicate a systemic autoimmune disorder or connective tissue disease, but are not conclusive. We will see this in rheumatoid arthritis, lupus and scleroderma. Of course the reason that connective tissue disease is in this chapter is that it too is an impersonator/imposter of fibromyalgia. Symptoms include any and all that I have and will discuss throughout the book. However, in addition, the following appear to be unique to CTD:

- Weak blood vessels
- Bleeding gums
- Problems with the lungs, heart valves, or digestion
- Blue or gray tint to the whites of the eyes
- Thin skin
- Curved spine
- Breathing problems
- Hearing loss
- Teeth that break easily

Reflex Sympathetic Dystrophy

Reflex sympathetic dystrophy syndrome (RSDS) has been known to go by many different names, such as:

- Algoneurodystrophy
- Causalgia Syndrome (Major)
- Reflex Neurovascular Dystrophy
- RSDS
- Sudeck's Atrophy
- Complex Regional Pain Syndrome

RSDS is considered to be a rare disorder of the sympathetic nervous system that is characterized by chronic, severe pain. Subluxation of the spine, when uncorrected, will lead to sympathetic nervous system dominance, a mini version or prelude to RSDS. The sympathetic nervous system is the part of the autonomic nervous system that regulates/moderates functions of the body that are involuntary, such as heart rate, and blood pressure. Excessive, exaggerated and/or distorted nerve signals of the sympathetic nervous system are thought to be responsible for chronic pain in the same way that we have discussed, with the chronic pain of fibromyalgia as a "central sensitivity" disease. Symptoms typically begin with burning pain, especially in the arms, fingers, hands, and/or shoulders. Symptoms may show up in one or both legs, possibly localized to one knee or hip. The skin over the affected area may become swollen and inflamed, sensitive to touch or temperature. Complex regional pain syndrome (CRPS) is considered an inflammatory and/or neuropathic condition that develops after trauma, most commonly seen following injury to a limb (Harden et al., 2007; Janig and Baron, 2003). The condition is characterized by various exaggerated painful sensations as time goes on and may be spontaneous and/or evoked, just like fibro.

RSDS, too, is frequently misdiagnosed as a local painful nerve injury in its early stages, and mimics severe migrating fibromyalgia pain with the additional distinctive characteristics as described above. Patients will frequently report symptoms coming on after injury, trauma, surgery, atherosclerotic cardiovascular disease, infection, radiation therapy, or after receiving some type of inoculation.

The diagnostic path tends to mirror that of fibromyalgia, lupus, and connective tissue disorders. Physical and neurological evaluations in respect to subluxations of the spine will frequently prove valuable to help manage symptoms. If subluxations are diagnosed, and therapy administered soon enough after an injury, the progression to RSDS may be avoided. This is a good reason to consult a chiropractor within 48 hours of even the most minor neck or back strain, sprain, or injury.

X-rays and MRIs may show changes in bone density. Nuclear bone scans will demonstrate abnormal patterns as well. Through specialized MRIs called diffusion-weighted (DW) magnetic resonance imaging, there can be seen evidence of pathological changes between gray and white matter within the brain. Many of the findings relate to areas that manage emotional and sympathetic communication with the rest of the body. This relates to our discussion about the way the body interprets pain through emotional centers, and helps explain the relationship between many of the autonomic, cognitive, emotional, and digestive disorders and how they link to chronic pain. This will bring objective confirmation of *central sensitivity*. I believe most readers will see this technology soon become the definitive diagnostic test that the fibromyalgia community has been waiting for.

You can expect to go through a process in an effort to differentially diagnose and eliminate most of the conditions that share symptoms with fibromyalgia, depending on your doctor's experience and intuitions. As of this writing, we still must accept that fibromyalgia is diagnosed by excluding other diseases. However, as we will discuss in later chapters, advanced imaging and neurobiological research will hopefully define specific diagnostic tests in the near future, as noted in the last paragraph.

CHAPTER 6

Fibro Men

Chapter Topics:
Men and Fibro
Physical Energy
The Big Why
Gulf War Syndrome
Post-Traumatic Stress Disorder

Men/Women

I suggest that women not skip over this section.

Men account for 12 to 20 percent of fibromyalgia sufferers. I suspect that in reality it's closer to the 20 to 30 percent range due to the fact that many cases don't get reported. While signs and symptoms mirror those of women, men will tend to deny, bite the bullet, or chalk up their aches and pains to the "stress and strains of life" or to "the old football injury." However, once fatigue and lack of sleep catch up with them, they will have no choice but to enter the fibro world.

Men will have all the same challenges, frustrations, and symptoms that women have. Men or women who are breadwinners will face additional pressure and pride issues—first, dealing with all the symptoms of fibro, and then having to search for their health team while earning a living.

As time goes on, fibro patients may need to tap into the Family and Medical Leave Act (see below). Subsequently, they may have to consider changing their careers in order to tolerate the physical and emotional components of fibromyalgia.

Additionally, as with women but maybe more so in men, there is a tendency to retreat from the family's domestic activities as well as social and sporting activities/hobbies. In my practice I see that the added emotional/pride pressure of being the breadwinner requires more emphasis on strategies that we'll discuss in our chapter on Emotions and Overwhelm.

* **The Family and Medical Leave Act was amended on January 28, 2008. Please visit <u>Wage and Hour web page</u> for additional information.**

Words

The Female Brain, by Louann Brizendine, clinical professor of psychiatry at the University of California in San Francisco, claims that men and women are different because their brains function differently (there's a surprise). One of the most interesting examples she comes up with is that women talk more: 20,000 words a day compared with 7,000 for the average man.

Men tend not to share their feelings as readily as women, at least not in words. But dealing with fibro is a time when men will benefit from stepping up to the plate, sharing feelings, and talking it out. Set aside the feelings of guilt or embarrassment as well as any feelings of inadequacy, and realize that fibro is every bit as serious and real as a heart condition, multiple sclerosis, or rheumatoid arthritis. Subsequently, your significant other/family will understand, support you, and know that "it's not your fault"—you got sick; you have a condition. You're no less of a man; it only feels that way sometimes.

Support Groups

Support groups—or just support in general—seem to be more crucial for men due to their need to cultivate and be encouraged to communicate. Men love camaraderie with other men—someone else in the foxhole with them to fight the battle. I emphasize men with other men. Most men like to participate in team sports or work together for a common cause or project. So a support group—a serious, productive, and educational team environment type of support group—is recommended. My advice is to find one ASAP, or create one yourself that is for men but may have female participation just in terms of education or to come in and give a lecture or something of that nature. But generally, the support should be men with men.

Support groups for men are unlikely to be conveniently available in a reasonable distance to where you live. You may have to reach out, or as aforementioned, start one yourself. Start by discussing this with members of your care team as well as checking the internet to see if there is already a group in your area. Some men will be more comfortable participating in support through online communities, blogs, chat rooms, or organizations. You can find a list of these types of opportunities on our website at www.fibro-doc.com. These are convenient links to help.

Social Support

Support groups don't have to consist of a group of men all suffering from fibromyalgia sitting in a circle that gets together on a regular basis. You may find that by hooking up with one or two guys who have fibro, or something close like chronic fatigue syndrome or possibly post-traumatic stress disorder, you can establish a social relationship that will work fine—even if that means something like shooting pool or just watching a baseball game together instead of playing golf, softball, or other activities that may aggravate your symptoms and drain your energy. Establishing what we'll call "fibro buddies" will open the door for family activities, such as barbecues or going on an outing with the kids. By doing so, sufferers, as well as their families, will feel that they have not been isolated and have not lost their whole family and social structure.

You don't want to create your own private world that you keep bottled up inside. If you do, you'll sabotage your life, your family, your health, and your future. You know the saying "step up to the plate"? Well, this is a plate that you have little to no reference to either understand or deal with. This will be a very unnatural time for you, but think about all the other battles fought and mountains climbed that started out as unnatural or unfamiliar. I recommend dealing with your personal emotions and the overwhelming issues first. Then begin to cultivate your support group or social support/fibro buddies. You'll find these two components will make things easier for you.

Remember

Remember your first day of football practice or when you first got to boot camp, your first job or starting college? Remember a home project that came off great (or almost great)? How about all the other challenges and things that you've accomplished in life that required change? So don't resist this. Accept and attack the challenge; change as you must. It won't be your last challenge, but it's likely to be one at this stage of your life that will be the most important for you and your family. See the ten points and 30-day challenge in Chapter 19. You may want to add an 11th point: "Change is empowering: I welcome it today."

Take Action

Taking action "now" is more important for a man's head and heart than for a woman's. It seems that men attach their identity more to "what they do"—so take action. There's another concept more specifically important for men that will help maintain "manliness and pride." There are two components to this, and two specific action steps that I recommend. One has to do with physical energy, and the other with what Tony Robbins calls "Your Big Why." Keep in mind that "manliness and pride" mostly mean the health of your relationship with significant others and feeling that you have hit the mark for them. This usually interpolates to physical intimacy for most men, but for most woman means emotional intimacy first. Man or woman, the more energy a person has, the better chance he or she will have to hit the mark.

Action Step #1: Physical Energy

Physical energy means that in spite of the aches and pains, you'll need to have the chutzpah, spark, and testosterone to fulfill your Big Why and to take the rest of your action steps. To do this, you'll want to first work closely with your medical doctor, your chiropractic doctor or naturopathic doctor to improve or acquire restful sleep.

Your medical doctor will be able to recommend medication to accomplish this. Your naturopathic doctor or chiropractic doctor can help via vitamins, minerals, nutrition, and diet. You'll want to pay attention to areas that we cover regarding nutrition, as well as our chapter on exercise to acquaint yourself with concepts and vocabulary to help you communicate with whichever doctor you find yourself working with.

Efforts to help you sleep better will either be helpful or not. Don't go on month after month without readdressing efforts with your doctor if you find things just aren't working and you're not sleeping any better. I'm amazed how frequently someone will tell me that he is taking XYZ for sleep and he has done so for two years but it really hasn't helped. Don't be one of those people. However, most likely there will be some trial and error, and that's ok. For long-term health, you'll want to regain sleep as naturally as possible. But again, if you're not getting the results you want, you'll want to change your medication, change your diet, and/or change supplementation accordingly. Many find that changing their doctor is the crucial step. If you're taking a pharmaceutical, you may find that you will do better by switching to highly absorbable calcium/magnesium product before bed. But the opposite can be true as well. Many people try supplements first, and subsequently revert to a prescription before sleep is under control. After making other changes in your life, you're likely to have the opportunity to then drop the prescription medication and find that natural supplementation will be more effective because you've made headway with your general health energy and pain management.

The bottom line: Keep trying, and don't just keep swinging the bat with the same doctors' recommendations over and over. Remember, you are going to need a team in place. Take advantage of the strengths and recognize the weaknesses of each doctor, stay involved, and help with the decisions about what to try next. That doesn't mean leaving any of the other doctors out of the loop; it just means that you're going to be the quarterback. Get your medication advice from your medical doctor and get your nutritional and dietary advice from your chiropractor or naturopath.

I mentioned that there are two considerations particular to men. One is the sleep issue, as we just discussed, to keep your energy up and meet physical demands as well as to inspire healing and help balance hormones. The second part of the energy equation is exercise. My best recommendation is to see Chapter 21 on exercise. Between improving sleep and participating in effective exercise, you'll have a better chance of managing energy, your attitude, work, and family responsibilities.

Action Step #2: The Big Why
The second action step specific for men—and possibly the most important action step—is coming up with your Big Why. Your Big Why has to do with things like supporting your family, taking care of an elderly parent, saving your job, maybe saving your relationship, taking care of a challenged child, or making sure that your children have all the advantages that you can provide for them. The part that we men don't naturally and inherently get is that supporting and taking care of things means meeting the emotional and spiritual needs of others—not just working harder or bringing home more money.

Your Big Why is a driving and passionate reason to live and not give up, the same passion and focus that drives a man to enter a burning building and save a cat, the same passion and focus that drives a man to fight with all he's got when only impossibility is seen by dispassionate eyes. Passion and focus are what we see in all of those guy flicks such as *Forrest Gump* when the hero carries a wounded comrade on his shoulder through napalm, saving his life. That's the hero every man would like to feel like. What's your Big Why?

I've seen many fibro patients who never come out of their man-box. They engulf themselves in work, thinking that working harder will solve all their problems. That kind doesn't work; it will ultimately lead to more pain, depression, and lack of energy. Please consider my recommendations no matter how childish, feminine, or unnecessary they may seem.

Day-Tight Compartments

Chunk your Big Whys down to a daily Big Why. Many success trainers break things down into small chunks that don't overwhelm and are easy to stay focused on. Dale Carnegie spoke about living in day-tight compartments. There's a corny saying: "Inch by inch life's a cinch; yard by yard life is hard." You get the point. So consider chunking life down day by day into your Big Why and daily purpose—or should I say daily target? Do it for the people you love and for those who depend on you. Accomplish this and you will maintain your pride and feel your family's pride in you. These are "must-do" concepts in order to feel like a king and hit the mark as a provider. This can't be accomplished by just working harder at what you already do. This will take a new consciousness and effort.

To find your Big Why, you may have to back off of focusing on doing and listening to the words echoing in your man-box and begin listening to others. You can than cultivate language that leads to effective communication, helping you to define your day-to-day Big Why, and then communicate, express, and execute it in terms that are important to your family. All we're really talking about is figuring out what will maintain you as an emotional and spiritual provider, as well as a financial provider, but doing it in terms of what the people you care about need to hear and feel, not what you think they need to hear and feel. This can be accomplished only by first listening.

Listening will shift your focus and attitudinal strength in spite of your pain, tiredness, irritable bowel syndrome, and depression. You must have a purpose, and need to meet that purpose daily. This doesn't mean that everyone in the family gets everything and anything that they want from you on a day-to-day basis. But it does mean that you don't miss the emotional needs of the people around you. When talking and sharing with them, as mentioned above, it must be meaningful. Meaningful means meaningful to them, meaningful to you, and then meaningful to your relationship. So listen for your future in day-tight compartments of passion and intention. Have one-on-one

powwows and chats with the people in your life, as well as family powwows and chats over a meal together or during an evening sitting in
the living room. It's the best chance you'll have to reveal what you are
going through. Share your feelings; make sure everyone knows what
you are going through so they don't feel detached. Otherwise they will
make up stuff in their own heads about why you are the way you are.

Discovery

Some of the things that you'll discover may surprise you. You may
find that the man-box of hard work that you used to concentrate on
before fibromyalgia kept you from realizing how important it was to
your daughter that you attend her soccer game; now you will. Or that
your son was sad because you weren't playing catch with him before
you had fibro, and you were so busy that you missed—or at least didn't
mention—the great job he did on the lawn. (What boy doesn't look for
recognition from his father?) And, you know, boys naturally have a boy-
box started in their own head. They won't share their feelings of how
disappointed they are when you didn't notice the lawn that they tried
to cut exactly the way you like. Your significant other may just need
more one-on-one talk time with you. Remember all those Saturdays you
played golf, went hunting, spent the day on the couch watching sports,
or helped a friend with the project that took you away from the family?

We could all use tuning up in this area, particularly when it comes
to relationships with our significant other. You may want to read or
reread *Men are from Mars and Women are from Venus* by John Gary Ph.D.

Gulf War Syndrome

In spite of the fact that the term Gulf War syndrome was coined
after the Gulf War in 1990, we can use it to describe almost any negative emotional aftermath of conflict.

The Oregon Health Science University conducted a study of Gulf
War veterans. One hundred and twenty five vets with symptoms similar to fibromyalgia were in the study. One hundred and four were
men, and 21 were women. The study found that 27 percent fell into the
category of chronic fatigue syndrome and 14 percent into the category
of fibromyalgia.

Gulf War vets would be somewhere in their forties about now—
exactly the time when fibromyalgia and similar complaints start to
become more obvious and less tolerable. Gulf War syndrome seems
to point to oddities of chronic fatigue syndrome and fibromyalgia as

part and parcel of or superimposed on post-traumatic stress disorder. Some officials suspect exposure to viral or bacterial agents as causative. Others feel that exposure to nitric oxide and/or vaccinations are contributory.

The Gulf War distinction was further noted by statistics that showed 50 percent of the people who served in the Gulf complained of symptoms such as fibromyalgia and chronic fatigue syndrome. Of military people serving at the same time but not in the Gulf region, only 15 percent reported symptoms. Obviously there are distinct additional stress factors to be considered when the person is in a war zone, but that doesn't diminish the suspicion of viral, bacterial, nitric oxide, or vaccination implications in fibromyalgia.

Hypothesis

Researchers have tried hard to correlate war-zone military service with the onset of fibromyalgia. However, there are no definitive studies correlating the two when compared to the general fibromyalgia civilian population. Some of the studies, as noted above, suggest a high probability that the relationship does exist—and further, that a war-zone environment with exaggerated physical and emotional stress compressed into a relatively short period of time is the perfect environment for a trigger.

Post-Traumatic Stress Disorder

Post-traumatic stress disorder (PTSD) has a classic relationship to military engagement. Experiencing fear, helplessness, and visual horrors within the context of frequently being physically and emotionally depleted makes for a perfect fibromyalgia trigger. What's interesting is that we see nonmilitary fibromyalgia cases that we can label as "civilian PTSD." Civilian PTSD develops more insidiously over time, caused by traumas such as relationship problems, car accidents, physical and emotional abuse, and the stresses of everyday life—in contrast to military stress, which is compressed into a short, intense period of time. Many psychologists and psychiatrists treat military PTSD as well as nonmilitary and cumulative post-traumatic stress disorder the exact same way. In general, as in all stress disorders, life management skills, counseling, family communication, understanding and support are crucial. When PTSD and fibromyalgia coexist, the sufferer may not have the wherewithal to manage stress and overwhelm on their own. There is also an issue of support system/caregiver burnout, which further raises the need for third-party counseling. Baby boomers experience similar burnout when caring for elderly parents.

Men vs Women

I'd like to note that there is no distinction between military post-traumatic stress disorders by gender. The sheer imbalance of the numbers of men versus the numbers of women in our military is the only reason that I've listed this disorder under the category of men. Certainly women in our military are every bit as much of a concern and every bit as susceptible as men. In some ways, women are more susceptible and sensitive to these factors and conditions that we've discussed.

> While most of the fibro picture is shared between men and women, there are hormonal, behavioral, and evolutionary distinctions. These distinctions call upon both genders to understand themselves and strive to be emotionally available to the nuances of feelings and needs through communication.

CHAPTER 7

Women and Children

Chapter Topics:

Children   Emotions
Invisible Disabilities   Family Leave Act
Allostatic Load   Obstetrician / Fertility
Diet + Nutrition   Back Pain
Genetics   Postpartum
Pregnancy

Children: The Challenge

Patient story: B & D, Hartford CT.

Bill, a patient of mine, talked to me about his son Collin. Bill explained that Collin had just turned 12. "He was kind of a wiry kid with lots of energy, or so we thought," he said. Everyone rationalized his behavior as "lots of energy." Bill explained, "He couldn't sit still and didn't sleep well; we chalked it up to kid stuff. And up until now, any time that he complained about aches and pains or headaches, we figured he was just trying to get attention or avoid having to go to school. He had plenty of friends and played with them okay, except he was always more aggressive and scrappy with his cousins. Over the past year the biggest change we've seen is that he doesn't seem to have that same scrappy energy; he still complains about aches, pains and headaches, but now we can't get him out of bed. His pediatrician diagnosed growing pains or possibly ADHD. Getting him to do his homework is like pulling teeth. That assumes he has even gone to school and has any homework. It wasn't until he started having diarrhea just after his twelfth birthday that his mother and I decided to take him to another doctor, but we didn't know whom to go to."

I had been treating Collin's father for a whiplash injury. When Bill told me about his son Collin, I recommended that he bring him into the office so we could take a look. Collin's mother's health was good, with no signs or symptoms that would suggest fibromyalgia. His father, other than the whiplash injury for which we were treating him, was in great shape. However, Collin's mom remembered that her mother was always complaining about being tired and having muscle soreness. She apparently spent a lot of time on the couch. In any event, after speaking with Collin and examining him, I felt that a diagnosis of fibromyalgia was very possible. This diagnosis could explain all his symptoms and behavior. I referred him to a rheumatologist for further tests. Subsequently we received confirmation of a fibromyalgia diagnosis. Not that this was such great news, but having a diagnosis was at least better than wondering every day. There was a certain amount of peace that Bill shared with me because he and his wife were becoming convinced that their parenting skills were at fault, and that had put a lot of strain on their relationship.

Perspective

Claudia Craig Marek reports interviewing many children with complaints that suggested fibromyalgia. She found that roughly 50 percent thought that something was different about them, but didn't know what. The other 50 percent thought that everyone felt the way they felt and that something was wrong with them because they weren't tough enough or brave enough to deal with the discomfort. Some said they just felt like they were complainers. They typically described themselves as having less energy than other kids, and they felt that they couldn't concentrate on things in the classroom. They were frequently frustrated and embarrassed about it, figuring they just weren't as smart as the other kids. If your child fits this category, you may need to bring it up to your pediatrician, who may up until this time have chalked up these complaints to growing pains and child socialization.

Pediatricians

Pediatricians are not rheumatologists and are unlikely even to feel the need to spend time researching rheumatologic problems; they're too busy with wellness-care visits and treating common childhood ailments. There's a good chance your pediatrician has never even come across a case of fibromyalgia. Consequently, coming up with a diagnosis will be more difficult and confusing for the parents. The parents who have fibromyalgia symptoms themselves--such as chronic fatigue, myofascial pain syndrome, or arthritis--will typically become suspicious and seek help sooner. Some parents have shared with me that even though they are in great shape, they remember their mother or grandmother spending a lot of time on the couch and always having aches and pains. These memories can frequently help bring a diagnosis sooner rather than later. The good news is that there are pediatric rheumatologists who are very familiar with conditions such as fibromyalgia. If your pediatrician doesn't think of referring you, you should bring up the question.

After the Diagnosis

Once the diagnosis is made, the clinical and treatment considerations for children are pretty much the same as with adults. Certainly medication, if necessary, would be adjusted to the size and weight of the child, with extra consideration to side effects. As a parent, you're likely to have additional challenges with other people in the family who already have observed the child's behavior and are now informed of the diagnosis; suddenly everyone becomes a doctor and wants to give you advice. This can make it more difficult for parents to control attitudes of friends and family, and may add confusion.

I recommend doing your homework and consider getting a recommendation for a child psychologist from a pediatric rheumatologist. I'm not convinced that the child actually has to go to counseling regularly, but in most cases we find that if parents can have the support and extra perspective, home management will be easier. And when I say home management I don't mean only the condition and the symptoms of the child, but rather the general household tension, attitude, and socialization.

The early years will be crucial to help your child cope and avoid complications down the road. More importantly, at this stage communication and your attitude will steer the ship. Remember that in spite of the fact that fibromyalgia is not a psychosomatic condition, there are depression, anxiety, and energy and behavioral problems that you'll need to deal with. You, your family, and the child will benefit from understanding cognitive behavioral techniques to avoid being overwhelmed and to help with normalizing everyday life.

Other Children

Counseling will also help your relationship and communication with other children in the house. Striking a balance will be difficult. You'll have to divide your attention and manage everyday life and family activities so as not to embarrass your fibro child or estrange any of the other children. Striving to provide an environment where they can all live as normally as possible, for the children as well as for Mom and Dad, is a challenge.

School

School, teachers, and friends become another challenge for the child with fibromyalgia. Discussing strategies and communication skills with a child psychologist before approaching your child's school or teachers would be wise. When the time comes, you'll likely be better off first approaching the highest level of educator in the school with whom you can get an audience. Also consider the principal and a counselor first, or possibly the school nurse, rather than going first to the child's teacher. Teachers, like all of us, may have attitudes and misconceptions that could single out or generally make the child's situation more uncomfortable both academically and socially. This especially holds true when a child has any condition that is termed "an invisible disability" such as fibro. Teachers and classmates will see no physical difference in your child, which may cause them to wonder, "How come Collin doesn't have to play soccer?" or "How come he takes so much time off from school?"

Invisible Disabilities

Being chronically sick with daily aches and pains, plus no energy, is difficult on relationships—particularly when the person looks normal and healthy. There is no bleeding, no disfigurement, and no physical accommodation is needed in everyday life. It has been estimated that over 125 million Americans have some type of chronic condition that renders them disabled to some degree without any visual signs. It's difficult for people around you to understand what you're going through and not suspect, at least a little, that you are just lazy. They may think, "She just doesn't even try," or "I have aches and pains all the time too, but I do what I need to do." Sometimes it's just hard for the people around you to be compassionate when it's hard for them to believe there's anything wrong with you because you look great. Children and adolescents have enough challenges under the best of circumstances. They are trying to negotiate their own bodies and understand their emotions, life, and relationships--all in a pool of changing hormones. Childhood and adolescent conditions are among the saddest and most invisible of the invisibly disabled.

Childhood Stress

Whenever we are under stress (physical, chemical, or emotional) our adrenal glands release a hormone called cortisol. Cortisol's job is to help us physically, chemically, and emotionally to deal with the stress. Adults and children alike maintain a certain baseline level of cortisol just for everyday functions. At times of excessive stress, extra cortisol is released. Children and their developing brains are more susceptible to spikes in cortisol and stress. Stress in early childhood could be anything from subtle abuse or neglect (such as letting a baby cry herself to sleep), to more obvious forms of stress and abuse such as spanking, rejection, or injury.

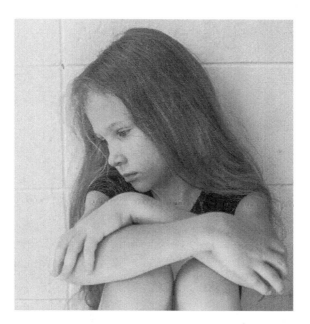

Allostatic Load

Introducing the term "allostatic load" might be a bit too much for this section; however, it helps to put stress, cortisol, and adrenal function into our brain bank for discussions to come as well as establishing general sensitivity to the level of stress that children go through. Frequently, as adults, we slough off the stress that children go through. Yet subsequently in adulthood many adrenal conditions that develop will, at least theoretically, correlate back to childhood stress.

Allostatic load is a term referring to the cost/burden that adaptive stress and adverse conditions put on the body and the brain. Although cortisol is a necessary hormone for healthy living, when overproduced, particularly in childhood, it can have a damaging effect on the brain. Cortisol's effect on the brain—specifically the part of the brain called the hippocampus—relates childhood stress and cortisol to the possibility of fibromyalgia expressing itself in later life. The reason is that the hippocampus is involved in memory, the perception of pain, and sleep regulation. In respect to fibromyalgia and "chronic pain," the developing brain is extremely sensitive to stress and the resulting high levels of cortisol, aka the allostatic load. Hippocampus abnormalities due to cortisol levels have been documented by MRI studies in fibromyalgia sufferers.

The hippocampus at this early development stage has the ability to sensitize itself in a way that effectively exaggerates the experience of pain, how it feels, and how a person should react. Further, it tells the rest of your brain and interpretation centers what you should experience when someone touches you or you flex a muscle. This directly relates to fibromyalgia. During the early stage of rapid brain development, these adaptations and learning skills in the brain (termed neuroplasticity) happen more rapidly than in an adult brain. As we get older, brain development slows down and what we've learned in early development is cemented in, frequently permanently. This is one of the very strong hypotheses about how fibromyalgia can develop from childhood, particularly in those who are predisposed via genetic links. General contentment has also been shown to help control cortisol levels as well as give the hippocampus a break. General contentment can include a positive atmosphere, humor, and pleasing music, to name a few.

It is said that an ounce of prevention is worth a pound of cure. In this case, a positive, happy, and fun environment that is nurturing emotionally and nutritionally is the best prevention—and possibly a cure if and when a problem is developing.

Diet and Nutrition
When discussing hypoglycemia (low blood sugar) we noted that high-carbohydrate diets and poor eating habits can cause chemical stress and increase cortisol. This raises the question of diet and nutrition's involvement. Meeting this challenge may require the incorporation of a naturopathic and/or chiropractic physician as part of your management team. Some of the considerations nutritionally will be to evaluate vitamin and mineral levels. For instance, magnesium supplementation has been shown to decrease serum cortisol levels after aerobic exercise. Omega-3 fats have been shown to help control cortisol as well, and have a corresponding positive impact on mental stress,

behavior, and attitude, whereas omega-6 fats have been shown to have a negative effect, as they generate inflammation and pain.

Genetics

Genetics, of course, can have a strong influence on any and all considerations. Whether there is a strong or relatively weak genetic link, stress factors can reach a critical point in bringing on fibromyalgia. The cortisol link would be an example of a neurochemical toxin. In another chapter we will expand on the influence of neurochemicals, with focus on the role of cortisol in the hypothalamic-pituitary-adrenal axis.

A child does not have to be genetically predisposed for fibromyalgia to develop. There can be a predisposition to other conditions such as chemical sensitivities, muscular and postural abnormalities, or neurological conditions that set the stage for fibromyalgia. Stressors, as we've discussed, can then lead to neurological changes and cause an organic development of fibromyalgia. This means that if a child is predisposed to chemical sensitivity, a vaccination or flu shot could overwhelm the system and push him toward the development of fibromyalgia. With a genetic predisposition to muscular and/or postural weaknesses, a seemingly innocuous injury or spinal alignment problem in childhood could neurologically challenge the hippocampus and subsequently help to develop central sensitivities, as we discussed in previous chapters, and subsequently trigger fibromyalgia.

For most readers, at least a portion of many chapters will include information that is less practical and more perspective-enriching, having little immediate application in helping a parent with her child. However, many of these points should be considered in overall family health strategy so as not to challenge the physiology of other children in the family—or the parents, for that matter. It's impossible to know for sure who has weakness or genetic predisposition to fibromyalgia and who doesn't. Having said that, contemporary science is making rapid progress in analyzing DNA with gene-snip testing. This test will become much more affordable and common as time goes on, offering a window into individual weaknesses and possibilities for developing disease. Soon we will see these tests as commonplace and encouraged, just as mammograms and colonoscopies are today. For more information you can call my office at 860- 745-7600 or email me at Fibro. EPC@comcast.net, or see the appendix.

In the meantime, give appropriate priority to family wellness care. Providing a physical, emotional, and nutritional environment that supports health and doesn't challenge possible genetic predispositions is wise for us all.

Pregnancy

Pregnancy is a game-changer for Fibros, but not as much as some may think. Pregnancy and two-to- six months postpartum will be much smoother for those who have worked their way through the strategies discussed in this book. Becoming your own advocate based on knowledge, and a having realistic perspective, along with preparation before pregnancy, will serve you best. You'll find that much of what has worked before you became pregnant will work just as well or better during pregnancy. Those who have been committed to Non-medical health care, such as chiropractic or naturopathic medicine, will need to sort out quickly who will be the right medical managers throughout their pregnancy. Ideally, you'll want an obstetrician who has experience with fibromyalgia pregnancies. On the other hand, if to this point you have had no Non-medical care, it's recommended that you discuss with your obstetrician the advisability of chiropractic co-management as your pregnancy progresses, for reasons that we will discuss in a moment.

Pregnancy will be a wake-up call for those women living busy lives who do not have a fibromyalgia management strategy in place. To put a strategy in place, you will want at least twelve months prior to becoming pregnant to establish a baseline of what works for you and what does not. Of course you might ask, "Why should I go through the trouble when everything's going change once I am pregnant?" But at least you will have a baseline to judge from, as well as a baseline to work your way back to after delivery.

Obviously it's not always possible to have everything sorted out and lined up before pregnancy. In any case, there will be a bit of scrambling to reprioritize, organize, and put together your health team. The primary care for your fibro may shift from your PCP or rheumatologist to your obstetrician. You'll want to find an obstetrician who is experienced with fibromyalgia pregnancies. Some of the medications that you've been taking up to this point may have to be reconsidered. If you're preparing for pregnancy, reconsidering medication sooner rather than later is important, as some medications will stay in a person's system for a long time. If your pregnancy is a surprise, your doctor may shift even your most effective medication to something considered more conservative and safer for your baby. Nutritional supplementation and herbal compounds will need to be discussed as well. You may be surprised to find out that those medications that the man in your life is taking need to be reconsidered as well. He could be taking something because he's the one who has fibromyalgia, or he's taking medication for other illnesses or conditions. In either case, the medication could affect his sperm. The chances of this are, admittedly, remote, but your medical doctor will surely consider the possibility even if it is not verbalized.

Preparation

Just as you prepare emotionally, physically, and financially for adding a little person to your life, you'll want to prepare for the shift in how you manage your fibro. Having a Non-medical physician in place to help you deal with pain and stiffness will be an advantage, as the choices for medication will become limited. Working with chiropractors, osteopaths, massage therapists, and participating in regular exercise may be an advantage. Keep in mind that just as it is important for you to find a PCP, rheumatologist, and obstetrician who has experience with fibro pregnancy, it's important to find a chiropractor, massage therapist, or exercise coach who has a lot of experience with fibromyalgia and pregnancy. The reason is obvious: there are nuances and special techniques that must be used during pregnancy, just as there are nuances and special considerations with any medication you might be taking.

Symptoms that you experience from time to time before pregnancy, such as depression, carbohydrate cravings, inappropriate tearfulness, feelings of anxiety, self-esteem issues, etc., may become exaggerated during pregnancy or postpartum. Ten percent of women develop clinical postpartum depression. The good news is that it is usually relatively short-lived.

Speaking of postpartum issues, you'll want to consider making arrangements for help after you deliver. It would be wonderful if someone could be there who is ready, willing, and able to help you and who has had specific experience with children as well as with fibromyalgia. But at least have someone in place to help keep up with household duties. Probably the first and most logical preparation is to make sure that your family (significant other as well as other children) are well-indoctrinated and capable of handling everyday activities around the house. Meals, organization, household chores, and being able to fend for themselves as much as possible will make things smoother physically and emotionally for you and for them. As Kristin Counts explains it: "Get some people lined up for the postpartum stage. You'll most likely need help. There will be two patients coming home from the hospital, you and your baby."

Most people will first consider their spouse as the default choice to take over everything. However, don't count on that working for you, even if he takes time off from work. If either one of you is consumed by household and family duties, that could affect parenting and your personal relationship. I'm not saying it can't work, as many families do make it work; I just wonder sometimes if it's as wise for their relationship as it might initially seem. Plus, once you have used up the time allowed off from work, you will likely still need some help. If you can afford to, you'll find that taking advantage of the Family Leave Act will be helpful for you, as well as for your spouse. Your obstetrician should have information for you but, if not, look up the Department of Labor, Family and Medical Leave Act (FMLA). Also check your state laws; some of them will include leave time for domestic partners, civil unions, and even other members of your family such as grandparents.

Overview:
   * **The Family and Medical Leave Act was amended on January 28, 2008. Please visit <u>Wage and Hour Web page</u> for additional information.**

The Family and Medical Leave Act (FMLA) provides an entitlement of up to twelve weeks of job-protected, unpaid leave during any twelve-month period to eligible, covered employees for the following reasons: 1) birth and care of the eligible employee's child, or placement for adoption or foster care of a child with the employee; 2) care of an immediate family member (spouse, child, parent) who has a serious health condition; or 3) care of the employee's own serious health condition. It also requires that employee's group health benefits be maintained during the leave. The FMLA is administered by the Employment Standards Administration's Wage and Hour Division within the U.S. Department of Labor. (http://www.dol.gov/compliance/laws/comp-fmla.htm)

Emotions and Fibro

In pregnancy, hormones will be changing radically, so you can expect some emotional surprises. Your mood, energy, brain fog, and patience will change. You are liable to experience new patterns of physical symptoms affecting muscles, tendons, and ligaments, as well as joints and flexibility. Aches and pains may begin to migrate and become exaggerated or confusing, as if it's not your body any longer. Patients tell us that early and late pregnancy feel the most uncomfortable, frequently mimicking PMS symptoms. However, most report that somewhere in the middle things seem to smooth out and they actually feel a little bit better than they did before the pregnancy.

If you don't already have a relationship with a psychologist, a productive support group, or at the very least a special non-spouse person to lean on, now would be a good time to hook up, even if you feel that you have gotten everything together.

A discussion with your doctor, a psychologist, or an advocate counselor could be helpful; your spouse/significant other should be included— and it may be advisable to include your other children as well, if applicable. Discussing symptoms—like mood swings, energy, and physical capabilities—will help make home life easier. You shouldn't have to go home and explain or defend your condition, symptoms, or capabilities every time you turn around. Have your family present so they can hear it from someone other than you; as it is said, "You can't be a prophet in your own land." Another effort (not as good as sitting down with the third party, however) would be to pick up a book, or select two or three sections of this book that you think would help your family understand what you're going through, and ask them to read it. Afterward, have a family discussion about what they've read.

Don't expect the people around you to "get it." This goes for fibro with or without pregnancy. They have no framework to understand what fibro sufferers go through. We can't forget that people around you can't feel what you feel physically or emotionally. Life goes on for them. Your other children will still have their own share of growing up and relationship problems; the adults around you won't stop having their everyday stresses at work, with finances, and their own health concerns. Roles may have to change from day to day. Everyone will have a turn at being a caregiver, being understanding and helpful. And everyone will have a turn at needing help and understanding.

Obstetrician Perspective and Fertility

There is research suggesting that fibromyalgia sufferers may be less fertile if they have myofascial pain syndrome. But there's no indication of an increase in miscarriages. When compared to the non-fibromyalgia population, there does seem to be a minor increase in concerns about getting pregnant if there has been a diagnosis of endometriosis as well. Also worth mentioning is that although there is a high correlation genetically to pass fibromyalgia on to a child, that risk in itself poses no danger and hence no reason to avoid pregnancy.

In a posting from the National Fibromyalgia Association, Dr. Brian Mason MD, a high- risk obstetrician (perinatologist), notes that there is a decrease in fertility amongst fibromyalgia patients, particularly if accompanied with myofascial pain syndrome. He noted that during pregnancy, non-drug options are the best and safest for pain relief. But this doesn't mean that patients and doctors should completely shy away from using medication, and should weigh risks against benefits at all times. He cites examples of non-drug options as meditation, aerobic activity, yoga, focused breathing, physical therapy, and certain forms of massage.

Unfortunately for his patients and readers, Dr. Mason is apparently unfamiliar with chiropractic or osteopathy. His unfamiliarity is one of our primary concerns when it comes to managing fibromyalgia— and, in this case, with the addition of pregnancy. Chiropractors and osteopaths, as well as medical doctors who have experience with fibromyalgia and pregnancy, will attenuate and adjust their techniques appropriately. The goal is to relieve symptoms and help to avoid drugs. Hopefully, a chiropractor or osteopath is already part of a woman's health team before she becomes pregnant. A PCP and obstetrician may know little to nothing about your posture and center of gravity's effect on your spine, joints, and muscles; more importantly, their medical education does not prepare them to make the correlation between the components mentioned and effects on your nervous system and possibly the pregnancy itself. During pregnancy, the radical change in weight, center of gravity, and changes in soft tissue due to hormones will play a major role in the comfort of a pregnancy.

Back Pain

As the pregnancy progresses, hormones will influence muscles, tendons, and ligaments in preparation for delivery. Mom's center of gravity begins to shift forward due to the weight of the baby. As a compensatory effort, this requires the upper body to shift weight and posture backwards. This all happens instinctively and automatically and would seem logical if all pregnant women ended up with back pain. But interestingly enough, many find that the compensation effort, which requires a sway in the low back, causes little to no back pain or aggravation of symptoms. And in some cases, it actually relieves pain. So while back muscles may have to work harder, the mechanical shift actually improves alignment and the neurology of low back joints, suggesting that subluxation within the low back predated the pregnancy, and that the pre-pregnancy low back pain was not due to fibromyalgia. When back pain does occur or is exaggerated due to pregnancy, chiropractic evaluation is necessary to avoid the common assumption that the increased discomfort is simply from pregnancy. Low back, pelvic alignment, and general conditioning will, in large part, dictate a mother's ability to successfully adapt to the changes. The bottom line is that a pre-pregnancy evaluation for subluxation by a board-certified chiropractor will be a great advantage. Additionally, we find that foot mechanics and any failure of the arch of the foot frequently encourages poor pelvic and low back adaptation; this causes a mom's low back to work even harder. Wearing flip-flops, sandals, or shoes with poor support can only make matters worse as weight increases during fetal growth.

Postpartum

Up to a year after delivery, moderate to severe depression may develop, although it most commonly occurs within the first three months. Postpartum depression—also termed "baby blues"—is usually short-lived. Men can experience postpartum depression as well. Baby blues can be quite debilitating, which makes a strong case for home preparations and help to be in place following delivery. Symptoms of postpartum depression are really not any different from depression at other times in life. I've seen no reports that fibromyalgia sufferers are any more prone to baby blues than anyone else. What does pose an extra challenge is getting adequate sleep, when generally fibro sufferers already have poorly restorative sleep. This will be a consideration when it comes to deciding whether or not you will breast- or bottle-feed. Dr. Mark Pellegrino MD reports that, due to sleep deprivation, many of his patients choose to bottle-feed during their second pregnancy, having learned the first time around that breast-feeding challenges quality sleep. Bottle-feeding may offer the benefit of enabling your partner to be more involved in nighttime feedings, which will help Mom get more rest.

In any event, depression raises general concern, and your doctor may want to do some tests to make sure that everything you've gone through has not triggered, complicated, or inspired another medical condition that needs to be addressed. If depression hits, don't put off consulting with your doctor.

> All of our chapters call for study and awareness. However, many of the topics in this chapter involve a limited yet crucial time frame, calling for increased diligence and preparation.

CHAPTER 8

Special Considerations

Chapter Topics:

Hypoglycemia / Diabetes

Glycemic Index / Glycemic Load

Cellular Energy

Sympathetic Dominance

Hypoglycemia

Breathing Right

Posture

ADD / ADHD and Diabetes

Menopause

Stress and Eating

Hypoglycemia and Diabetes

Hypoglycemia is defined as low blood sugar, whereas diabetes is considered a metabolic disease that causes high blood sugar.

At first glance, hypoglycemia sounds simple; it's a decrease in blood sugar. Diabetes, as a metabolic disease, is usually considered a more serious condition. While I don't mean to minimize the seriousness of diabetes, hypoglycemia is every bit as detrimental to a fibromyalgia sufferer or someone who is genetically predisposed to fibromyalgia.

In either case, blood-sugar management and its relationship to energy as well as inflammation is pivotal to understanding many other concepts of this book. It will put personal struggles into perspective. Understanding it will help manage emotions, diet and exercise, control the sense of being overwhelmed, and help in all considerations of general health.

Please don't be impatient with this section; read it carefully even if you don't think you have diabetes or hypoglycemia. It will help you to understand diet strategies and hypoglycemia which, as a fibro person, you are much more likely to be suffering from whether you know it or not. Symptoms such as confusion, visual disturbances, fatigue, anxiety, headaches, cravings, sleepiness, and poor muscle recovery can all be signs of hypoglycemia. But they are not necessarily signs of fibromyalgia, in spite of the fact that they frequently coexist with and/or complicate fibromyalgia.

Dr. St. Amand has compiled statistics to show that 75 percent of fibromyalgia patients have a blood-sugar management problem. We have found in our work that if we are to prevent, control, or reverse fibromyalgia, blood-sugar management is job number one nutritionally and behaviorally. For conditions such as chronic fatigue syndrome, myofascial trigger points, and idiopathic pain, blood sugar management must be of prime clinical concern; if not, all other clinical efforts will be less effective than they should be.

Glycemic Index

The glycemic index, simply put, is a frame of reference. It puts into perspective the speed at which a carbohydrate-containing food is processed into sugar and enters the bloodstream, hence becoming available for energy.

The body breaks foods down for energy and nutrition. The energy part of the breakdown ends up as sugar (Sugar or blood sugar is a colloquialism. The proper term is blood glucose; however, you'll hear the terms used interchangeably). Glucose in the bloodstream signals the pancreas to secrete the hormones insulin and glucagon. The body tries to keep a constant supply of glucose for cells by maintaining a constant glucose concentration in the blood—otherwise cells would have too much glucose right after a meal and then starve in between meals and overnight. When you have more blood glucose than you need for energy, the body uses insulin to process it out of the blood and store it in the liver, muscles, and fat. When there's not enough glucose circulating, the body uses the hormone glucagon to increase circulating glucose by pulling glucose out of its stores in the liver, muscle and fat, thereby maintaining energy. Insulin is a key management hormone for all food groups (fats, proteins, and carbohydrates). We will be focusing on carbohydrates.

Cells can become resistant to the action of insulin for several reasons: genetics, decreased activity which reduces the need for energy, and obesity. Although there is a question as to whether obesity is caused by insulin resistance or the insulin resistance is exacerbated by obesity, let's accept for now that they are reciprocal. In the past, one could draw a logical metabolic conclusion that cells could become resistant simply from being overly exposed to insulin and basically shut down. More recently, studies have helped us to understand that cells become resistant to insulin to protect the cell from becoming toxic as it works harder and harder to process the glucose. This means that insulin resistance, as commonly seen in diabetes, while not desirable, is a protective mechanism confirming sugar excess and cellular toxicity. Cellular toxicity becomes ubiquitous, encouraging systemic inflammation, and is likely to play a role in all disease processes—including, of course, fibromyalgia.[36]

To compensate for cells' being resistant to insulin, the pancreas works harder and secretes more insulin. People with this syndrome have higher levels of insulin in their blood as a marker of the disease rather than a cause. Over time, people with insulin resistance are likely to develop high glucose levels in the blood, or diabetes, as the pancreas can no longer meet the demand for insulin; it too then shuts down. It basically wears out.

The Signs of Insulin Resistance Syndrome[36]

- **Impaired fasting blood sugar, impaired glucose tolerance, or Type II diabetes.** This occurs because the pancreas is unable to turn out enough insulin to overcome the insulin resistance of cells. Blood sugar levels rise and the person becomes pre-diabetic, if not diabetic.
- **Abnormal cholesterol levels.** The typical good cholesterol levels (HDL) of a person with insulin resistance are low. Bad cholesterol levels and triglycerides are high.
- **Heart disease.** An insulin-resistance syndrome can result in atherosclerosis (hardening of the arteries) and an increased risk of blood clots.
- **Obesity,** especially abdominal obesity or belly fat. Obesity promotes insulin resistance and negatively impacts insulin responsiveness.
- **Stroke.** Cerebrovascular insults encourage ischemic injury and poor clinical outcomes.
- **Disease.** Any inflammatory disease or pain syndrome.

To give you an idea of how various foods rank on the glycemic index, here are a few foods along with their average GI ranking: 55 or less is considered "low," 56-69 is considered "medium," and 70-100 is considered "high." Non-carbohydrate or low-carbohydrate foods (protein, meat, fat, nuts, oil, etc.) have a "low" glycemic index.

Food	Glycemic Index	Food	Glycemic Index
Peanuts	8	All-Bran cereal	55
Agave nectar	11	Cliff Bar	57
Dark chocolate	23	Power Bar	58
Cashews	25	Soda	59
Grapefruit	25	Honey	61
Chickpeas	28	French fries	63
Apricots	31	Green beans	63
Lentils	32	Sweet potato	63
Tomato juice	33	Raisins	64
Soy milk	34	Popcorn, plain	65
Pizza	35	Fruit punch	67
Apple	36	Brown rice	68
Skim milk	37	Baked potato	69
Baked beans	40	White bagel	69
Apple juice	41	White rice	73
Fruit yogurt	41	Doughnut	75
Orange	43	White bread	75
Snickers bar	43	Watermelon	76
Milk chocolate	45	Chocolate chip granola bar	78
Corn tortilla	46	Gatorade	78
Meat lasagna	47	Instant oatmeal	79
Vegetable soup	48	Corn flakes	81
Orange juice	50	Caramel rice cake	82
Banana	51	Pretzels	83
Ice cream	51	Rice milk	86
Sweet corn	52		
Potato chips	54		

Think of a glycemic index this way: sugar goes into your blood stream at a speed of 100 mph. So, as an example, if you eat a piece of sugar candy, it will spike your blood sugar at 100 miles an hour. A doughnut turns to sugar and will be in your blood stream at approximately 75 mph, chickpeas at 28 mph, and peanuts at 8 mph.

The amount of fiber and/or fats that a substance has in it will influence the glycemic index. Carbohydrates with more fiber and more fat are said to be more "complex" carbohydrates. Typically, the more refined or less complex the food is, the faster it will turn to sugar (a higher glycemic index) and be more detrimental. When we overwhelm our bodies with high-glycemic index foods, our bodies have to either burn the sugar immediately or store it as fat. It turns into fat by becoming a triglyceride in the bloodstream first. When you have blood tests, you'll notice that you have total cholesterol read as well as good cholesterol (HDL), bad cholesterol (LDL), and triglycerides. Triglycerides are an indication of circulating fat in the bloodstream and will potentially lead to fat storage. PBS aired a documentary on carbohydrates showing that high levels of circulating triglycerides will make circulating blood look like pink cream. And while these triglycerides may end up in fat cells, making you look plump and pink, it could be worse. If it goes on too long, depending on some genetic factors, you could end up with Type II diabetes. So the moral is that low glycemic index foods are better for you. However, there are other factors, because some foods have a higher glycemic index but are still beneficial. Let's take their benefits into consideration. You'll see the term "glycemic load." It is felt that this is a much more resourceful evaluation tool. We touched on this concept when speaking of complex carbohydrates.

Glycemic Load

Glycemic load refers to how much work or energy must be expended in order to break down a food or a meal into sugar (let's change gears now and refer to "feedings" rather than a food). The more fat, fiber and protein in a feeding, the more load—aka effort and time it takes the body to break the feeding down into sugar.

I'm not going to offer a lot of examples or detail in reference to glycemic load because frequently a person will use this information to rationalize eating donuts, pancakes, and spaghetti where the glycemic load number is lower than the glycemic index number. Or a meal with fried foods may seem to be a convenient choice, having a lower glycemic load due to the fat. The way to wisely use the glycemic load concept is in structuring meals/feedings. For instance: rice has a relatively high-glycemic index and high-glycemic load. Now let's add some stir-fried vegetables. This adds fiber and many nutrients, which together with the rice lowers the glycemic load. If we want to tweak the load even further, at the same time improving nutrition and adding anti-inflammatory qualities to the meal, we could sprinkle some cold-pressed virgin olive oil on top. And why not add some raw nuts for more good fats and protein? So now we have a high glycemic index base of rice, considered to be a relatively simple (75ish) carbohydrate; however, we've turned it into a complex carbohydrate (45ish) meal with a low glycemic load. This would be a wise strategy for everyone, whether it's felt that there is a carbohydrate metabolism challenge or not, in helping to control blood sugar and enhance energy and general health.

The bottom line: control blood sugar and you'll go a long way toward controlling inflammation and some of the aches and pains, soreness, and fatigue that are common to fibromyalgia. Further, we'll set the stage for any other therapeutic effort to be that much more effective because cells will be healthier and more capable of healing. Remember Dr. St. Amand's guaifenesin protocol? It appears to be minimally helpful without tending to blood-sugar management. Blood-sugar management also plays a crucial role in brain chemistry and the cells' ability to communicate with each other; we will discuss this in more detail shortly.

Let's discuss the basic perspective of both hypoglycemia and diabetes. Then we'll tie this into what you may be experiencing, or that which you may be unaware of as a blood-sugar issue. Then we'll discuss diabetes in a little more detail and work our way back to hypoglycemia, surprising you with some considerations that few patients have been made aware of by their doctors. There are some aspects of hypoglycemia and diabetes that your doctor may not have told you about. A common theme of this book is "Your doctor doesn't know what your doctor doesn't know." But you must know this, in order to help yourself.

Cellular Energy

A study reported in 1999 by Swedish researchers Dr. Bengetsson and Dr. Hendrickson found a 20 percent reduction in muscle energy in those suffering from fibromyalgia. The energy that this is referring to is ATP (adenosine triphosphate), which is produced by a specialized function of all cells.

Poor blood-sugar management can reduce or even stop the production of energy (ATP). This can be caused by nutrient deficiency or nutrient excess, as discussed above. But as long as a healthy amount of oxygen and sugar (glucose) are provided to the cell, energy production will usually keep up with a body's demand. This assumes no other cellular encumbrances exist. While there are many factors that can reduce cellular energy, we're going to discuss three special situations that can cause or perpetuate fibromyalgia—and which, as aforementioned, your doctor most likely will never tell you about. Consequently, you'll go about your business never knowing how negatively these are affecting your health. They are:

1. Physical and emotional stress. We all know that stress comes in many different flavors. Stressors challenge the hypothalamic adrenal pituitary axis (HPA) and keep us in a constant state of sympathetic dominance. This challenges blood-sugar management, even if a person has a great diet.
2. Chemical stress, aka diet, challenges the pancreas's ability to manage insulin; this means blood-sugar deregulation. Too much blood sugar or too little blood sugar leads to cellular energy deficit.
3. Breathing, oxygen, and hypoxia. If oxygen availability is reduced, tissues will become toxic and create free radicals, reducing the cells' ability to produce energy.

Reduced energy/ATP production encourages cravings, an increase in appetite, tight muscles, poor stamina, and weight gain, possibly leading to increased blood pressure and increased bad cholesterol (LDL) levels along with triglycerides, and working its way to excess body fat and a compromised immune system. Being in this state is bad news for fibromyalgia sufferers. When cellular energy is down, our body energy is down. Muscles get tired and sore, movement can be painful, mood and attitude suffer, and brain fog becomes a way of life.

Stress: Physical and Emotional

Sympathetic Dominance

Recurrent physical or emotional stress will make its way to sympathetic dominance. This is when the sympathetic and parasympathetic nervous system are out of balance. The sympathetic portion becomes overly active, which excites physiology and upsets the balance between the brain and the adrenals into a term called "flight or fight," aka hyper-arousal physiology. During the early stages of recurrent stress the body does its best to cope, resetting itself back to a healthy baseline after a stressful event. Men seem to recover/reset their systems faster than women, bringing the hypothalamic/pituitary axis back to a healthy baseline. This may help to explain at least one component of why women are more susceptible to fibromyalgia. Women, for emotional and hormonal reasons, have more lingering effects from a stressed state and consequently have an increased challenge with blood sugar/energy management.

When stress persists, imbalance persists with a constant flow of stress hormones. One group of stress hormones is called cannabinoids. Cannabinoids exist to help us combat stress, but can lead to diabetes and obesity. Released during stress, they block insulin from doing its job of getting glucose into cells; this includes muscles or brain cells.

Stimulation of the cannabinoid system is something that many baby boomers are familiar with, having experienced the munchies or mellowness after smoking marijuana. The body tries to overcome the situation by increasing insulin in an attempt to push more glucose into the cells. Cells can handle only so much, so they literally resist. In turn, the pancreas puts out more and more insulin and cells become more and more resistant to it. This is the same scenario as insulin resistance that we discussed above—however, for a different reason. As above, sugar will build up in the blood. Secondly, muscles and brain cells will lose energy, obviously causing weakness—and, if nothing else, brain fog. Little by little you may begin to notice that you get more frequent headaches and you're a little more tired than usual. Your neck, shoulders, between your shoulders and maybe your lower back will frequently feel tight and not tolerate any one prolonged position or activity. You may notice that your allergies are just a little more intrusive. You may have mood swings and digestive disturbances. This scenario is of great concern, as it is of epidemic proportions in just about all modern societies and cultures.

Daily stressors also cause adrenals to overreact. In the early stages, adrenals will make the same effort as the pancreas; they recover when stress abates. But as time goes on and stress persists, they will become exhausted as well. This too reduces cellular energy and will negatively affect other organs, systems and hormones, corrupting the hypothalamic/adrenal/pituitary axis (HPA axis). Over time, this may encourage the transition from hypoglycemia to diabetes; this is theoretically proposed as the common denominator of many fibro and chronic fatigue symptoms, demonstrating more inflammation and pain, allergies, and a whole host of other problems.

Diabetes
Diabetes affects five percent of the population in industrialized nations. Type I is called diabetes mellitus. It usually shows up in children due to autoimmune destruction of specialized cells in the pancreas. Type II, which is more common, is considered an adult-onset

condition due to progressive insulin resistance and/or a relative deficiency of insulin secretion, leading first to overt hyperglycemia. Adult onset or developmental diabetes is most likely in those who are genetically predisposed. "Predisposed," however, is a relative term because even someone considered to be non-predisposed genetically, and unlikely to become diabetic, could live a lifestyle overwhelming their system and still develop diabetes. Some researchers and clinicians are suggesting that there is a third type of diabetes; namely Alzheimer's disease. This is due to its relationship to carbohydrate consumption and the encouragement of chronic inflammation within the brain. It remains to be seen how this will play out within the healthcare community. Clearly we should all strive to live a lifestyle that does not challenge our genetic makeup, because you never know how susceptible you might be. However, research is moving quickly to unravel genetic codes, hoping to predetermine genetic concerns.

Genetics

When genetically coded as a Type I diabetic, children are likely to require insulin injections. More common to fibromyalgia is Type II/adult diabetes. Acquiring Type II means your genetics have prevailed, possibly in spite of a relatively good diet, or there is little to no predisposition, yet the diet is so poor that the pancreas simply can't handle what you eat and diabetes develops.

Even if you have no suspicion or family history of diabetes, this chapter is likely to hit home with symptoms and similarities in how you feel. It is important to gain perspective and to correct/reverse any threat that your diet or lifestyle may pose to blood-sugar management and genetics.

Chemical Stress

Basically, we've already covered this, revolving primarily around diet, but a couple more nuances won't hurt. Your health will benefit by considering yourself pre-diabetic if you have the slightest degree of hypoglycemia or carbohydrate sensitivity; in which case you should consider sugar look-alikes such as sugar substitutes as well as carbohydrates and overeating a threat. Fibromyalgia sufferers are most likely going to be carbohydrate-sensitive if not hypoglycemic. Weight management could be difficult in that the body may continue to store fat and malfunction in spite of carbohydrate management. This speaks to an urgency to manage blood sugar.

What to Do

1. Consult your medical doctor for a definitive diagnosis.
2. Discuss options with your doctor about non-drug efforts that are proactive.
3. Get some coaching about "universal truths." A universal truth would be something like the benefit of simply walking for 30 minutes a day. This is universally accepted as a truth and something all will agree can improve your health (assuming you're capable). An effort like this will improve almost any health condition. But, as with other recommendations, suggestions, or thoughts in this book or any other writing, you should consult your doctor before undertaking any changes in diet or medication. In any event, these 30 minutes of walking will stimulate endorphins and, at least for the short term, will help you feel a little better, improve your outlook on life and help to reduce pain.

   In the initial stages, you'll want to keep exercise extremely modest, and, although there will be short-term symptom improvement due to endorphin stimulation as aforementioned, progressing too quickly may challenge your body's ability to deal with exercise toxins such as lactic acid and work against you in the long run. See Chapter 21 on exercise for more details.

4. Consult a naturopathic or chiropractic physician for nutritional considerations having to do with diet, toxicity, lifestyle, and/or supplementation such as ginseng, cinnamon, and chromium. When consulting your naturopathic or chiropractic physician, consider discussing adrenal tests, as adrenal stress can sabotage the HPA axis and lead to pancreas stress.
5. Keep a regular schedule to monitor lab findings, and when you start to feel better, don't feel as if monitoring is no longer necessary.
6. Stay in tune with what you're feeling. How do your shoulders and neck feel? What does it feel like in your mid-upper back between your shoulder blades? Tightening up in those areas could be a sign of sympathetic dominance brewing. You'll feel tension and you will be aware of and distracted by those muscles pulling up into your neck, possibly feeling like a headache. Osteopathic or

chiropractic therapy will go a long way to help mitigate sympathetic dominance for most, and may be the only way for some. The relief you feel will not only help to reset your body-brain/brain to body communication, but will help improve sympathetic and parasympathetic balance, enabling you to exercise and have the will to pay more attention to your diet.

7. Monitor blood pressure. You'll most likely find that if your blood pressure is going up, your energy will be going down. Behind the scenes you'll be creating and holding on to more inflammation than your body can handle, which will increase your fibromyalgia symptoms.

Hypoglycemia

Carbohydrate sensitivity and hypoglycemia are basically the most subtle/insidious versions of diabetes. They are frequently undetected and undermine every health effort undertaken.

The line between diabetes and hypoglycemia is best seen as a gray area. Let's say you don't really have any of the associated conditions as mentioned above, but you have noticed that you have stiffness, painful movement and fatigue (you know, aches and pains and feeling older than you should). You don't seem to have any sleep problems, yet you never really feel rested. Have you noticed that once you start eating, you want to keep eating? Do you have trouble controlling your weight? Do you have a general lack of enthusiasm? Would you rather stay on the couch watching TV than be active? Would you rather sit rather than stand? Are you unable to think as clearly as you'd like? Are you noticing that you have anxiety from time to time? Do you have light sensitivity or sensitivity to sound? If you answer yes to any of these, you are likely to be knocking on the door of prediabetes and presently could be a full-blown hypoglycemic Fibro.

Fibroglycemia

I love the word fibroglycemia (fibromyalgia and hypoglycemia).[66] Fibroglycemia was coined by Dr. St. Amand to describe the special and common relationship of blood sugar to fibromyalgia. And, as we've discussed, you as a Fibro are very likely to fall into this category.

With a good understanding of blood-sugar management, you'll not only be able to self-diagnose, but will greatly increase your ability to manage your symptoms and your energy. More fundamentally, you'll be in a better position to understand foods, nutrition, and lifestyle issues in a way that will empower you to diagnose and manipulate your lifestyle as well as manage your recovery. No doctor can do this for you.

Early Stages

As we have already established, in the early stages of hypoglycemia we may simply be carbohydrate-sensitive. This early stage can be complicated and encouraged by poor breathing habits, poor posture, and a host of other issues. These are subtleties that defy clinical consideration by most doctors' and patients' logic, issues that undermine health and encourage hypoglycemia. They literally set the stage for and increase susceptibility to fibromyalgia, perpetuating or complicating it. These issues apply whether or not you are genetically predisposed.

We'll cover three basic issues:

1. Eating habits
2. Breathing habits
3. Posture/physical stress

Eating habits are easily understood as part of the picture; too much sugar and too many simple carbohydrates are a prescription for trouble. But the idea that breathing and posture could play a role is a bit of a stretch for most patients. Some MDs will be aware of the breathing connection, yet unlikely to recognize the posture connection. One reason is that MDs think in term of chemistry. The other reason is that the posture/neurology connection can be subtle and lurk below the radar. Doctors, unaware of or untrained to investigate those aspects, are unlikely to consider them as a possibility to help you. Let's emphasize once again the importance of patient education and confident self-advocacy, and consider that our health care system is 90 percent a disease-care system, and breathing habits would not be considered a concern until a full-blown respiratory problem is diagnosed. Posture would not come into question either, until you have a back pain, a disc problem, or a radical distortion such as scoliosis, and even scoliosis may be considered a concern only for vanity.

Why Is That?

Without getting too far off track, let me briefly list some of the reasons that we ignore wellness-care, most of which are no secret, but are simply not part of Western medical culture.

1. Most Americans are too busy to ask for wellness-care. In this conversation, wellness-care does not mean a checkup

to find out if you have a disease. Wellness-care means to investigate and address behavioral and lifestyle issues that eventually might sabotage health and speed up the aging process. Wellness-care means to improve health. Health is defined as "...*a state of optimal physical, mental, and social well-being, and not merely the absence of disease and infirmity.*"[25] Adult consciousness/priorities are serendipitous leftovers from a "bullet-proof" consciousness as young people. We don't believe anything can hurt us until it does. We take more chances and abuse ourselves more than we should. Consequently, true health care is not at the foreground of the average person's mind until there are health problems.

2. We turn to doctors and health coaches only after we're in trouble.

3. Big money (pharmaceutical and technology money) promotes the quick fix, usually meaning "knock out the symptoms," and because of number one above, we "buy into it." We proceed to live it until some problem catches up with us and covering up the symptoms isn't working any longer.

4. Wellness-care takes a lot more time. Wellness-care costs too much for insurance companies, and they will pay for wellness-care only if they see that it could save their shareholders money. Pharmaceutical and technology companies support their effort—for instance, paying for a colonoscopy rather than paying for colon cancer surgery/care. I'm not saying this isn't smart; I'm simply saying that it's not wellness-care/health consciousness. It is insurance company economics 101.

5. Only a small percentage of our medical community has the interest and the education in the subtleties of health. Rather, they have a great education and interest in disease and trauma. This should not be looked at as a flaw in the practice of medicine, and I don't mention it or any other recurrent theme to disparage the integrity, the value, or the ability of the medical community. It is, after all, the way it was designed, intended, and what we certainly need. The missing link is acknowledging the unintentional lie that indoctrinates the lay public to believe that Western medicine, the pharmaceutical industry, and insurance companies are aligned with health as I am more broadly defining it here.

6. There are other disciplines that have a paradigm interest and philosophy in steering health's subtleties, leaving

disease and trauma in the hands of those who are trained and focused on it (the medical community). Other disciplines/physicians are sometimes termed alternatives, meaning "alternative to Western medicine." So-called alternative practitioners are osteopathic physicians, naturopathic physicians, chiropractic physicians, and some specialties in physical therapy and nutrition.

7. In our current socio-political and economic environment, doctors won't be paid to spend the time necessary to address the nuances of health. They can, however, get paid to look for disease, order tests, and execute procedures, as well as treat disease and injury. However, even these efforts are being squeezed by the insurance companies— which ironically enough were designed and are managed by their own medical colleagues. Generally, insurance companies bring in alternative physicians only when the public demand is high enough that if they didn't they would be unable to sell the big policies to municipalities, big companies, and organized political structures and organizations.

8. Saving lives makes great news headlines and makes for dynamic politics, as well as making pharmaceutical companies and technology companies lots of money. Alternative health care (non-drug/non-surgical) offers little to no financial gain for pharmaceutical and technology companies and only vanilla headlines for the media.

Alternative care works with lives and conditions in the "invisible disability" category, and yet these conditions can claim the lives of sufferers and families. Treatment of invisible disabilities rarely makes good news headlines or dynamic political issues.

Breathing

Breathing badly is usually a habit[32] in the same way that bad posture may be a habit. Bad habits feel normal; therefore they self-perpetuate. The consequences may never point back to the bad habit that caused them, meaning bodies do the best they can to compensate for bad habits, yet pay the price over time, showing up as seemingly unassociated symptoms or causing a disease that eventually will create symptoms of its own.

Modern life, with all its time-saving technology and benefits, has not decreased stress. Stress causes us to tighten up. You may have noticed how your shoulders get tight and seem to be sucked up to the base of your skull, causing your neck to tighten. Or you have knots in your shoulders, maybe your head feels heavy, or you have a low-grade headache. These may indicate upper chest breathing, aka apical breathing; it is shallow and poorly efficient, decreasing oxygenation of blood, vs. full lung and diaphragmatic breathing, which is six to seven times more efficient. Full lung breathing is also more efficient in encouraging healthy flow of lymphatic fluids—which, as you'll recall, is considered part of the circulatory system and has great responsibility in detoxification as well as distribution of nutrients to cells. The lymphatic systems volume is twice that of blood; however it is on its own to circulate because it has no heart pump as blood does. Lymph circulates by muscle contraction and proper breathing.

Upper-chest breathing encourages a mild/subtle state of hyperventilation, aka over-breathing. We find that most fibromyalgia sufferers tend to hyperventilate slightly. Another consequence of hyperventilation is overeating, especially triggering carbohydrate desires as blood sugar drops and energy drops.

Hyperventilation / Over-Breathing
The body is always struggling to balance the flow of oxygen and carbon dioxide to assist in balancing acid and alkaline body chemistry. Maintaining proper amounts of carbon dioxide helps to relax muscles, decrease anxiety, and generally calm the nervous system; modest exertion can help with deeper breathing and actually relax muscles. But if a person has poor breathing habits, meaning breathing mostly from the upper chest, which is inherently shallow, this can cause carbon dioxide to be over-expelled, which, in turn, increases blood pH, over-alkalizing body chemistry.

Under this condition, blood vessels will constrict, reducing blood flow to the heart and brain, hence losing oxygen. Pain thresholds will lower, causing more experience of sensitivity/pain. This scenario can takes place in reverse also, when someone is under constant emotional stress and tension first, causing muscles to tighten up in the neck, shoulders and upper back. This scenario leads to relatively shallow breathing from the upper chest, once again creating an imbalance between carbon dioxide and oxygen. The effects that this will have on the nervous system include:

- Nerve sensitivity that increases, consequently causing pain.
- Light and sound sensitivity that increases.

- Muscles become tighter.
- Decreased circulation to the brain affecting mood and concentration levels, aka brain fog.
- Anxiety is exacerbated.
- Emotions are challenged.
- A negative vision of the world and a person's life are likely.

Obviously these scenarios will add to stress, and a vicious cycle ensues.

Overeating / Emotional Eating

We have all heard of comfort foods or people who are emotional eaters. This helps to relax and increase the depth of breathing patterns. Anxious people and people who are under a high stress load—as in most family and business situations these days—have a tendency to consume more food than necessary. The overeating is likely to be carbohydrates, with poor intake throughout the day of minerals, proteins, and fats that help stabilize blood sugar and satisfy hunger centers in the brain. However short-lived it may be (approximately an hour), overeating at least temporarily appears to calm the nervous system, relaxes muscles, and reduces anxiety and stress. Sometime between one and two hours after a large meal, as the stomach gets closer to being empty, breathing works its way back toward upper chest and shallow hyperventilation once again.

Dr. Konstantin Pavlovich Buteyko found that eating fruits and vegetables nets less of an impact on ventilation due to the availability of digestive enzymes in live foods, hence making their digestion easier. Dr. Russell Jaffe's work adds perspective that the increase in minerals through more natural live foods serves up minerals necessary in controlling pH and respiration.

A diet high in cooked proteins, fats, and simple carbohydrates will drop pH (cause more acidity). The body will make an effort to normalize pH by increasing respiration to push out more carbon dioxide, thereby raising pH and balancing the acidic effects of proteins, fats, and simple carbohydrates. An added insult is that the cooking of foods destroys most enzymes, which is another reason that most of the meats, fats, and carbohydrates that we eat cause our blood to be more acidic. This is a bad scenario, not only in managing blood sugar but also in managing chronic pain, fatigue, and various other symptoms.

Conclusion

For these reasons among others, more alkaline diets—eating live foods such as raw vegetables and fruits—are generally considered healthier. You can see that it's not just a matter of calories. We recommend that patients who are incorporating animal proteins and plenty of healthy fats and nuts also attempt to over-consume live vegetables and eat a very, very modest quantity of whole grains and legumes (assuming tolerance). Meals should be complex with an emphasis on vegetables.

I'd like to offer one other perspective. It's naïve to believe that balancing diet has to do only with foods consumed and/or eliminated. Our activities and physiological demand must be considered too. This speaks to the need for diet customization, to say nothing of considering genetics and other variables. We'll talk more about this in other parts of the book but, just as an example, a person who lives a relatively sedentary life with little to no exercise may have blood sugar/energy issues and carbohydrate intolerance not because the digestive system can't handle him carbohydrates but because physiological demand does not call for more carbohydrates. Someone who lives a more active life and participates in strenuous exercise may do himself a disservice by eating too few carbohydrates. In either case, proper breathing will actually help to curb appetite as well as manage physical and emotional stress. This is a simple self-management method of helping to control blood sugar; in addition, you may notice that some of the symptoms of fibromyalgia and chronic fatigue improve.

Posture

Posture is one of the missing links in fibro management. It will affect blood sugar, energy, breathing, and nerves. Also, general posture considerations and ergonomics of work and domestic environment will play a role in muscle fatigue and the propensity to hyperventilate. Above and beyond that, there are neurological issues that arise when spinal dynamics are compromised

Poor posture becomes a habit, not only from the over-breathing/hypoglycemic standpoint, as we discussed, but from the irritation of spinal nerves, which help control metabolism and the insulin responsibilities of the pancreas. These issues are not addressed medically; rather, they are handled by alternative physicians, ideally in a wellness-care model to avoid creating disease. However, posture usually is not addressed until after blood sugar, posture, back pain, and/or breathing problems have become apparent. The scenario is, as discussed above, in reference to energy and pain. However, it is from a different causative factor: posture and the spine. Nine out of ten times the scenario begins with mid-back discomfort; the shoulders become tight and pull up into the neck. This will progress to low-grade headaches, neck pain, and pain between the shoulder blades, at which point a second opinion/co-management by an osteopathic or chiropractic physician would be in order.

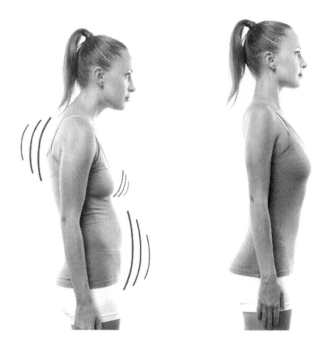

The more a person's posture deviates from ideal, the lower a person's general health score becomes. The journal *Spine* explains it this way: "*Negative health effects are linear and correlate with postural deviation from normal. There is a high degree of correlation between posture, health scores and chronic pain.*" The Journal *Spine*, September 15, 2005; 30 (18): 20 24–9

Posture Counts!

ADD/ADHD

One in every 10 American children is diagnosed with attention deficit hyperactivity disorder ADHD. And more than 3.5 million children between the ages of 4 and 17 are taking a drug to control their behavior, according to a study by the Centers for Disease Control and Prevention.

Some research suggests that ADD/ADHD and fibro are related, each being a manifestation of Autonomic Nervous System Dysfunction (ANSD). There are many similarities in symptoms; however, these symptoms are expressed differently at different ages. ADD is most often diagnosed in childhood, while fibro is diagnosed in adulthood. There doesn't appear to be any value in evaluating ADD patients for fibromyalgia, however. Dr. Glenda H. Davis and Patricia Stephens, CNC, suggest that fibro patients meeting ADD criteria and treated accordingly may improve markedly. However, the stimulants that are commonly prescribed for ADD have not been cleared to treat fibromyalgia.

Neurologist Dr. Richard Saul echoes the Autonomic Nervous System Dysfunction (ANSD) theory. He reports that ADHD is a collection of symptoms, rather than a specific disease. He explains that there are over 20 different conditions that mimic the signs and symptoms of ADHD. Therefore, hyperactivity labeled as a disease based primarily on behavior might cause doctors to miss underlying conditions that could be causing the symptoms. This is not dissimilar to some of the controversy that exists as to whether fibromyalgia is a disease or simply a constellation of symptoms. Dr. Saul calls true ADHD a "neurochemical impulsive distractable" condition. And only this condition requires treatment such as Ritalin. There's no reason for Fibros not to be evaluated for ADD; it may prove interesting depending on the case.[34]

There was an interesting study conducted in Sweden and published in *JAMA Psychiatry*. The study's findings correlated an increase in mental illness and ADHD in children who were fathered by men over 45. Apparently, middle-aged men have a high number of spontaneous DNA mutations. I have not seen any research attempting to correlate fibromyalgia with parental age. Considering the suspicion of ADHD/ADD being related to fibro, we are now conducting our own study and would love to hear from you. If you have fibro, please let us know the age of your paternal parents at your birth. If you have a child, with fibro please lets us know the age of both parents at the birth. Please go to Fibro-doc.com and send us an e-mail. Thank you.

Menopause

Menopause poses an extra challenge to fibro sufferers. The earlier there is a reduction in estrogen, the more chance there is of aggravating fibro symptoms.[48] Any upset in hormones will generally leave someone susceptible to increased sensitivity to pain. During menopause, estrogen, progesterone, and testosterone levels will drop, all of which contribute to aggravating fibro. Menopause and perimenopause are stressful, which brings into play cortisol levels. Between increased cortisol and decreased estrogen, weight gain is likely. This can further upset hormone levels that are already challenged.

As ovaries produce less estrogen, the body will look elsewhere to replace it. It looks to fat cells for help; yes, fat cells produce estrogen to help make up for decreased ovary production. The body begins to stockpile fat to help, encouraging weight gain.

As testosterone lowers during menopause, lean muscle decreases and metabolism slows. Fibro sufferers already have low energy production, so while this scenario also helps to increase fat, it lowers energy, further aggravating symptoms. Progesterone also drops during menopause. This doesn't help energy production and doesn't help to produce more fat cells; however, it will encourage water retention and bloating. Bloating will cause clothes to fit tighter, make a person feel more sluggish, and take a toll on self-esteem and emotions. This sounds all too familiar to many readers, I'm sure. I bring it up simply because it's normal and I encourage you to tend to menopausal and perimenopausal concerns ASAP through nutrition and lifestyle. If you begin working with a naturopath or functional-medicine doctor early enough, you may be able to avoid some of these pitfalls, which include having to take hormone replacements. By doing so, your menopausal years will be smoother. Additionally, I encourage you to read Dr. Christiane Northrup's book; *The Wisdom of Menopause.*

> The fundamentals of diet and body chemistry are synonymous with the fundamentals of blood-sugar management and improved clinical outcomes for Fibros. Life becomes easier, and discomfort and stress become more manageable, when diet supports physiological balance. Don't get caught up in letting life just happen to you; study and take control. You know; that proactive stuff.

INSIGHT #2

PLATFORM FOR RECOVERY

The platform from which health springs is an understanding of principles, tools, and commitments which all else will spring from.

—Author Unknown

CHAPTER 9

It's All in Your Head

Chapter Topics:

Pathways to rhe Brain	*Chronic Pain*
Endorphins	*Rx Where/Why*
Controlling Pain	*Music?*
Glial Cells	

Pathways to the Brain

Let's begin by understanding what happens to nerve impulses when there is an injury, using a leg injury as an example. The damage causes direct and/or toxic triggering of pain receptors, which initiate electrical impulses at a rate of 400 mph. The goal of the signals is to reach the brain for your awareness and response.

The electrical impulse/signal that began in the leg must be transferred to nerve pathways in the spinal cord to make its ascent to the brain. The transfer from one nerve to another takes place at a synapse (common space) where things slow down. Unlike electrical nerve transmission, synapses are sites for chemical transmission/communicators (neurotransmitters). Neurotransmitters either excite or inhibit the signal. This is a site of opportunity for the body to begin to control/modulate the information and disseminate it to other tissues and locations that must be alerted to the damage in the leg. One of the first neurotransmitters called to action are endorphins.

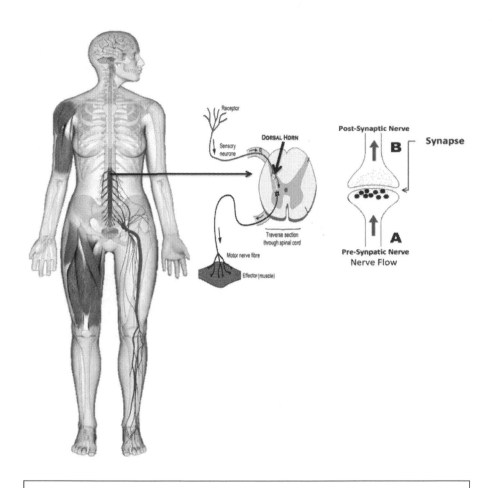

Damage of the leg begins its ascent to the brain. When entering the spinal cord at the Dorsal Horn, the body will have an opportunity to adjust the signal (increase, decrease, or stop) before the signal proceeds to the brain.

Endorphins

Endorphins are neurotransmitters produced in the pituitary gland and the hypothalamus. However, some research is pointing to cells in the spinal cord and brain as playing an important role in producing endorphins as well.[64]

An injury is not the only way to stimulate endorphins. They are stimulated by a chiropractic adjustment, acupuncture, exercise, excitement, pain, making love, and stress; even spicy foods and great music can stimulate endorphins. The word comes from combining endogenous (within our own body) and morphine (because morphine acts as a natural opiate).

Endorphins are released throughout the body, as well as into the spinal cord and the brain, and help to regulate and modulate pain signals, improving mood and optimism. However, receptor sites can be fooled. Substances like nicotine and marijuana (cannabis) are accepted and basically fool the receptor site, in effect blocking the body's endogenous endorphins from doing their job, which is to modulate pain. Other chemicals that cause a similar response are morphine and heroin. There are also prescription drugs that can take the place of our own natural endorphins, such as steroids, naloxone, and naltrexone. Some of these drugs are used in drug rehab/detox therapy, taking advantage of a feedback loop mechanism to help control the production of endorphins as well as other natural opiates as a person's system is reconditioned off street or prescription drugs,

Endorphins attempt to block the pain signal at its source first, and then once again attempting not to allow the signal to enter the spinal cord. This happens at the synapse, effectively dampening and possibly completely blocking the signal from continuing its path to the brain.

Much of the scientific community, and many people in the general public, encourage the legal use of marijuana for its pain-blocking ability that comes from its ability to mimic endorphins. There are, however, two components to marijuana: one component bends the mind and accounts for its social pleasures, the second is its ability to block pain. It will be legalized without prescription dispensaries the second that marijuana can be cleaved to clone a plant that maintains only the pain-blocking components. Marijuana is not the only substance that mimics endorphins. Hemp interestingly enough is rich in cannabis with few if any psychogenic properties.

When the body experiences severe or intense pain, endorphins will be released into the bloodstream. The more severe the insult, the more endorphins will be released. This doesn't mean that the job is always complete; any fibromyalgia patient will testify to this. However, it's not uncommon to hear of people having their finger cut off or having a leg shot off in war who say that they had no pain. This is primarily due to a dramatic infusion of endorphins at the time of injury.

Some of the therapeutic value of exercise, massage, acupuncture, osteopathic and chiropractic manipulation, placebos, medical procedures, and emotional therapy can be accounted for by their ability to stimulate endorphins. So we can see why doctors and fibro literature frequently encourage exercise. We also find that more contemporary open-minded physicians will consider acupuncture, chiropractic, and osteopathy for their manipulative value in stimulating endorphins, thereby decreasing the need for OTC/Rx drugs. In later chapters, we will discuss the specifics in the application as well as the drawbacks of these efforts for fibro sufferers.

An interesting aspect of these natural efforts to stimulate endorphins and influence the health of our nervous system specifically in controlling the pain of fibromyalgia is that endorphins must be stimulated regularly—meaning daily—to sustain healthy levels. Regular endorphin stimulation, to hit the "stay healthy and control pain" mark, requires a conscious and proactive effort. A sedentary life won't do; we must increase our activities as well as participate in the well-care aspects of the natural therapies as mentioned above. So we find that the body has an ongoing monitoring and application system of chemicals—endorphins—to manage and balance inflammation, pain signals, mood, and energy. When participating in these activities and therapies, we are participating in true health management and wellness-care—I think of this as neurological nutrition. We are ultimately protecting and managing brain chemistry, physiological set-points and, in large part, the brain's ability to interpret and manage many aspects of life above and beyond pain.

Traditional Western medicine and certainly insurance companies have not fully appreciated these aspects of health care. Rather, they are fixated on disease care. In and of itself, disease care is not a bad thing. The point is not what they're doing right (most of which we definitely need), it's what they're leaving out that accounts for so many non-life-threatening invisible disabilities. I suspect that due to such a strong historic medical paradigm, the direction of health care has little chance of shifting in time for those reading this text. When it does shift and they do "get it," we will find that lifelong well-care participation in the therapeutics of acupuncture, chiropractic, massage, and exercise will be encouraged with understanding and open interdisciplinary referrals. Ironically, however, as general health will improve, the masses with chronic pain will be reduced and pharmaceutical companies will lose money. So, we can see how they could continue to work against the acceptance of natural efforts. Of course if they could figure out how to put together a capsule that, taken three times a day, supplies us with the recommended daily allowance of exercise, chiropractic, and acupuncture, then things would change.

Endorphin Deficiency

There are conditions—congenital as well as behavioral—that can cause a deficiency in endorphins. A congenital deficiency needs no explanation; a person can be genetically coded to simply be deficient in production of endorphins, setting the stage for reduced tolerance to pain as well as encouraging depressed mood and attitude. In fact, a deficiency of endorphins is frequently misdiagnosed as clinical depression and treated as such.

Behaviorally, a person taking drugs by prescription or socially, or self-medicating through behavior (this may also include exercise addicts or adrenaline junkies) can cause the natural production of endorphins to be diminished. This can happen via a feedback mechanism affecting other neurotransmitters such as dopamine, subsequently throwing off the balance of endorphins.

This mechanism also helps explain addictions and confirms that many addictions are in fact physiological and not simply a matter of willpower and behavior.

Stimulate Endorphins Naturally

As aforementioned, therapeutic efforts directed at one of the symptoms or conditions a person is suffering from (such as back pain) are intended to release endorphins for their effect at the site of pain. However, the effort understandably has a ubiquitous effect due to stimulating endorphins in the brain and central nervous system. As we've mentioned, these natural efforts would include chiropractic, osteopathic manipulation, acupuncture, and massage, as well as participation in physical activities such as exercise, tai chi, yoga, or Qigong. As a side note, not all of the natural physical efforts to stimulate endorphins are tolerated well by Fibros. Frequently there are preliminary clinical/therapeutic steps that need to be taken to improve a person's physiological tolerance before they can reap the benefits of natural endorphin stimulation. The initial and most conservative efforts may involve subtle endorphin stimulators such as listening to your favorite music, watching a funny movie, having some fun with friends, and getting adequate sunlight. Comprehensive nutrition, of course, is a factor in all health considerations. Foods such as chocolate and spicy foods—especially those containing capsaicin, like chili peppers—and complete protein sources will help also.

Tonight try a funny movie while sipping fresh lemonade (no sugar, use Stevia) with some cayenne pepper sprinkled in it, while a loved one is massaging your shoulders. Tomorrow morning, get out there for a modest walk in bright sunlight while listening to your favorite music.

Controlling pain

There are five opportunities the body has to control or eliminate pain before it becomes chronic and challenges the system, threatening to trigger or exacerbate fibro.

1. Stop the causative factor, aka the irritation at the site of insult (a burn, broken leg, whiplash, subluxation, or emotional trauma such as abuse).
2. Stop the inflammation at the site of injury, usually by some type of anesthetic, possibly ibuprofen or any number of other anti-inflammatory drugs/herbs, etc.
3. Also it's possible to block the signal peripherally before synapsing / entering the spinal cord. Medication, fascial work, laser therapy, and other adjuncts may help.
4. Block the pain signal at the synapse just before it enters the spinal cord. This could be done with endorphins or drugs like naltrexone, which as of this writing is still in experimental stages.
5. If it actually synapses with pain nerves in the spinal cord, the message/signal is on its way to the brain. The next opportunity would be to affect the brain directly via nerves and *glial cells* with cognitive therapies or anesthetics such as nitric oxide or naloxone, etc.

Glial Cells and Pain

For the purpose of this chapter we're going to focus on glial cells, as in number four above, because they are the least obvious solution and hold great potential with evolving science and opportunity.

Glial cells, once thought to be helpers or a type of housekeeping cell within the brain, were historically neglected by researchers. Most recently, science has been amazed to realize that glial cells make up approximately 85 percent of brain matter; they communicate with each other, sense electrical activity, and control brain function.[18] Brain glial cells are where most research has taken place. Glial cells help to control response as well as produce cytokines. Recently scientific researchers have been amazed to find that glial cells are influenced by endorphins and cannabinoids.

After an injury to the body or an infection, whether viral or bacterial, cells involved in the body's defense and healing mechanism release chemicals called inflammatory cytokines and chemokines.[18] Inflammation, as we have discussed, is a healthy physiological response; however, the body can overreact, or a person's tolerance to inflammation might be low. In either case, something like ibuprofen or aspirin can bring relief by blocking the action of the cytokines. Glial cells have the ability to control their response, increasing their normal sensitivity when appropriate. However, the heightened sensitivity and awareness in the area of inflammation may cause more pain. This improves/sharpens reflexes and consciousness, to help protect the area. But when this happens, there's potential to not reset/recover back to the original baseline of sensitivity. The body may literally lock itself into a hypersensitive protective mode as a primitive protective effort. So now we have a protective mechanism that has become a disease in and of itself. Pain may now be perpetuated even after the threat or the injury has passed—as in fibromyalgia, when there is pain and sensitivity for no apparent reason.

So where do these cytokines come from? Cytokines are produced by glial cells which, therefore, leads us to believe that glial cells may play a more direct role in pain management.

Chronic Unrelenting Pain

When one or more of the possible controlling mechanisms has lost its effectiveness, pain will surpass its original protective responsibility and become a disease termed *neuropathic pain*.

Nerves become relentlessly overexcited and neurotransmitters flow without adequate regulation, allowing hyperalgesia (an increased sensitivity to pain), if not allodynia (pain from a stimuli that would not normally cause pain), will prevail. Think of the advantages of having an electric stove with the ability to control the heat and time to cook your Sunday turkey dinner perfectly. But when the turkey's cooked, instead of being able to turn the heat off, the stove locks itself into cooking mode. Neither you nor the stove has the ability to stop the cooking.

Why?

How does this happen? Why does the body lose control? Much of the scientific community explains this glitch by pointing the finger at inflammation. It's clear that drugs like ibuprofen and aspirin bring relief by reducing inflammation and helping to protect nerves from being further stimulated, in turn reducing the threat to trigger fibromyalgia. This issue may be the most valuable and valid reason to use anti-inflammatories immediately after an injury even if you have only minimal pain, especially if you have any reason to believe that your nervous system is already challenged genetically, chemically, physically, or emotionally. However, taking medications and then going about your life as usual is not advised. We suggest taking whatever medication is needed so you can sleep well and function safely during the day, but not assume that medication and reduced pain means that the damage has healed or the danger has passed. Healing and repair are taking place behind the scenes.

All injury triggers high-alert status; the nervous system becomes hypersensitive/on-guard. The neurological sensitivity that develops is not only at the site of injury, where the pain, swelling and redness are--the entire body is reacting.

The Nervous System

In a classic sense, neurophysiologists and neurobiologists have traditionally focused their attention on "nerves." Nerves were considered to be conduits of electrical impulses. The "neuron doctrine"[53] would dictate that all functions of the nervous system are the result of activity along nerves/neurons. And via nerves, all integration of brain function takes place—and whole body functions, for that matter—primarily due to the interconnectivity of these nerves. The work of Oschman, Becker, and Fields has helped to confirm that the "neuron doctrine" is an inadequate view of the nervous system's workings, and further, that the nervous system in fact includes glial cells, as mentioned above, which constitute the majority of the brain.

Robert O. Becker refers to a "dual nervous system" consisting of the classic work of nerves (neuron doctrine) and the perineural (cells/tissue around nerves to assist and protect) network of cells that regulates wound healing and tissue repair as part of the brain. More recently, Dr. R. Douglas Fields, PhD, refers to the perineural system, aka glial cells, as "The Other Brain."

The neuron doctrine speaks primarily to a "point-to-point" transmission of very specific cause-and-effect signals. However, the perineural/glial system does not have specificity. Instead, it cascades its information throughout the entire body, helping to integrate and regulate all processes.[31] In our subject, this information is primarily the propagation, interpretation, and experience of pain.

The glial system helps us to understand how an initial pain-related event can cause a person to have headaches or be unable to eat, have bowel disturbances or sensitivity to light or to noise. So we begin to understand how an injury that seems to be isolated to one area—like whiplash injury to the neck, for instance—could disturb the nervous system, triggering a fibromyalgia state, including a plethora of signs and symptoms that seem to be unrelated. Unfortunately, many doctors--and certainly insurance companies--don't understand the correlation between a regional injury and the central nervous system. It would not be surprising if 10, 20, 30 years from now we realize that there is yet another major component to the brain and central nervous system. But for now, we realize that glial cells and neurons are intimately related, and it appears that nerves are more dependent on glial cells than glial cells are dependent on nerves.

Dr. Fields describes glial cells as not communicating in a straight line but rather broadcasting their signals in every direction. This allows glial cells to communicate and stimulate other glial cells in every direction simultaneously. This summons other glial cells to come to the area of injury and begin to release excitotoxins that are meant to protect. In normal function, this response will resolve after a period of time when the injury and threat are gone. But in some cases, as in fibromyalgia, the chemicals that are released linger. There are other factors involved with this condition such as genetics, lifestyle, allostatic load, nutrition and structural integrity, particularly as it applies to the alignment and movement of the spine. Let's not forget that the pain nerve fibers are primarily located in the spine, spinal joints, and between the bones, discs, and surrounding tissue. We will talk more about this shortly.

Findings and studies reported by University of Colorado, Boulder, as well as Mueller and colleagues at the University of Ohio and Dr. Fields, have reported that chronic pain can be reduced by suppressing/limiting the action of glial cells. The ideal solution would be to find a medication that could block the proliferation and dumping of excitotoxins that perpetuate pain without negating the benefits that glial cells provide. This is a work in progress.

The Future

So as we look to the future, what are some of the new possibilities—real possibilities—for controlling pain?

Control Glial Cells, Control Pain

In discussing pain there are two distinctions I'd like to make. The distinctions are between allodynia and hyperalgesia. Allodynia is pain that is inappropriate, meaning that a person might feel pain when lightly touched with pressure that would not normally cause any pain at all. This type of inappropriate pain can be triggered by temperature, physical contact, stretching, motion and sound. The glitch or misinterpretation by the nervous system is very much part of fibromyalgia and is not only triggered by physical, chemical, or emotional insult but by thought and mere anticipation of a touch, chemical or emotional event. In contrast, hyperalgesia is an overreaction to a stimulus that is expected to be painful. So while hyperalgesia is simply an overreaction to a painful stimulus, allodynia is a painful reaction to a non-painful stimulus.

No Pain

As a side note, there is a condition that is a congenital insensitivity to pain with anhidrosis (CIPA). This is a rare inherited disorder of the nervous system that seems to be accounted for by a genetic mutation. There are likely to be no more than 24 to 30 of these cases in the United States. A person with CIPA will feel no pain and little if any heat or cold. Additionally, the person may have an inability to sweat (anhidrosis). Due to their inability to feel pain, heat, or cold, they are very susceptible to injury and infection and frequently will die before age 30. Some reports speak of babies with this condition who never cry. As the child gets older, the only indication of any injury is the visible damage. It is necessary to physically see a burn, broken skin, or blood. An older child may run to his parents joyfully pointing out a dangling arm that had just been broken. Obviously this poses a huge danger. As a person gets older, there is no protective mechanism to understand that there's pain in the person's stomach due to disease, or pain and fever due to appendicitis, for instance. However, some of these children have been reported to have the ability to feel emotional pain or empathy. This is an interesting area of science, to say the least.

The reason I make a point of this condition is that in the long run, the ability to feel pain is a blessing. So whether pain feels like a blessing or a curse, it does protect us and help us to evaluate and adapt to our external and internal environment. When we have pain, the body will normally control it. However, as we know, chronic pain can ensue and the protective mechanisms fail, leading to allodynia and hyperalgesia. Medication is the first line of defense, at least in an MD's office. Regardless of how effective the Rx appears to be, it would be best if looked at as a temporary solution. Frequently these drugs will reduce the body's innate ability to participate in pain control, requiring higher dosages of medication to get the same result. This sets the stage for addiction and the subsequent side effects that complicate chronic pain. The moral is to use only necessary medication and in a timely manner.

Stop the Pain #1

It always comes as a surprise to me that pain receptors are not located in the brain. It's merely the interpretation and evaluation of the signals that take place in the brain. Pain receptors themselves are located in the spinal column. This is a protective mechanism to help you to understand if you are safe and how your body is moving. Pain receptors are located between the bones of your spine, in the joints, in discs, and in surrounding tissue. It's impossible to have a discussion about the central nervous system and pain management without clarifying the intimacy among the spine, spinal cord, and brain.

It's felt that even though eons have gone by since we've walked on all fours, we still have not fully adapted as two-legged creatures with an ability to tolerate gravity as well as we should. When considering poor body mechanics and the accumulation of small insults over months and years of everyday activities, it's no surprise that we have a nearly 100 percent chance of having some type of spinal pain, back pain, neck pain, or pay the price of emotional stress, all of which is sure to take its toll on the spine. This can cause, perpetuate, or compromise pain-management mechanisms.

When pain receptors are triggered in and around the spine, the signal moves along the nerve fibers and enters the spinal column to reach the Dorsal-Horn (graphic pg98) portions of the spinal cord with the goal of communicating with the brain, as well as putting on alert other nerves above and below the level of entry. There are also nerve signals that are sent out to the skin and muscles as well as the cascade of perineural/glial communication as discussed above.

When a pain signal reaches the brain, it enters an area called the thalamus, which is a major switching station to disseminate and communicate information with the cerebral cortex, and simultaneously with emotional centers in the brain. So we can see that pain is perceived, evaluated, and interpreted in emotional centers of the brain. The state of heightened sensitivity in these emotional centers is why it's so difficult for a person to communicate his or her level of pain or suffering to another. It's emotionally subjective, much like beauty, love, or fear. It also poses a social and clinical problem for family, friends, and physicians to understand what a Fibro is going through.

The most effective way to stop pain is to stop the nerve impulses as close to the source as possible. This calls for working with spinal joints, alignment, muscles, tendons, and ligaments as soon as possible, assuming no contraindications such as broken bones or disease. If caught in time, home management may be possible. However, most conditions will instantaneously involve the spine and most likely will require passive non-drug chiropractic or osteopathic treatment if we are to minimize and or possibly eliminate the need for medication. The effort is to short-circuit the pain signal so it doesn't succeed in reaching other areas in and around the spine, or enter the spinal cord on its way to the brain. As a practical clinical matter, this rarely happens, simply due to the logistics of not getting to a chiropractor or osteopath quickly enough to stimulate enough endorphins and short-circuit pain-signal propagation. Therefore, frequently-- and particularly with chronic pain--medication or local anesthetic becomes necessary, targeting spinal levels.

Now let's assume that local/spinal level attempts fail. The next opportunity would be to influence the signal after it gets into the spinal cord. Women are very familiar with this practice, where the pain of childbirth is blocked by a "spinal block," which literally blocks pain signals from continuing their path to the brain. However, there is another possibility that research is focusing on.

Stop the Pain #2

From the concept of an injury evolving to chronic pain, researchers are focusing on glial cells. A quote from *The Other Brain* by Dr. R. Douglas Fields: "We have two methods of attacking against micro glial induced spinal cord pain: 1. Block the receptors on the micro glial, 2. Block the release of the substances from the micro glial which makes the neurons hyperactive. These new drug approaches are not based on the old narcotic pathway to pain relief and could help patients avoid medical and social toil that narcotic drugs can exact."

While the science and management of glial cells is still in its infancy, the possibilities are inspiring and hold application in curing fibromyalgia. It has application to infections and viruses, curing cancer, mental health, and solving a dilemma of neurodegenerative disorders, aging, and many other conditions. Additionally, management of micro glial cells could improve the quality of life through improving memory, neurological function, cognitive skills, and more.[31]

If this subject interests you, consider reading *The Other Brain* by author R. Douglas Fields, PhD, published by Simon and Schuster.

Why and Where Rx and Treatment Work

Recently, while watching the Summer Olympics, I was thinking about how many things we take for granted. We take things for granted via the brain's ability to preprogram itself with instinctive or cumulative knowledge. Imagine someone arriving on the earth from another planet. Let's assume their planet has no water. How comfortable do you think someone would be jumping off an Olympic diving platform, and landing on this glistening transparent substance 32 feet below? Let's add that when hitting he seems to be swallowed whole by it and lives—pretty scary. Our brains need a lot of information before we can be committed, comfortable, and confident in participating in something new. That prerequisite information is instinctive and cumulative. Once we understand what water is and that the disappearance into it is only temporary and that magically we will reappear on the surface unharmed, it's much easier to participate and follow through. So what could this possibly have to do with taking medication, specialized nutrition, or receiving a spinal adjustment?

Fibromyalgia and chronic fatigue threaten a person's life in many ways. However, as far as we know, they're not life-threatening in terms of "death." When the need for medication is to save a person's life, it's easy to remember to take it. However, long-term follow-through becomes more difficult when it's not a matter of life or death. We've found that the more understanding a patient has about the anatomy, physiology, mechanism, need, and benefit of an Rx/treatment, the more likely he is to follow through and benefit from it.

Let's agree that that Rx and OTC medication, nutrition, spinal adjustments and exercise, etc., collectively can be referred to as a *treatment.* We will go over some of the more common treatments, what they do in the body, and where they do it. Hopefully this will help readers have more confidence in and compliance with treatment. With more clarity, there will be improved communication with caregivers, whether they are medical doctors, chiropractors, or naturopaths prescribing nutrition.

Many treatments affect more than one part of the body, meaning they could act on a muscle, joint, and circulation as well as within the central nervous system, including the brain and spinal cord. However, for the sake of our illustrations, we will note the most effective and common site that the treatment is intended to target.

All that we note has been shown to be helpful, but not for every person and every case. The specifics will need to be discussed with your doctor. Therapeutic solutions, whether pharmacological, natural, or physical medicine, have unique applications as well as contraindications, side effects, and clinical failures. This is just one more realization of the extraordinary multidimensional and multifaceted complexity of fibro, necessitating multidisciplinary understanding and perspective for the best possible clinical outcome. Our illustration below is far from complete, but I hope that it will help with the most common therapeutic efforts.

What's not noted in this section is the clinical value of laboratory tests (blood, sputum, urine, fecal). Tests can, of course, be very valuable, but an air of caution should prevail. Values measured in the upper or lower limits of normal should be of concern; also, let's consider that the tests are at a moment in time value--a snapshot of the time the specimen is acquired. Therefore, clinical relevance must be interpolated, considering all other factors in the case. Retesting may be required to confirm the necessity for intervention before prescribing or refilling. This includes tests for vitamin, mineral, and enzyme levels as well as common/routine blood tests.

Frequently, in a clinical setting, treatment is rendered anecdotally regardless of the objective data, for reasons as noted above. Therefore treatment/prescriptions for drugs are likely to be written with a "let's try this first" pen.

In a medical doctor's world, there's little to go on nutritionally without depending on objective lab work, due to the lack of education in nutrition in medical school. Non-medical doctors have extensive nutritional and functional biology education in school, hence nutraceuticals may be prescribed with relative confidence. Regardless of the type of doctor you are working with, or if the choice is drug or nutraceuticals, there is an unspoken acceptance of trial and error. Each approach has its flaws. In shooting for the first best step, I would put most faith in the non-medical doctor's nutritional recommendations.

Let's first cover the three drugs that are currently approved by the FDA for the treatment of fibromyalgia. They are: Lyrica (pregabalin), Cymbalta (duloxetine), and Savella (milnacipran).

Lyrica (Pregabalin)

The way in which Lyrica works is not fully understood. It is thought to work by binding to calcium channels found on nerve cells in the brain and spinal cord. Lyrica is thought to reduce the release of neurotransmitters called glutamate, noradrenaline, and Substance P. I say "thought to reduce" because it does not clearly fit in the scientific parameters of understanding. Like many treatments in the medical as well as non-medical professions, there is significant clinical application without concrete scientific understanding. Nevertheless, its mechanism appears to block pain signals at pain synapses in the spinal cord as well as various nerve transmissions in the brain.

Cymbalta (duloxetine) and Savella (milnacipran) oral selective serotonin and norepinephrine reuptake inhibitor (SSNRI), are typically used to treat depression, anxiety disorders, and some musculoskeletal pain. They are FDA-cleared for insomnia. They're meant to help serotonin in the brain and nerve synapses linger longer than the normal reuptake cycle. Talk to your doctor about timing: if either medication makes you tired, you may need to take it at night. If it gives you a little zip, take it in the morning. **Escitalopram (lexapro)** may also be prescribed for insomnia; however, it is not specifically cleared for fibromyalgia.

Warnings

With all prescriptions/medication, over-the-counter medication, nutraceuticals and nutritional concoctions (vitamins, minerals, enzymes, and herbs) your doctor will want a thorough understanding of your history and current health status. From your doctor you will want an explanation for the intent of the prescription, its side effects, precautions, and administration. Then you could complement your understanding by speaking to your pharmacist when filling the prescription or seek manufacturer's information. For vitamins, herbs, and nutraceuticals, contact the US Pharmacopeia, USP at **www.usp. org/usp.../usp**

Looking at the graphic below, please note to the left, medication Rx, and to the right natural/physical and OTC treatment. The goal/ treatment of choice will vary depending on the case; however, consider the right side your first line of defense/treatment and move to the left as an alternative or temporary effort. For Fibros, consider getting a Chiropractic spinal adjustment and or taking medication ASAP after a new injury to mitigate pain before it has a chance to over-sensitize nerves and add to allodynia and/or hyperalgesia any more than it has to.

The arrows point to the target of the treatment: either the spine, muscles, or brain. Regardless of the target site, the ultimate intent is to control nerves and neurotransmitters.

Along the bottom you will find headings: Nerves, (NSAIDS), Endorphins and how to Increase Cellular Energy:

<u>NSAIDS</u>—nonsteroidal anti-inflammatories to help control pain by decreasing inflammation.

<u>Endorphins</u> can be stimulated by chiropractic adjustments, exercise, orgasms, massage, etc.

<u>Cellular Energy</u> can be increased by, but not limited to, the list provided.

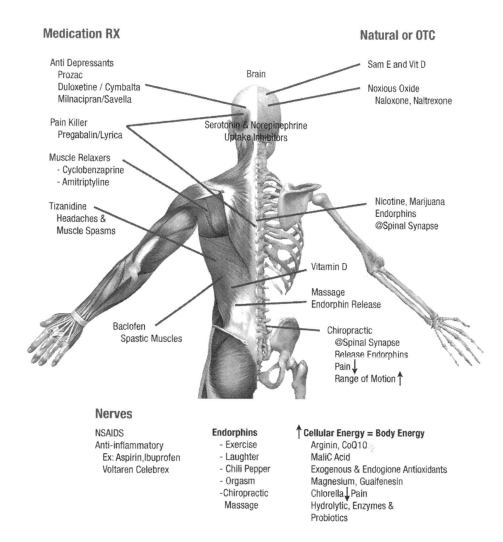

Medication RX

Anti Depressants
Prozac
Duloxetine / Cymbalta
Milnacipran/Savella

Pain Killer
Pregabalin/Lyrica

Muscle Relaxers
- Cyclobenzaprine
- Amitriptyline

Tizanidine
Headaches &
Muscle Spasms

Baclofen
Spastic Muscles

Brain

Serotonin & Norepinephrine
Uptake Inhibitors

Vitamin D

Natural or OTC

Sam E and Vit D

Noxious Oxide
Naloxone, Naltrexone

Nicotine, Marijuana
Endorphins
@Spinal Synapse

Massage
Endorphin Release

Chiropractic
@Spinal Synapse
Release Endorphins
Pain ↓
Range of Motion ↑

Nerves

NSAIDS
Anti-inflammatory
Ex: Aspirin,Ibuprofen
Voltaren Celebrex

Endorphins
- Exercise
- Laughter
- Chili Pepper
- Orgasm
-Chiropractic
Massage

↑ **Cellular Energy = Body Energy**
Arginin, CoQ10
MaliC Acid
Exogenous & Endogione Antioxidants
Magnesium, Guaifenesin
Chlorella ↓ Pain
Hydrolytic, Enzymes &
Probiotics

Music to Reduce Pain?

Holly Corbett in *Prevention* Magazine reported that studies have shown music to be a powerful pain reliever. Corbett goes on to note that previous studies have found that listening to music helps people do things like exercise more and be able to put their hands in ice water for a longer period of time. This can also be accomplished by concentrating on literature, a movie, or any number of physical activities or thoughts. Activating higher centers of the brain inhibit/distract pain signals.

Dr. David Bradshaw, PhD, of the Pain Research Center at the University of Utah, had people listen to specific children's songs that they knew well, such as "Mary Had a Little Lamb." Their task was to identify deviations in this song such as noting a jump in pitch or octave. At the same time they were being administered shocks that would cause pain. He found that brainwaves were altered, netting a decrease in pain.

So how does this work? Many of the same pathways that mediate pain also mediate music. When the music signals get to the brain they compete with pain signals within emotional centers. This shifts the emotional integration of pain to the emotional integration of music thereby reducing pain. There is some question as to whether this approach is more effective for acute pain or chronic pain.

We've all experienced some type of pain or headache that seems to go away when we get busy during the day, unless we're reminded of it—and bingo, it's there again. So distracting the nervous system, either physically or emotionally, changes our experience of pain. The most important aspect for being distracted—whether with music, activity, or conversation—is that you must be fully engaged and interested in what you're doing. It must have emotional value to override your brain's default perceptions based on past experience. This goes back to the concept of being of service to others as a tool to improve the quality of life; it lifts spirits and alters circuit firing. In my practice we find that we can accomplish a similar outcome by having people meditate, pray or participate in "self-talk" or psycho cybernetics two or three times a day, focusing on a particular topic. This effectively tweaks default interpretations by the brain. As the day goes on, pain signals have competition for attention.

We can compound the effectiveness by using these techniques not only to help reprogram your perception of pain but your belief system about the pain and your condition in general. For instance, someone who feels like a victim has no hope and believes the pain is never going to end will experience more pain and more suffering given the same level of pain than a person who believes that he is not a victim; he is in control and has hope that there's a solution. How? By working toward that solution and utilizing choice to actively channel neurological interpretation and experience--anytime, anywhere.

Understanding how the brain and central nervous system work brings new perspective and importance to spinal health, mobility, and posture. Pain pathways are negotiated through the spine, and at that level a major opportunity is at hand to manage pain without drugs. When tended to soon enough, you may spare the brain from toxicity, permanent remapping, and encouraging unrelenting pain.

CHAPTER 10
Intangible Perspectives and Non-Drug Solutions

Chapter Topics:

Introduction to Chronic Pain   *Depression*
Emotions/Pain Management   *PTSD*
Alternative Medicine   *Relation Therapy*
Emotional Freedom Technique   *Mental Imagery*
Psychotherapy   *Biofeedback*
Anxiety   *Hypnosis*

Introduction to Chronic Pain
Hyperalgesia: Exaggerated pain.

Allodynia: Pain for no apparent reason.

Medicine: The practice of diagnosing and treating disease, primarily through pharmaceuticals/surgery.

Functional Medicine: A shift from traditional disease-centered medical practice, believing that disease is a manifestation of chronic dysfunction and accordingly should be treated from a cause perspective as naturally as possible.

Integrative Medicine: A functional medicine model with more emphasis on using all appropriate therapeutic approaches, health care professionals, and disciplines, tempering use of pharmaceuticals.

Chiropractic: An integrative medicine model that specializes in the brain and central nervous system's responsibility in managing physiology/function by primarily addressing spinal integrity.

Healthy Perspective
With neuropathic pain (as in allodynia and hyperalgesia) it's resourceful to look at neurological mapping as a neurological habit. Having the pain doesn't mean that it is causing more damage. Let's say you have a habit of putting your feet up on the coffee table and watching

television. The more you do it, the more it patterns your behavior, hence becoming more of a habit. But you're not really making anything worse every time you do it, other than the habit itself cementing in the pattern, allowing it to continue more predictably. When visiting a friend's house, you may inappropriately put your feet on his coffee table, because it's automatic. There is nothing wrong with you as a person. It's not going to kill you. So helping to change this habit or this pattern of your central nervous system is what this chapter is really all about. You can choose to help your nervous system learn a new habit, a new pattern that reduces pain and will help you to be happier, healthier, more productive, and have more fulfilling relationships with your loved ones; this is a healthy, optimistic perspective that's doable even if you could never break the habit of putting your feet on the coffee table.

As we expand our vocabulary and perspective and create greater possibilities to advocate our own path with confidence, we find "language" and "words" to be of major concern. Their usage and context can make all the difference in the world. Your clarity and understanding will help to unclutter the thoughts and recommendations that others will use to try to influence you. We're talking about the friends, neighbors, and caregivers who will offer you advice at every turn. Have you ever noticed that when you have a health problem, everyone around you turns into a doctor who wants to diagnose and advise you? We want to prepare you to keep your wits about you. In doing so, you will be able to ask better questions and avoid confusion. Of particular concern is your ability to formulate and pose questions in the language of the people you look to for help. This of course will help you get better answers and direct your recovery.

Before we agree on a few definitions, let's keep in mind the two most important abilities you'll have in your recovery:

1. Understanding and controlling your emotions and feelings so as not to become overwhelmed.
2. Choosing the best doctor for you, one who will be a good doctor, coach, and teammate to help you negotiate your journey and meet the challenges as your path evolves.

Emotions and Pain Management

The importance of managing emotions and stress goes far beyond common understandings and normal clinical protocols in managing pain.

Wall & Melzack's *Textbook of Pain* helps us to understand that when pain signals begin their journey to the brain they must enter the spinal cord at the "Dorsal Horn." Within the Dorsal Horn, normal signals are routinely amplified and facilitated to aid in setting up communication as discussed on page 107, before proceeding to the brain. They found this to be true not only due to physical stimulation, but also from emotional events. Emotionally charged physical events had a higher degree of priority, amplification, and facilitation. What this means is that before a signal makes it all the way up through the spinal cord to the brain, the neurons of the Dorsal Horn do the following:

1. Reduce the pain threshold, meaning cells become more sensitive and reactive.
2. Become more efficient in their response.
3. Recruit/involve surrounding nerves with complimentary responsibilities.
4. Increase the size of the responsive nerves.
5. Distribute pain to uninjured sites.

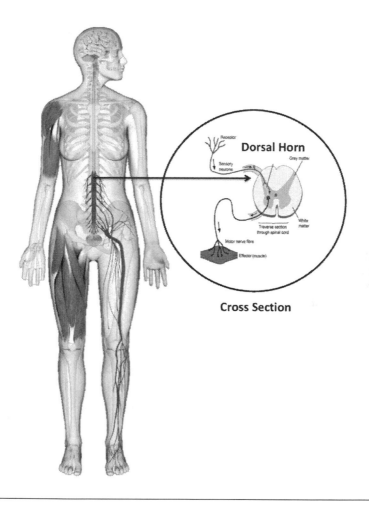

Dorsal Horn

Receptor

Sensory neurone

Grey matter

White matter

Traverse section through spinal cord

Motor nerve fibre

Effector (muscle)

Cross Section

Diagram shows a cross section of the spinal cord. Nerve signals enter the cord at the Dorsal Horn and, after amplification and enhancement, track up the cord to the brain. This happens at every spinal level.

You can see that if all of this is taking place before the signal even gets to the brain, intervening and attempting to control pain at the spinal level is crucial. Along with medications there are emotional and spinal manipulative techniques that are designed to control pain at this level; these are the focus of this chapter.

Dr Frederick Wolf reported that when emotionally charged signals reach the brain, anxiety and objective judgment disorders may precipitate. The disorders become amplified and endure long after the stress has passed (hypersensitivity). When the brain is in this state of hypersensitivity it can anticipate pain and actually trigger the experience of pain before it happens. Worse yet the triggered experience can be worse than when it originally happened.

Dr. Gorr and Associates, in 1947, experimented with other senses in respect to Wolf's findings. They used sudden loud noise and verbal stimulation—such as an embarrassing question, or bad news—and found in all cases that nerve facilitation took place in the spine first and that one of the first reactions was the over-activity of muscles (muscle tension). Further, these regions were the last to subside when the stimulus passed. This is one of the reasons for muscle trigger points and myofascial pain that persist.

Dr. Leon Chaitow notes research as far back as 1993 that showed that in people who are highly emotional or people who experienced an initial injury under highly emotional circumstances (such as fear during a car crash or some type of physical or sexual abuse) the central nervous system would have more of a tendency to lock in the experience of pain, causing a more permanent and exaggerated imprint in the brain. Consequently, in the future this enables the brain, with less provocation, not only to feel pain but to exaggerate/amplify it. So we see that allodynia or central sensitization can be brought about by physical/emotional abuse as well as emotionally charged injuries, and not only by prolonged repetitive/chronic pain as it is usually defined.

Emotionally Charged

A highly emotional person tends to feed or load (frequently overload) an area of the brain called the limbic system. The limbic system helps to manage emotions and behavior.

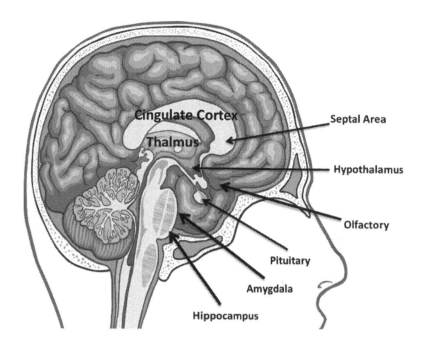

> The limbic system is not really a system, although most still refer to it as such. Rather, it is an acknowledgement of the total brain integration of functions and regions cooperating to create an individual's reality of such things as emotions, behavior, motivation, and memory.

Managing emotions and behavior also means the management and relationship between beliefs and feelings, thoughts, and other areas of the brain. Let's review: emotions can sensitize the brain to interpret pain as being worse than it is (termed hyperalgesia), or possibly react and cause you to experience pain when nothing happens that would trigger pain at all, yet the brain creates the pain all on its own (allodynia), similar to the way you could have jealousy or fear when there's no reason for it. One of my favorite examples is the experience of fear when seeing an angry lion on a movie screen, or a movie that brings you to tears with grief. We would agree that the fear or the grief is contrived; we are in no danger and have nothing to grieve. But emotional centers of the brain do not always make that distinction between fabrication and reality. Some of us are more inclined to react this way to movies or real life, depending on how our limbic system is loaded or innately pre-wired.

Definitions

Thoughts: The result of deliberate brain activity producing ideas, concepts, and judgments that formulate action ultimately influencing beliefs, feelings, and emotions.

Emotions: To a neuroscientist, emotions are a reaction to stimuli. Stimuli can be physical or from mindful thought (with intention). Or they can be auto-generated by the nervous system.

Feelings: Feelings are the perceived/experiential awareness in every cell of the body as a result of emotions—non-intellectual, non-thought mechanism (autonomic, inherent).

Beliefs: Ideas that mind accepts as true and valid; something you feel you know for certain and can count on.

You may be agreeing or disagreeing with these definitions one way or the other; your assessment will be based on your beliefs. Beliefs are variable based on past thoughts, experiences, and emotions behind them. For example, we "believed" that consuming fats would be harmful. Why? Because we were told so! We were told so by people whom we "believed" to know the truth. (They were wrong, by the way. We all know now that we must have fats in our diets.) Yet based on what we "believed," we stayed away from fats for two decades. Medical and pharmaceutical money/voices when combined are hard not to "believe". We accepted it as proof, hence it continued to support and direct what we believed. Subsequently, this notion/directive has done harm to the structure of cells, hormone levels, and metabolism. Further, this belief in large part is in large part responsible for the epidemic of vitamin D deficiency that we are now seeing.

What does this have to do with fibromyalgia? It has everything to do with fibromyalgia and our ability to change and control our beliefs that are reciprocal with our thoughts, emotions, and feelings. So here's the real message:

By selectively changing beliefs, we can begin to control the brain and neurological mappings within it—hence, how pain is experienced.

Herein lies another opportunity to erase pain by improving our skills in controlling thoughts, emotions, feelings, and beliefs. These "things"— thoughts, emotions, feelings and beliefs—are every bit as real to and influential on our nervous system and our experience of pain as a whip-lash injury, mononucleosis, a tick bite, back injury, or the physical and emotional abuse that many fibromyalgia patients report. It's all taking place automatically inside our heads, and it can be controlled.

Doctor Antonio D'Amasio, chairman of the University of Iowa's neurology department, during an interview reported in *Scientific America* explains, "In everyday language we often use the terms inter-changeably (emotions and feelings). This shows how closely connected emotions are to feelings. But for a neuroscientist emotions are more or less a complex reaction to certain stimuli."

When a person is afraid of something, the heart begins to race, the mouth becomes dry, the skin turns pale and muscles tighten up. This emotional reaction occurs automatically and unconsciously. Feelings, on the other hand, occur only after the brain becomes aware of such physical changes. Only then do we experience feelings—in this case, fear. Interestingly enough, not all feelings result from the body's emo-tional reaction to physical changes. Sometimes feelings arise within the brain from brain mapping that already exists and is poised to help us integrate and understand seemingly unrelated stimuli--for exam-ple, when we feel sympathy for a person who is sick. The emotion was already programmed/mapped, and was simply waiting for the con-scious stimuli of another person who is sick to trigger the emotion.

Also, mapping of our physical state is not exact or stagnant. Under times of extreme stress or extreme fear, even physical pain can be dismissed emotionally, resulting in either no pain or greatly reduced pain; the brain ignores the signals. We've all experienced an all-day headache that's a killer if you think about it, yet may be completely dismissed if you're busy and distracted.

We'll explain how this can be done by intent through MRI imag-ing in the chapter on "New Science, Real Hope." But for now, I want to discuss on a practical level how in your own life you can begin to control and influence your experience of pain/fibromyalgia while you work toward complete recovery.

While Dr. D'Amasio's studies are interesting, we don't want to get caught up with too much distinction between feelings and emotions.

For our purposes, let's go ahead and consider them as one and the same. Just understand that they are real neurological and physiological activities of the brain and body, not esoteric or voodoo concepts.

Fibromyalgia sufferers know all too well that there are mood and emotional swings, depression, and feelings of vulnerability. Some feel like victims. Some actually are victims, as in the case of physical or emotional abuse. Whether you are able to trace back what you believe to be a cause or a trigger of your fibromyalgia, or if you think you have cumulative insidious insults over time, you can bet that emotions will be part of the fibro condition and will need to be dealt with. If you believe that physically and emotionally you have a pristine history, you can be assured that pain, lack of sleep, and other coexisting symptoms and conditions of fibromyalgia will challenge your moods and emotions. So one way or the other, fibromyalgia sufferers will have to deal with emotional issues. And then the sufferer will have to deal with the emotional/physical ups and downs, financial challenges, job, relationships, etc., of everyday life. It is difficult at times to decipher fibromyalgia emotions from everyday emotions. Where does fibro start; where does every-day life begin?

It may be impossible to distinguish between the two, except to acknowledge that whatever you're going through, there is a good bet it is amplified and exaggerated when compared to the general non-fibro person.

What to Do and Believe

Thousands of people have been helped, regardless of whether they have fibro, by using some of the considerations on "Avoiding Overwhelm" as covered in our Chapter 19. But for now, consider this.

Having a diagnosis labeled fibromyalgia will bring the emotion/feeling of a sense of relief, at least for a moment or two. The diagnosis tells you you're not crazy; you don't have cancer or some horrible autoimmune disease. That doesn't mean you won't have real problems, however. No matter what the diagnosis, you are still left with the emotional struggle. Knowing that you're not alone and you're not crazy helps to support your spirit and smooth out everyday emotions.

Emotions, after enjoying the relief of having a diagnosis, may run the gamut. Anger, fear, sadness, and questions about whether or not you'll ever be the same again may be experienced. Keep in perspective that you have had other challenges, physical and emotional, that you've overcome. Your family has had challenges, met them, and adapted. The healthiest and most productive medicine at this point is to accept and not deny your condition. The good news is that you already have, in a way, accepted your diagnosis or you wouldn't be reading this book, so congratulations.

Thea, a 43-year-old patient, wrote:

Coming to a diagnosis of fibromyalgia helped me to accept myself. Then sharing it with my family was one of the best things that I've ever done for myself. It helped us all to understand, and instead of striving for a life completely free of pain, I would set my goals on living a full life, focusing on the things that I could do rather than the things that I could not do. It's hard to maintain self-acceptance when people around you don't feel what you feel. My husband became discouraged because he couldn't fix things for me. I asked him to read your book and that really helped--if nothing else, it gave us a starting point for conversations. I then felt more whole and in control.

Dr. Reinhold Niebuhr, of the Union Theological Seminary, New York, offers the following prayer:

God grant me the serenity
To accept the things I cannot change,
The courage to change the things I can
And the wisdom to know the difference.

This is a healthy mantra to avoid living with anger or denial of fibromyalgia. This book, however, is more to the contrary from that point on. We don't want to accept dogma, authority, or paradigms in health care without first having the courage to believe that healthier answers are out there and all things change with time. And we want to have the serenity to know that acquired wisdom can make a difference. In other words, you may accept the diagnosis--but don't give up on finding a solution.

The Path
Your path to get to this point, whether or not you've had a clear diagnosis of fibro, has most likely been a long one. At least you now know you're not crazy. You can stop questioning your own perceptions (Is this pain real? How come she has energy to take her kids to the soccer

game and I don't? Why don't I want intimacy? I used to love getting together with my friends.) So now you know why: You have fibromyalgia.

At every turn your emotions will recycle even though you thought you had a handle on them. It can be frustrating when you're the one who has to nurture and take care of your family members because of their lack of understanding of what you're going through. Why should you have to, anyway? After all, you're the patient. You may think, "It's my life that has changed, not theirs." The truth is, their life has changed too and will continue to change along with yours. Here are some recommendations that might help:

1. When we work with fibromyalgia patients, we believe it's the entire family that has fibro and we do our best to treat accordingly. Patients wonder how they can begin to deal with emotions and care for their families and themselves all at the same time. We encourage patients to first bring their significant other into the office so that he or she can hear directly from the doctor what they are going through. Whether your pivotal doctor is a medical doctor, a chiropractor, or a naturopath, look for their willingness to spend extra time with you and your family.

2. You could pick out two or three chapters from this book and encourage your family members to read them. Better yet, send me an email at Fibro-epc@cmcast.net and I will put you on an email list and inform you of upcoming webinars, pod-casts, and or trainings as they arise. They will help you and your family understand what to expect to go through in the future.

3. Ask family members to attend counseling sessions, or at least re-evaluations and pivotal conversations that you'll have with your doctors. You will reduce stress by helping the people closest to you not to feel in the dark and helpless; keep them in the loop.

4. You and your significant other could attend what's called "The Forum," designed and presented through Landmark Education. (See chapter 19 on Avoiding Overwhelm.)

5. If you're lucky enough to find a real support group, ask your family to attend with you, although not necessarily every meeting. Also make sure you've attended the support group yourself enough to know that it's truly a "support group" and not just a session of sitting around complaining. Support groups should meet regularly, have a

chairperson, and bring in educational material and guests of different disciplines to speak about different aspects of fibromyalgia and evolving theories, science, and day-to-day helpful hints.

6. Seek to meet and find other people or families who have a Fibro in them with whom you could socialize. It makes for great interaction. No one feels left out, deprived, or held back. You can sit in the sun, have a cup of tea, or take a walk with the other family's Fibro, and your family or significant other can participate with the other family member in any manner, sport, or activity that they would like.

The Science

Let's not forget that emotions have to do with neurology, biochemistry, and our perception of pain, as we discussed earlier. Let's also remember that emotions are no longer locked into some esoteric or pseudoscientific voodoo that equates to something that is "not real." We now understand scientifically that the body (perception of pain and physical symptoms), the mind (thought, cognitive processing, judging, evaluating) and behavior are the integration of all existing brain maps waiting to be utilized, similar to the way a computer has all its programs sitting there waiting to be utilized. It's through emotional mapping that we negotiate life and relationships.

Toxicity

Sometimes we hear things like "emotions can be toxic," "emotions are things," or a symptom is being diagnosed to be "emotional." This isn't the '60s, when a person's ailment could be passed off as being "emotional" and just left at that as if there were no basis in reality for the complaint and nothing to do about it. Baldry, in 1993, proved that emotions (positive or negative) are real and negative emotions, in particular, are toxic to cells and the nervous system. Toxic means they have a negative effect, causing the nervous system to be hypersensitive, and can lead to inappropriate mapping, perception, and future interpretation of signals—in this case misinterpretation of pain, causing an exaggerated and amplified experience of pain.

Why Tell Me This Now?

Dealing with this component of life is crucial for us all, but in particular for Fibros. Don't forget, generally we already consider Fibros to be more susceptible and sensitive neurologically than the average person. As a Fibro, you can use all the help and perspective that you can get. And most of the recommendations, whether in this chapter or the chapter on "overwhelm," are meant to empower you personally to help deal with and steer your course. They cost little to nothing to institute and cultivate, and are guaranteed to help your muscles and emotions.

Osteopaths, chiropractors, and neurobiologists have documented that the same overactive or hyper-reactivity can occur in the brain with plan old physical problem. Most commonly seen when joints, muscles, tendons, ligaments, and fascia, of the spine are repetitively irritated. Basically I am talking about the combination of abnormal spinal joint alignment, movement and posture together with our discussion about emotions creating a neurological soup that can corrupt and distort just about every bodily function as well as all our perceptions, judgments and beliefs in life aka Subluxation.

Dr. D. Korr, an osteopath used the term "facilitation" to describe Subluxaton. Dr. David Seaman, a chiropractor, has advanced the concept, terming it "Segmental Dys-afferentation." In any event, the disruption of spinal joints cause an emotionally and physically heighted neurological state at the spinal level in turn influences the brain to literally remap itself. The natural function of the body in accomplishing this is called "neuroplasticity." The brain is literally being retrained/reprogrammed/remapped—for better or for worse—depending on the health of the spine.

This condition is all too well known by a fibromyalgia patient as a vicious cycle of aches and pains creating myofascial trigger points, muscle pain, weakness, and contact tenderness as well as mood and energy swings. By addressing spinal conditions, we can influence a broad spectrum of emotions and pain. Physical medicine is sometimes looked at as "alterative medicine".

Alternative Medicine?
Now that it's clear that science is consistent through medical/non-medical and allopathic/alternative medicine, I'd like to address the term "alternative medicine." To suggest that emotions should be dealt with only by counseling or medication is scientifically naïve. Stepping away from the naïveté requires an alternative to medicine. I find the whole concept and interpretation of "alternative medicine" to be bizarre. What does alternative mean? Does it mean that anything that is not part of the majority is considered alternative? Does alternative have to do with natural and unnatural? Is the herb boswellia an alternative to aspirin? Or is aspirin an alternative to boswellia? (Both have

anti-inflammatory applications.) If you needed to relax, and you had to choose between Valium or chamomile tea, which would you consider the alternative—and why? Can we label something alternative because it's not scientific? Which one is more scientific, by the way, chamomile or Valium? Somehow, in spite of the fact that they both started out as being natural, the powers that be, the big money and the big influence (AMA and pharmaceutical companies) have gotten most of us to believe that the medication Valium would not be considered an alternative, but chamomile would. And the same perspective holds true when comparing physical medicine to chemical medicine, as in prescribing painkillers for back pain vs. physical medicine such as some form of osteopathy, physical therapy, or chiropractic for back pain. Physical medicine will frequently be pointed to as an alternative. It seems to me that as you depart from the natural, it becomes more of an alternative. So, for instance, surgery would be considered the most severe form of alternative medicine. The takeaway is that we have been socialized to believe that "alternative medicine" is anything other than a strict allopathic paradigm; which most frequently involves pharmaceuticals.

Contemporary neurobiology is in the foreground of realizing that the most intangible pain or treatment, such as a placebo effect, is a call to respect and study disciplines, theories, and procedures that have yet to be understood. The placebo effect, to a neurobiologist, is every bit as neurologically real as the evidence on an X-ray.

Remember when we spoke of beliefs? Beliefs are chosen and hung on to; they are hand-me-down communication, experience, and the powerful influences of mentorship. The same people who would pooh-pooh traditional Chinese medicine, the placebo effect, therapeutic nutrition, chiropractic, and acupuncture (the list goes on) are the same people who put themselves on a pedestal convincing us that Thalidomide, hormone therapy, eliminating fats from our diet, and taking statins are safe and necessary. (By the way, all these concepts have been found to be questionable if not disproven—an example of how beliefs and science change. What's real today may not be real tomorrow.)

So-called "alternatives" exist because mainstream medicine cannot hit the mark with everyone all the time. You're not reading this book because mainstream has all the answers or because you don't need more help; you're reading it because you believe there are better answers. A great case in point is Emotional Freedom Technique. If you're not feeling the way you'd like and you believe you can do better, then you have the opportunity to keep searching.

Emotional Freedom Technique

Emotional freedom technique (EFT—sometimes termed emotional release technique), is a form of counseling intervention. EFT draws upon various therapies that might be termed alternative medicine. It includes aspects of acupuncture, neuro-linguistic programming, energy medicine, and thought-field therapy. The results can be quite profound in helping to control emotions and the way people deal with fibro symptoms.

Again, because of a misunderstanding, many of us have been misdirected and discouraged from participating in so-called "alternatives." Some have suggested that the benefits of emotional freedom technique are due to the placebo effect, desensitization, or distraction rather than mechanisms proposed by its practitioners. The amazing thing is that the neurology of chronic pain and hyper-sensitization, the placebo effect and desensitization are exactly what anyone with chronic pain will be looking for in a medication or physical medicine; further, such results would be considered a success. People with chronic pain, fibromyalgia, reflex sympathetic dystrophy, rheumatoid arthritis, and a myriad of other chronic pain conditions may benefit from emotional freedom technique and avoid medication.

During a session of EFT, the client focuses on specific emotional issues while participating in something called tapping, a process that stimulates the endpoints of acupuncture meridians, as the studies of traditional Chinese medicine dictates. The patient can be taught to do this at home.

Western medicine/science points out that based on Western medicine and science there is no evidence that acupuncture points, meridians, or traditional Chinese medicine concepts are valid. Yet it is demonstrably true that our bodies have positive and negative charges and these charges flow throughout the body. It just hasn't been proven in Western terms, most likely because it hasn't been considered to be significant or important enough to drum up financial backing to conduct studies. Besides, if this is a self-help effort, there's little to no chance that usual and customary funding could be found via pharmaceutical or technology companies. So too the government is unlikely to spend the money to help prove the validity/science of another country's health approach.

Scientific vs. Anecdotal

Don't get caught up in the argument that some methods are scientific and others aren't, or that evidence-based medicine has any more chance of helping you than anecdotal treatment. If a method like emotional release helps you, it doesn't matter how it's labeled. Embrace it. When making a decision on what techniques you'll use, go back to our original definitions. Allow your emotions, feelings, and experience to shape your thoughts and beliefs. Don't allow negative campaigns to dissuade you from something that could change your life and that statistically is as safe as or safer than aspirin.

Therapists

Psychiatrist: a medical doctor specializing in mental disorders.

Psychologist: a professional who studies the way the mind works, how people think, act, react, and interact. They're concerned with all aspects of behavior, thought, feelings, and motivation that underlie behavior.

Psychotherapist: may be a psychiatrist, psychologist, or mental health professional. They work with individuals, groups, couples, and families to help them overcome stress, emotional, and relationship problems, and troublesome events.

Working with a psychologist or psychotherapist may be of great help. They don't prescribe drugs. They have at least a master's degree, if not a PhD. In contrast, psychiatrists are medical doctors who can and do prescribe drugs. They generally don't participate in the kinds of noninvasive therapies that are meant to empower patients and help them to understand their plight or how to control pain and emotions. With time constraints and managed care, it seems that the pharmaceutical side of their education prevails.

Psychotherapy

The best avenue to find a psychologist who specializes in pain management is to discuss with your doctor who he or she knows to be such a therapist in your geographic area. You'll find it will be invaluable to have a Non-medical-biased teammate whom you can talk to openly and who has the tools to help you control emotions, life perspective and pain. They are more likely to integrate meditation, emotional freedom technique, acupuncture, nutrition and chiropractic and/or massage into the conversation, helping you to avoid medication when possible.

Keep in mind that when first interviewing or meeting your psychologist you're looking for what we call enthusiastic believers in fibromyalgia. This should be relatively easy, because you probably already chose the doctor who will be your captain to quarterback your efforts, so your doctor's referral will most likely be someone who works with chronic pain and fibromyalgia patients frequently. Keep an eye out for someone who understands the peripheral and central sensitization aspects of pain, emotions, and behavior as it relates to chronic pain. That will dovetail best with the challenges ahead and the information and understanding that you'll be acquiring throughout this text.

You don't have to have been diagnosed with depression, anxiety, or post-traumatic stress disorder to be under the care of a psychologist. If you follow through, it's all but guaranteed to help you with no negative side effects. You will have to consider the financial challenge, however, depending how your insurance policy is set up. But the good news is that the tools you acquire can be self-implemented; you can use them for a lifetime.

In a sense, the tools that you'll learn will be a Western version of what Buddha, Gandhi, and yoga masters accomplish with meditation, tai chi, Qigong, and other practices.

A few of the possible techniques are as simple as:

Relaxation therapy
Mental imagery
Biofeedback
Hypnosis
Cognitive behavioral therapy
Emotional release therapy

Anxiety
Chronic pain is very likely to cause anxiety. However, feeling in charge and empowering yourself to understand and control pain will reduce that anxiety. Generally, anxiety causes a feeling of panic and confusion, has aspects of irrational thinking, and has an unproductive, unhealthy perspective on your life and conditions. Worry and fear can cause a self-perpetuating process that taxes your adrenals. If you've ever had anxiety or a panic attack, you'll notice that you may

feel almost faint or lightheaded, experience heart palpitations, or break out into a sweat. Chronic pain will increase the chances of your having anxiety, and anxiety will increase pain because of its effect on your brain and nervous system. This is similar to our discussion regarding people who are "emotionally charged," when we noted that one can experience fear when seeing an angry lion on a movie screen, or a movie that brings you to tears with grief. The fear or the grief is contrived; we are in no danger and have nothing to grieve. But the brain does not always make that distinction, in the same way anxiety is created within the wiring of the brain. Under the guidance of the right psychologist it is manageable.

Depression

Most people have experienced depression to one degree or other. There is minor depression and major depression. Minor depression is experienced from time to time by most people, and with fibromyalgia you're pretty much guaranteed you're going to have more than your share. The therapies that we're discussing in this section will go a long way to control and minimize your experiences of depression. However, if major depression has been diagnosed, you now have a medical condition that will need to be treated accordingly. You are likely to need medication first, which will then set the stage for your patience, open-mindedness, and will to participate in the techniques and training that follow (assuming that you have your doctor's blessing). Experiencing anxiety, depression, or post-traumatic stress disorder is likely to make pain worse. When you add the likelihood of non-restorative sleep, chances of recovery diminish. As we discussed earlier, having friends or a support group and other people around you who have fibromyalgia, or fibro-like conditions, will help you not to feel like a victim or that you are alone on your path; this in itself is a great stress reliever. I have mentioned before that support groups, or socializing with others/families that have a chronic pain/fibro person, can be resourceful. However, be careful not to be pulled down by negativity. When encountered try out your wings as a teacher and coach. If it seem unlikely that you could turn attitudes around, move on; you can't afford to go backwards.

Post-Traumatic Stress Disorder

Post-traumatic stress disorder (PTSD) is anxiety that is caused by some type of trauma, whether physical or emotional. It can be triggered by one major event or by cumulative events that have a strong emotional component such as emotional or physical abuse, a horrific accident, a natural disaster, or participation in military action. When anxiety is of the post-traumatic stress disorder variety, it's considered more serious. And, as with anxiety, there can be distorted, irrational, and unfounded thoughts as well as worry and fear. Sufferers may complain of bad dreams and memories, loneliness, and feeling out of place even among their closest loved ones. It can also sabotage restorative sleep.

Treatment

Most commonly, medication will revolve around serotonin. Serotonin is a neurotransmitter, meaning it helps the body to communicate with itself. Most serotonin is found in the gut in specialized cells that help regulate intestinal movement. This is an important factor with fibromyalgia, due to the large percentage of people who have gut/bowel and digestive problems. Serotonin is also synthesized in special cells within the central nervous system where they help to regulate mood and appetite. It plays a role in the way we think, including memory and learning.

Through research presented in *BioDrugs* 2001, Dr. Dirk Van West and Dr. Michael Maze explain a very interesting hypothesis that fibromyalgia is related to dysfunction of peripheral and central turnover of serotonin, meaning if serotonin is able to linger long enough to do its job, it will:

- Improve REM sleep
- Improve the effectiveness of analgesics. Analgesics are basically pain killers used in conditions such fibromyalgia, rheumatoid arthritis, and other types of neuropathic pain. The most popular is acetaminophen. Serotonin also enhances the action of nonsteroidal anti-inflammatory and opiate drugs such as morphine and opium.
- Help to reduce inflammation by helping to control cytokines (chemicals that help to control immune and inflammatory responses).

Therefore, research is showing that the addition of antidepressants in the management of fibromyalgia and other chronic pain conditions (regardless of anxiety, depression, or post-traumatic stress syndrome) is resourceful. It almost sounds like antidepressants are a type of multivitamin for fibromyalgia sufferers.

When I first started working with fibromyalgia patients, antidepressants were the treatment of choice even though at that time there were very few physicians who actually believed in fibromyalgia. The clinical presentation was frequently not termed fibromyalgia, but rather might have been referred to as myofascial pain syndrome, fibromyositis, fibrositis, or was just generally chalked up to depression. Depression was frequently the overwhelming recognizable symptom at the time. Consequently, prescribing antidepressants was the treatment of choice. Physicians at the time had no idea of the wide reach and therapeutic value that antidepressants could have on the fundamentals of fibromyalgia. Nevertheless, they were prescribed and worked effectively. It wasn't until many years later that doctors really understood the impact of antidepressants in controlling serotonin levels and their influence on managing inflammation and pain in fibromyalgia. So in retrospect, in the earlier days ('60s,'70s and,'80s) administering antidepressants would have been considered pseudo-science and anecdotal. As a physician, it's encouraging to me to note how many times in our history of evolving health care and science that what was once considered pseudoscience/anecdotal subsequently rose to real science and real hope. Physicians with many contact hours with patients in chronic pain can recall successful anecdotal efforts that were not understood at the time, yet were a valued part of the nature of evolving science.

Non-Drug Treatments

Relaxation Therapy

Relaxing muscles, tendons, ligaments, and the mind helps to calm nerves and sets the stage for helping to control pain and breaking the neurological pattern/mapping, aka neurological habit of pain. Meditation is a form of relaxation therapy in which a person might use body positions, music or sounds, mental imagery or special breathing to help relax the body. Tibetan monks have done this successfully for centuries. Chinese practices such as tai chi and Qigong, and yoga, which originated in India, are other methods of calming the nervous system (body, mind, and spirit). In the Western world where we're uncomfortable with anything that can't be documented by objective data or technology, we call this pseudoscience or anecdotal. However, biofeedback can be used to electronically confirm and hopefully control nerve electricity (energy), equating to relaxation. Biofeedback is a tool to train and emotionally confirm that a person is accomplishing the relaxation he is attempting to achieve.

Mental Imagery

Mental imagery is related to daydreaming, where we want to escape mentally to our favorite beach or hiking trail, or to an event (even if contrived) that makes us feel particularly relaxed, happy, and tranquil. Many people use a form of this to sleep at night, possibly assisted by white noise, pictures, or aromatherapy that help bring them emotionally and mentally to another place. Another example of distraction is desensitization that functions as pattern-interrupt of the habitual firing of nerve pathways within the brain. But all of these techniques, no matter how effective or healthy they might be for you, take more effort than simply popping a pill.

Biofeedback

Biofeedback, as we touched on earlier, is an electronic training method to help a person relax and control stress reactions. Basically, a person is hooked up to electrodes that relay electrical signals within the brain to a computer. Then physical/mental manipulations are performed, watching for signals from the electrodes to be transformed into sounds or images displayed on a computer screen.

An example of physical manipulation would be something like simply relaxing your shoulders and taking the grimace off your face. A mental example is imagining your favorite sunny spot by a babbling stream. These conscious manipulations correlate with representative sound or visual display on a computer that helps you to reinforce the accomplishment of relaxing. Biofeedback can also measure your success of relaxing by measuring blood pressure, heart rate, sweat gland output, muscle tension, and skin temperature. As with relaxation therapy and mental imagery, things were accomplished naturally without devices by yoga masters, Tibetan monks, and Qigong and tai chi practitioners. The takeaway is that these techniques can help chronic pain patients monitor their bodies to reduce tension and the physical and emotional impact of everyday life. Ultimately this helps to re-pattern and break neurological habits that generate pain.

Cognitive Behavioral Therapy

Cognitive Behavioral Therapy (CBT) is great training to help a person cope, putting into perspective how their behavior, thoughts, beliefs, and values can affect pain and emotions. We know neurologically that the better we can control these things, the better chance we have of controlling pain. CBT is basically learned coping skills.

Cognitive behavioral therapy puts a little more pressure and responsibility on the participant to delve into areas that might feel threatening, taking an introspective look at self, not only to relax the nervous system but to unravel emotional baggage, determining what's real and what isn't. We will discuss other aspects of this in Chapter 19 when we look at how and where our values and beliefs come from. In CBT, the participant works to replace negative and learned baggage by seeing things through the eyes of who they are today. Both negative and resourceful thoughts, behavior, or beliefs are strongly embedded in our hearts and our heads. It's a little of the glass is half full or half empty analogy. If you're naturally a glass-is-half-full person, or a glass-is-half-empty person, it's hard to change how you're wired and how you see things. Your thoughts and feelings are your thoughts and feelings in spite of the fact that you realize they are negative, possibly invalid, and likely holding you back from improving your health. Your so-called negative thoughts simply generate more negative feelings, negative behaviors, and negative emotions, leading to more depression, anxiety, pain, and a likely withdrawal from relationships. Cognitive behavioral therapy is an opportunity to change that.

During this process there will be an attempt to identify any irrational, non-resourceful, and unproductive thoughts and replace them with more productive, inspiring, and positive thoughts. The problem is that whatever feelings we have, we usually believe them to be real, valid, and necessary, so the first step is to realize that we have the ability to decide what has meaning and what no longer has meaning, what's real and what's not real, and whether we're going to look at the glass as being half full or half empty.

Hypnosis

Hypnosis is a neurological relaxation process that is aided by the words and instructions of another person. Again, this is something that many would consider a pseudoscience. However, new technology is documenting the effects of successful hypnosis on the central nervous system and, in particular, pain as it relates to fibromyalgia. As with the other methods we discussed, a person can be taught to self-induce a hypnotic state. As the nervous system relaxes, not only does it help to interrupt patterns and neurological habits in attempting to reduce pain, but it also opens cognitive pathways to help rethink and reorganize thoughts and perspective about your condition as well as opportunities to empower and control your life better. And it can be used in conjunction with CBT.

Trial and Error

Everything we've discussed in this section has little to no downside, but each tool has the potential to help you feel better and be happier. While I'm generally an advocate of doing as much as possible without medication, the research is overwhelming in support of anti-depressants being a wise addition to almost any chronic-pain condition. Figuring out which approach is best for you is a matter of trial and error. The team of doctors that you put together will guide you.

I would like to add, however, that the ultimate goal should be to reorganize life's reset opportunities and push in the direction of sustainability. Consider improving your nutrition and being better informed about food choices. Adopt neuromuscular-skeletal well-care habits to reduce spinal stress on the nervous system. Include conservative exercise as well as possibly yoga, massage, chiropractic, and other approaches that from a wellness-care and healing standpoint to reduce the need for antidepressants. The problem is that these efforts are more of a lifestyle versus a moment-in-time treatment and many readers will be well served to participate in antidepressant medication sooner rather than later, while their transformations of lifestyle, non-drug interventions, and self-help tools are cultivated.

While instituting antidepressants early in your care may be highly effective and possibly necessary throughout your care, there is an opportunity to wean off of them through diet and supplementation as you and your body become more proficient at controlling stress and emotions. We will be discussing nutritional and dietary considerations throughout the book. However, it's unlikely you will be able to implement this information on your own. Consider seeking out an appropriate doctor to help guide you. A chiropractor, nurse practitioner, naturopath, osteopath, or MD are possible choices, but they must specialize in nutrition and/or functional medicine.

> Fibromyalgia, chronic pain, and chronic fatigue syndrome, as well as almost all coexisting and fibro look-alike conditions, are multidimensional causally. Consequently, they require a multidisciplinary approach. While gaining perspective as to where the pain comes from, self-help techniques will help settle the mind, brain, and pain nerves.

CHAPTER 11
Contemporary Insights

Chapter Topics:

The Future	*The Spine*
Cognitive Therapy	*Myofascial Trigger Points*
Placebo Effect	*Upper/Lower Cross Syndrome*
Glial Cells	*Substance P*
NSAIDs	*Myofascial Pain Syndrome*
Lower Back Pain	*Wind UP*

Fibro Myths

A myth is a traditional story that attempts to explain a phenomenon, a custom—something generally unproven or fictitious in the light of reason. However, sometimes myths have common threads of perceived reality, such as tricks of Mother Nature and of our own perception.

In the study of fibromyalgia, I believe that most researchers and clinicians who have many contact hours with fibromyalgia sufferers proceed with myth-influenced science. Doctors who have the interest to unravel the condition have perpetuated their personal or shared observations, anecdotes, and isolated triumphs as science. Commonly these amount to little more than opinion. While this is the foundation for evolving science, it must be acknowledged for what it is in the moment so as not to slow progress.

The Future

Is there real hope for fibromyalgia sufferers, or are we doomed to a trial and error pursuit riddled with unfounded opinion? Will we spend the next 20 years with misunderstood talk therapy, esoteric placebos, and a quagmire of medical prescriptions targeting symptoms? Will the big money of pharmaceutical and technological companies control our future? Are we being misled by the relief and hope of human touch by chiropractors, and massage and physical therapists? Or is there real hope and a real opportunity to understand the common denominators of all these efforts, and could we be on the brink of the so-called 100th monkey? Are we at the same precipice with fibromyalgia as we were in 1985 when the electronic computer revolution was about to explode through the minds and genius of people such as Bill Gates and Steve Jobs?

I believe that the future is here and we're in the midst of linking together all we know through the study of neuroscience, neurobiology, and functional medicine. This chapter will help explain in more depth the science behind previous chapters.

Functional medicine addresses the underlying causes of disease. It forms a partnership between doctor and patient, stepping away from a traditional disease-care model to a patient- centered approach, addressing the whole person as opposed to an isolated set of symptoms. The terms neuroscience and neurobiology are generally interchangeable. Neuroscience is a term that is a little more general, encompassing the science of the whole nervous system, whereas neurobiology is more specific to the living chemistry of the nervous system, especially the brain.

If you're interested in following any of these thought processes and studies, you'll see terms like molecular biology, electrophysiology, and computational neuroscience. You'll find organizations of neuroscientists and educators who share ideas through The International Brain Research Organization, founded in 1960; The International Society of Neuroscience, founded in 1963; The European Brain and Behavioral Society, founded in 1968; and the Society of Neuroscience, founded in 1969.

Cognitive and Behavioral Neuroscience
Cognitive neuroscience has given us an opportunity to understand the moldable plastic talents that our brain has to adapt, for better or for worse, to the experiences and perceptions that the senses conjure up. The brain sorts these experiences and literally starts to change how it functions and how we perceive things—things such as chronic pain. Now that we have specialized neuroimaging such as MRIs, PET scans, and SPECT scans, along with electrophysiology and human genetic analysis, we've been able to confirm that fibromyalgia is truly all in your head. These types of imaging have allowed cognitive psychology to be able to map brain activity and explain emotions and perceptions. This in itself has been healing for fibromyalgia patients. It confirms that fibromyalgia is not some esoteric or emotional freak show. Doctors who are unwilling to accept fibromyalgia as a diagnosis and discussion it as a very real syndrome have lost touch with research and science.

The Placebo Effect

One real hope for the future is the study of the placebo effect. The placebo effect refers to a phenomenon in which people feel better and their symptoms diminish after being subjected to an idea, therapy or biological agent that they believe offers them hope to feel better. This seems to be particularly obvious in relation to conditions of pain or depression. It can actually be documented to some degree in all diseases and conditions.

The placebo effect works both ways, meaning if you believe something will help you, it then has a potential to literally help you feel better and reduce pain. If you believe something will cause pain, it is more likely to cause pain. It has been proven that belief in your doctor or therapist comes into play also. Documented physiological and neurological changes are more obvious when both doctor and patient believe that the substance or the activity is going to be beneficial. The opposite holds true as well. If one of the participants does not believe that it's real and will help, then the body's response is reduced. If you believe you're receiving something that will cause the pain to be worse, then it will likely be worse.

One of the most important things is to find a doctor whom you believe in and trust. This will be one of the most important steps to take advantage of the placebo effect that will in fact make a difference: choosing the right doctor. By the same token, the doctor has to be truly engaged in fibromyalgia, understand it to the best degree he or she can, and have a belief that their therapeutic efforts will be productive. So, you have to believe in your doctor—but your doctor has to believe in himself and fibromyalgia for best results

Continuing with the placebo effect and its relationship to controlling pain, let's talk about an area of the brain called the amygdala. The amygdala is an area of the brain that stores memory and emotional data. The data is then communicated and integrated into other areas of the brain. The amygdala basically matches emotions such as fear with stimulus such as pain.

The brain, orchestrated by the amygdala, molds itself with chemicals and circuitry and then neurologically remembers the pattern and the relationship between, for instance, the "fear" and the "pain" that it imprints. The brain then uses the information, circuits/mapping/imprints over and over again in the same way a golfer patterns a swing by practicing it over and over at the driving range so that it imprints his body and his coordination, speed, and accuracy to execute a reproducible swing. It becomes easier, faster, and more efficient. The body does the same thing with its experience of pain and fear.

Now the fear or the pain related to the newly learned pattern becomes easier to access. We become better at responding with efficient reproducible pain. At the same time, it can become amplified as the sensitivity in the awareness of the circuits is queued-up to respond. By now the redundancy of this theme must be obvious, but its importance cannot be overstated. It is essentially about what fibromyalgia is as about. To be able to use this science, we must be comfortable with the understanding.

So we confirm once again that the brain becomes sensitized. The technical term for this is "potentiation" or as referred to in the past, hypersensitivity; the ready state of the nervous system to experience pain faster and easier. This holds true with simple anticipation, being touched lightly or moving a certain way causing inappropriate pain. Remember we're linking/combining emotions (frequently fear) with pain.

Have you ever been going about your everyday business or just relaxing and someone drops a spoon or closes a cabinet door, or maybe says hello to you when you didn't expect it? Do you remember being startled and almost jumping out of your skin? This is an example of your nervous system being overly sensitized, most likely due to accumulation of stress. It's that same type of sensitization that causes a fibromyalgia patient to overreact to a light touch on the leg, or to moving an arm. The brain is so good at learning and developing these new imprints that MRI scans have proven that the experience of pain actually begins before the fibromyalgia patient is even touched. Not only has the brain mapped out the experience of pain, but also the circuit/mapping is hypersensitive, ready to fire easily/instantaneous. Worse yet, you could be accused of being a hypochondriac. The person touching you is thinking, "That's ridiculous; I barely touched her and she tells me there's pain?" I know, it sounds crazy. But once the circuits are primed, just knowing a loved one or doctor's hand is going to touch you, especially in an area that has been painful in the past, will cause the brain to react and of course, there it is, pain. An analogy you may find easier to accept is the way your mouth begins to secrete saliva just anticipating that you're going to eat a slice of warm bread and butter. Plus, behind the scenes, your pancreas anticipates the bread and begins to secrete insulin.

Why Don't Doctors Know?

In our section on "New Science, Real Hope," and "Finding the Right Doctor," you'll find several reasons why doctors don't know about fibromyalgia pain. Some of these hopeful neurobiological findings are not yet in textbooks. Unless a doctor has a particular desire to understand the latest research on managing chronic pain, he or she will not find this information until it becomes public knowledge.

Doctors are generally too busy with their practices to stay abreast of the latest research in all areas of clinical concern. In large part they depend on information via the same source that the general public does: the media. Some doctors will read journals specific to their discipline, or general journals such as the *New England Journal of Medicine*. But very likely they do not read from cover to cover; they'll gravitate to articles that directly relate to their interest and their practice.

Science does not usually make its way to textbooks until there is enough interest to generate funding and research in a particular area. Neuroscience/neurobiology is still working toward getting more funding to bring revolutionary science into everyday practice.

Glial Cells

Please recall that we talked about glial cells in Chapter 9. They make up 85 percent of all brain cells and communicate primarily by point-to-point transmission of very specific cause-and-effect signals. However, the glial system does not have specificity; instead, it cascades its information ubiquitously throughout the entire body, helping to integrate and regulate all processes, or primarily the propagation, interpretation, and experience of pain.[53]

Einstein's brain was studied and it was found that there were no more nerves or brain matter in his head than there is in anyone else's. But they did find that he had an amazing increase of glial cells.

Let's take a look at glial cells and synaptic clefts within the brain in relationship to pain.

Inflammation of peripheral structures (muscles, joints, ligaments, etc.) helps us understand that neural inflammation is a double-edged sword within the brain. It begins as a self-defense reaction, attempting to eliminate and protect the injured tissue, subsequently to repair tissue. But at the same time it contributes to tissue damage when it is excessive.

At the juncture where one nerve meets another along its path there are little spaces—at these little switching stations, or synaptic clefts, neurotransmitters would be deposited causing the signal to jump over the space to the next nerve, continuing its journey within the brain for full communication/information integration. In some cases there is a glitch; the action of the neurotransmitters does not stop even when the pain signal is no longer being sent. The term for this, as we touched on earlier, is allodynia. allodynia is pain due to some type of stimulus that does not normally cause pain, after there was once legitimate pain. So allodynia describes a central neurological aberration or misstep/glitch that allows the brain to continue to believe there is pain when there is not. When this happens, pain is considered to be a disease in and of itself.

Non-Steroidal Anti-inflammatory Drugs (NSAIDs)

Until recently it was thought that anti-inflammatory drugs like ibuprofen or steroids would have little or no effect on fibromyalgia itself, other than on how they might affect an inflammatory condition that coexists with fibromyalgia; therefore, the fibromyalgia patient would feel better. But the decrease in inflammation really had no effect on the perpetuated allodynia within the brain and the cycle that fibromyalgia patients live with.

In 2010 the *Journal Pharmaceutical Sciences* reported that NSAIDs, in fact, cross the blood-brain barrier quite efficiently. They assert an anti-inflammatory effect on glial cells and associated synapses. However, there is no less controversy about the safety of long-term use of NSAIDs in the brain than there is in peripheral tissues, because they have a negative effect on the gastrointestinal tract and kidneys. This obviously poses clinical limits to their use. An article in the *New England Journal of Medicine* reported that prescription pain drugs cause bleeding and take 16,500 lives each year. Over-the-counter drugs take another 20,000 lives. In spite of the pain-modulating benefits in the brain, NSAIDs will ultimately be detrimental and inhibit the activity of glial organic activation. This means the drugs simply won't allow the body to do its job naturally. Along with other problems, NSAIDs are the second most common cause of leaky gut syndrome, after antibiotics.

Developing drugs hold the promise of managing glial cells and re-regulating them to manage the synapses between nerves properly.

However, covering up the symptoms with drugs, or intervening at the glial level, should be only a last resort, especially when we consider that physical medicine, such as chiropractic and physical therapy, as well as nutrition and psychological support--will all help to reorganize and regroup the brain's interpretation of the stimulus we call pain, hopefully without the assistance of drugs.

We get some insight to triggering and perpetuating mechanisms by noting that a large percentage of pain that fibromyalgia patients report is in the neck and low back. But why would neck and low back be so common? The answer lies in the neurology of spinal joints and their effect on nerves.

Low Back Pain
Sixty-three percent of Fibros responding to questionnaires about their pain admitted that low back pain was their primary discomfort. Additionally, many respondents associated conditions revolving around the neurology of the low back (dysmenorrhea, irritable bowel syndrome, and restless leg syndrome, to name a few). We're going to look at the possibilities of mechanics and neurology of low back joints as being contributory to these symptoms, along with the their relationship to central mismanagement that includes discussing glial cells a little more along with neuroplasticity and the amygdala's learned and cumulative memory, which is the backdrop of pain interpretation once a pain signal gets to the brain.

Simply put, as mechanical beings, we struggle to deal with gravity and the bodily movements of everyday life. The low back and neck, their nerves and spinal bones, are challenged and stressed beyond healthy limitations, causing us to have pain. This happens frequently enough to irritate nerves and cause inflammation, encouraging misinterpretation by our brain, leading to chronic pain and subsequently the disease of "pain."

The Spine
Spinal joints offer insight into understanding central sensitivity and the nervous system's ability or inability to manage our perception and interpretation of pain. When spinal joints are not functioning properly, they will irritate nerves due to abnormalities in the mechanics (too much or too little joint movement). The resulting ramping-up of glial and inflammation can trigger pain signals. Together they not only can account for physical symptoms such as joint, muscle, and nerve pain, but will also irritate nerves going to and from the brain.

Once irritated, a feedback loop generates distorted signals to organ and systems that can be recognized as dysmenorrhea, irritable bowel syndrome, restless leg, hypoglycemia or hyperglycemia, etc.

This scenario snowballs, leading to repetitive firing of pain nerves, taking its toll on different areas of the brain, causing them to become overly sensitive (central sensitivity syndrome). This helps explain how so many coexisting symptoms such as nausea, vertigo, anxiety, and brain fog are related to fibro.[41]

The osteopathic and chiropractic community diagnose these conditions regularly. As we have previously discussed, the chiropractic term for joint dysfunction with neurological consequence is subluxation. The osteopathic term is somatic dysfunction.

Unfortunately, most clinical efforts revolve around taking some type of medication first. And although medication may help with the symptoms, there is danger of the subluxation persisting while medication masks the symptom. Frequently this will lead to chronic and recurrent episodes, as well as the use of prescription or OTC medications which, as we've discussed above, is a health hazard in itself. Only about 10-12 percent of the population will first consult a chiropractor to correct the cause. The question is: "How would you know if you needed to see a chiropractor or osteopath or take medication?" For approximately 90 percent of the population who don't see chiropractors, the answer is simple: they try medication first. When symptoms persist, an alternative medication is tried; then another medical doctor is consulted. After it becomes clear that pain will be a way of life with or without medication, abnormal spinal joint function and neurological consequences (subluxation) will come into question and require osteopathic or chiropractic evaluation. However, your MD will not have been schooled in these aspects of spinal neurology; consequently it will often be up to you to seek an opinion. Further, due to MDs' focus on "medicine," they may discourage you from seeking an opinion about something they don't know about. Younger MDs and foreign-schooled MDs will be more attuned to spinal/neuro considerations and value diverse efforts so as not to deny you greater possibilities to improve.

Myofascial Trigger Points and Myofascial Pain Syndrome
Myofascial pain syndrome is not fibromyalgia, and fibromyalgia does not cause myofascial pain syndrome. However, it's clear that they can coexist and frequently do.

The interesting thing is that fibromyalgia and central sensitivity can be inspired, complicated by, and/or perpetuated by myofascial trigger points.

Myofascial trigger points increase excitability of local and spinal nerve pools, sensitizing their pathways. When chronic, the central nervous system becomes vulnerable and overly excited. As the inflammation becomes chronic, there are specialized cells that actually change their characteristics and their behavior to adapt to this inflammatory condition and begin to release Substance P. Substance P appears to play a role in pain and a major role in fibromyalgia.

So before a person graduates to full-blown fibromyalgia, myofascial trigger points should be treated. This of course would require some type of well-care examination periodically to know that these sites exist, assuming the person has not already begun to experience symptoms.[16,69] The professions that deal with these myofascial trigger points are chiropractors, osteopaths, neurologists, physical therapists, and massage therapists.

There is an added bonus when seeing a chiropractor or osteopath for a well-care checkup, in that they will also be able to also recognize spinal-joint abnormalities before chronic pain ensues.

To review, myofascial trigger points can cause pain on movement, tingling, numbness, and muscular asymmetry. All these symptoms can be exaggerated by physical and emotional stress. Janet Travell's research has confirmed that the following factors maintain and exaggerate myofascial trigger points:

- Nutritional deficiencies
- Hormonal imbalances
- Infections (bacterial, viral, or yeast)
- Allergies (most commonly wheat and dairy)
- Low oxygenation of tissue (aggravated by tension, stress, inactivity, and poor respiration)

These points relate to levels of toxicity in tissue, as well as overstimulation of the sympathetic nervous system, which encourages trigger points. The common denominator she has left out is subluxation of the spine.

Myofascial Trigger Points vs. Fibromyalgia Tender Points

The acknowledgment of myofascial trigger points and fibromyalgia tender points is a superficial attempt to define and understand fibromyalgia. It's my opinion that treating these points, while seemingly satisfying to the patient, will be of little or no productive value in sustained improvement.

The primary muscles in which trigger points are found are postural muscles. These muscles come in two varieties, typically termed tonic muscles and phasic muscles. Tonic muscles are meant to sustain contractions and sustain activity. Phasic muscles are meant for more rapid contraction, but are not meant to sustain contraction over a long period of time. Where this comes into play is that when a person's center of gravity/posture is off, phasic muscles are called upon to do more work than they were intended to do. Tonic muscles then compete with them, causing more complication to body mechanics and circulation, and encouraging inflammation. This scenario means that some muscles will be forced to overwork and others will become lazy and weaker. It's usually the overworked muscles that will develop trigger points. It's easy to see that treating the trigger points without treating the postural abnormality that inspired the trigger points is futile.

Upper Cross Syndrome

Upper cross syndrome may be demonstrated by persons carrying their head forward of their shoulders. These are very common postural characteristics, especially these days with people spending so much time on computers and leaning over work stations.

Upper cross syndrome typically shows a tightening of the muscles of the neck, shoulder, and upper back (trapezius and levator scapula muscles); at the same time a weakening of the rhomboids and stratus anterior muscles between the shoulder blades occurs. The reverse takes place in the front of the body, with weakening of the deep neck flexors and tightening of the chest muscles (pectoral group).

This syndrome can be noticed when the person's shoulders are seen to rise up and roll forward. The overworked muscles, particularly in the neck/shoulder area between the shoulder blades, will be overworked and develop trigger points. This condition leads to muscular imbalance and encourages myofascial trigger points, neurotoxins, and movement problems, ultimately tightening muscles more, perpetuating abnormal posture, muscle/spinal malfunction, and subsequently, pain.

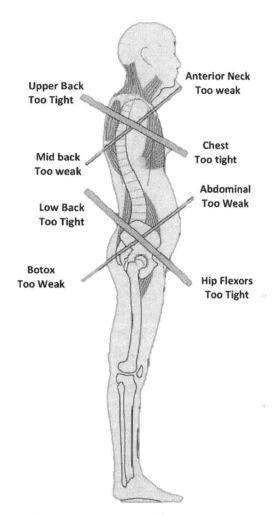

**Upper Back
Too Tight**

**Anterior Neck
Too weak**

**Mid back
Too weak**

**Chest
Too tight**

**Low Back
Too Tight**

**Abdominal
Too Weak**

**Botox
Too Weak**

**Hip Flexors
Too Tight**

Upper and Lower Cross Syndrome

Lower Cross Syndrome

In lower cross syndrome we have the same pattern of weak muscles and overly tightened muscles. We note that the abdominal muscles become weak, along with the muscles of the buttocks, while back muscles and deep muscles of the hip and front of the leg become tight in an effort to make up for the imbalance caused by the weak muscles. Lower cross syndrome is a common finding with low back pain and sciatica. We commonly find that people with a history of low back trouble have weak muscles in the buttocks, as well as the abdomen and tight muscles in the back of the legs and hips.[16, 69] These people can be seen to have postural changes of the pelvis tilting forward and an increased curve in their low back—possibly the lumbar spine shifting to one side or the other, or a leg that tends to rotate out, or knees that have a tendency to flex backwards. This is a perfect setting to cause abnormal joint function of the low back, leading to pain.

Each of these abnormal postures will create specific pain patterns that will develop trigger points and spinal-joint pain, leading to disc irritation or nerve root irritation. Referred pain for myofascial trigger points can mimic conditions such as thoracic outlet syndrome, angina, and trigeminal neuralgia, to name a few. In our practice we see that the greatest danger of not correcting posture at its root causes sets the stage for fibromyalgia and countless other problems that subsequently lead to mismanaged medical care and progressive malfunction.

These conditions are subtle. They develop over a period of time. A patient will be able to tolerate the abnormalities and compensate for them, consciously and/or unconsciously. Nevertheless, they create more areas of fatigue, irritation, and inflammation. Patients will tend to reduce their activities, encouraging more weakness, imbalance, and vulnerability to future injury with very little provocation.

Substance P

Substance P is a neurotransmitter and has been implicated as a major contributor to fibromyalgia. It can be released from almost any tissue within the body—mostly skin, muscles and joints. Substance P is thought to play a role in everything from psoriasis and asthma to migraines, fibromyalgia, and chemical sensitivities.

As a neurotransmitter, Substance P helps with transmitting different stimuli from nerve to nerve into the spinal cord and up to the brain for interpretation. It's found in its greatest quantities in areas that regulate emotions (hypothalamus and amygdala).

When Substance P occurs in high quantities in areas that control emotions, there is a stronger memory and consciousness that endures/imprints the initial pain. This sensitizes emotional centers and inspires anxiety and fear when combined with pain, cumulatively turning chronic pain into chronic suffering.[16] The relatively relentless anxiety, pain, and suffering on a daily basis force sufferers to reduce activities of daily living, which further encourages the cycle to repeat itself, perpetuating the pain and suffering. As things get worse, depression and further disability become obvious.

Substance P is influenced by the thyroid, and depletion of the mineral magnesium. For this reason, many nutritional companies have formulated fibromyalgia-specific supplements with high magnesium. Substance P is reduced by treatment with capsaicin (cayenne pepper), hence reducing pain. We find this to work with some patients; including cayenne pepper with fresh-squeezed lemon in water, when taken daily, will help with pain. Cayenne pepper helps to reduce Substance P, and the fresh lemon provides vitamin C and helps to control inflammation by alkalizing body chemistry.

Trigger Points and Substance P

For our discussion, we'll talk about categorizing trigger points as active and latent. Active trigger points are likely to demonstrate pain upon movement. Latent trigger points generally do not demonstrate pain (unless palpated) but influence muscle activation patterns, which can result in poorer muscle coordination and subsequently encourage these points to become active over time.

Active trigger points have been shown to have increased amounts of neurotoxins such as Substance P, serotonin, calcitonin, bradykinin, and norepinephrine. These toxins cause hypersensitivity to the nerves and surrounding tissue by stimulation of specialized nerve receptors called "nociceptors." The process of stimulating these pain endings and generating pain is called "nociception." Nociceptors can be stimulated and generate pain by other things such as heat, cold, or pressure. This condition in itself can cause localized hyperalgesia, leading to stress on the central nervous system—first where it enters the spinal cord and then up the spinal cord into the brain, causing central sensitivity, leading to idiopathic pain or allodynia.

Allow me to add a little perspective relating neurotransmitters to neurotoxins. You'll note that I called Substance P a neurotransmitter, and then in the paragraph above I referred to it as a neurotoxin. Neurotransmitters are endogenous communicators within the body, such as Substance P. We also have endogenous neurotoxins, such as calcitonin and bradykinin. They also have a necessary function in reference to communication and protection. When endogenous neurotransmitters like Substance P overreact, are poorly controlled, or linger too long, their influence becomes an irritation—they become toxins. This is the case with Substance P. It's felt to overstay its benefit; it becomes a neurotoxin and perpetuates pain.

It appears that these localized areas of increased toxins are created to put the body on alert and protect the area and the body in general from further damage. After the danger has passed, these areas are supposed to at least go back to a resting state of non-active or latent trigger points. However, when the irritation and the stress stay high, the muscles cannot recover; hence neurotransmitters become toxins. Stress can be from temperature change, overuse (as in upper/ lower cross syndrome, or can be triggered by chemical toxins from other sources, such as joint malfunction/inflammation in the area. Regardless of the cause, when this happens the heightened sensitive state in the area may not go away, and, in fact, may become chronic or permanent because the brain at that point would be convinced it must stay in that state to protect itself. At this point clinically, we start to look at this trigger-point area as a disease and a condition in and of itself that needs to be dealt with.

Let's talk a little bit more about what happens at the site of a trigger point area. It's similar to any other site of damage like a strain, sprain, being hit, breaking a bone, or a chronic repetitive insult. There is always a physical and emotional component. Remember that pain is interpreted primarily in emotional centers of the brain. This creates a relationship between the two and cements/links the emotions (fear and anxiety) to the pain, which encourages perpetuation and/or amplification of the pain, fibro style. If the fear/anxiety component is controlled or reduced, there is a better chance of reducing pain and short-circuiting its potential to perpetuate. One of the ways to help is by improving posture, joint movement, and spinal alignment, as well as building up endurance and confidence in activities. Confidence sends a signal to the brain that it's okay to be less protective—less protective means there is no need to be hypersensitive. While the chemistry is complicated, the concept is simple. Almost anything we do or experience in life is easier and less stressful, emotionally and physically, if our confidence is high and we don't have any anxiety or fear about the activity.

So how does the body try to defend itself and tolerate trigger points or an area that's developing trigger points? First, there is a homeostatic/inherent response that attempts to neutralize the toxins locally in the muscle. Keep in mind that once they're there, they have already started the communication process of the pain signals working their way into the spinal column, attempting to get to the brain.

Nevertheless, locally the body will try to neutralize the toxins and reduce the pain. If the body loses that battle and nociceptors fire, the signal will proceed into the spinal cord, where the body will make its next attempt to turn off or neutralize the effect of the toxins.

As an example, after suffering even the most mild and seemingly innocuous whiplash injury, trigger points will begin to develop in the neck and shoulders and attempt to tell the brain what's going on by getting the signals into the spinal cord. At the whiplashed spinal joints in the neck where irritated nerves enter and exit, the body will try to turn off the toxins to slow down or stop the flow of this communication up the spinal cord to the brain (Walker and Hohman 2005). If it is successful, things usually turn out pretty well. However, if it's not, the signals may become excessive and chronic, leading to hypersensitivity within brain circuits via cellular memory (pain and emotional patterning). Myofascial trigger points and pain are now likely to continue for two reasons: one, neck bones/joints, soft tissue, and nerves have been disrupted, causing subluxation; and two, central sensitivity is threatening, all related to the myofascial condition. You'll see this relationship over and over in this book. With each example, I'll try to reinforce a familiar concept that clarifies a multitude of symptoms and clinical efforts that might be undertaken. When the redundancy annoys you, you'll know you've got it.

Wind-Up

You may hear or read the turn "wind-up" from time to time. It is simply another term to describe the hypersensitivity and hair-trigger response that a person may feel when being touched. The neurology is basically the same as we've discussed above. A person in this state may jump off his seat with a big "Ouch, don't do that!" when someone tries to rub his shoulders, compared to the general population that would simply sit there calmly and say "Oooh, yeah, that's tender."

This phenomena holds true not just with myofascial trigger points/ pain syndrome, but with fibromyalgia sufferers as well. As I said, the neurology is the same, but it is sometimes difficult to distinguish between myofascial pain syndrome/trigger points and fibromyalgia unless you're thoroughly familiar with each.

Your Brain

We've discussed the first two defense mechanisms, and we've also explained how the body attempts to defend itself at the tissue level and then defend itself at the spinal-cord level before the pain goes to the brain. Once it is in the brain, yet another attempt will be made to try to understand the hypersensitivity that's in progress and get the central nervous system to literally forget the stimulus and stop the cycle. It is well-known that after a severe injury—severing a finger, gunshot, industrial accident—a person may report no pain when the event initially happens. This is an example of the mechanism we've been speaking of working at its best. The body shuts off the pain, fear, and anxiety that are taking place.

Data that is accepted as science and is reliable today is likely to be not much more than a stepping stone on the way to the next reliable scientific belief. That doesn't make contemporary insights any less valuable. These are the best building blocks available for today's understanding and for the diagnosis, treatment, and science of tomorrow. Use today's science to bring hope and ask better questions.

INSIGHT # 3

PERTINENT AND PERSONAL

With knowledge and awareness come responsibility

and great potential.

Nathan Fay, LMT

CHAPTER 12

Toxins, Free Radicals, and You

Chapter Topics:

Allostatic Load	Heavy Metals	Vaccinations
Excitotoxins	Detoxification	Gulf War Syndrome
Low Blood Sugar	Dental Fillings	Cytokines
MSG, Children/Toxins	Glutamate	German measles
Fibro-Brain/Fibro-Fog	Amalgam Removal	Inflammation
Environmental Toxins	Heavy Meal Testing	
Radiation	Thiol Testing	

In this chapter we will cover many of the issues, pertinent and personal, that sabotage health, both knowingly and unknowingly. For instance, diet and environment pose an extra challenge to Fibros, making it necessary to understand the nuances of cumulative and compounding exposure to toxins when living in a progressive society—the likes of which, as Dr. Russell Jaffe has noted— impose a human cost of reducing the life span of the average person by 8.8 years… or approximately a 10 percent biological tax on lifespan. While the body has an innate ability to detoxify as well as excrete toxins, resilience can be reduced over time with increased allostatic load.

Many times the more we hear or use the same words over and over we become unaffected by them. Words like stress, fatigue, arthritis, pollen…even saying "heart disease" may become easy to ignore, until the condition/factor becomes so imposing that one has no choice but to deal with what it really means to our ability to function. The word "toxins" I believe fall into this category. When we use the word *toxin*, we mean something that is attaching the nervous system, killing nerve cells—killing the brain. Toxicity means cells are fighting to stay alive. This is not a word to become unaffected by.

Allostatic Load

I want to cover the term "allostatic load" in a little more detail than previously, as you are liable to come in contact with the term in other writings. It was first coined by B.S. McEwen and Spellar in 1993. It comes from the word "allostasis," meaning balance, stability, and homeostasis. The concept of allostatic load was proposed to help put into perspective our bodies' response to stress as either adaptive or damaging, and the physiological consequences thereof. In other areas of the book we'll be more specific about the adaptive changes within the brain (hippocampus, amygdala, and prefrontal cortex) due to chronic stress. Keep in mind that chronic stress forces areas of the brain to restructure/remodel themselves to adapt. This is referred to as neuroplasticity. Neuroplasticity may cause alteration in behavior and physiological response, as well as perception and interpretation, such as being touched lightly on the shoulder or leg and feeling more pain than is appropriate.

Many bio gerontologists (the study of biological, psychological, and sociological phenomena associated with old age and aging) believe that toxins or stressors that cause damage throughout life are not really the ultimate cause of aging. Rather, they believe that aging is a result of progressive loss of our DNA's ability to repair the damage when it does occur. This is good news for fibromyalgia sufferers, because it provides hope that damage due to toxic exposures can be mitigated. At the end of this section we will explain plasma thiol testing, which is used to help measure human health status and estimates our DNA's ability to repair.

There are of course physical, chemical, and emotional stressors in life. In this section we are discussing chemical stressors, aka toxins. Toxicity is a constant problem for our bodies to deal with, creating neurological and physiological stress via free radicals, subsequently leading to disease. We're exposed to toxins at every turn, whether it is the air we breathe or the water we drink, the foods we eat, exposure to cleaning products, or even health efforts such as prescriptions, over-the-counter drugs, and supplements. All of these can add to our allostatic load. Some toxins are picked up by our senses and we have a better chance to manage them. They may put off an odor, taste funny, or may burn. But most often they are silent, and they are painless. They pollute muscles and affect hormones and the nervous system. They can cause everything from poor memory and brain fog to mood swings and digestive problems. While there are many detoxification systems and tissues in our body, the main organ is the liver. We'll discuss this in more detail shortly.

Excitotoxins

Excitotoxins are any substance that overly stimulates neurotransmitters. While it's mostly discussed in reference to brain/central nervous system neurology, excitotoxins can take their toll on peripheral neurology as well.

Excitotoxins set in motion a pathological process by which nerve cells are damaged and functionally corrupted, possibly leading to cell death. One such excitotoxin is glutamate, which can cause cumulative damage to the nervous system and reach toxic levels insidiously due to food additives such as monosodium glutamate (MSG). I'll mention two other causes of excessive glutamate concentrations: one is hypoglycemia; the other is status epilepticus (seizures). For our purposes we will not discuss status epilepticus.[9] Rather, we'll focus on dietary considerations and their more direct relationship to fibromyalgia.

Low Blood Sugar

When blood sugar is low, we're said to have hypoglycemia. The brain can also become hypoglycemic. Interestingly enough, brain hypoglycemia may exist independently from systemic low-body blood sugar. This means that during an annual physical, blood sugar tests could register perfectly normal at the same time that the brain is suffering from hypoglycemia. When blood sugar is low, not only do people find that they become sleepy and sluggish physically and sleepy, but their mental capabilities become fuzzy. This can cause the nerves in the brain as well as in and around the spine to fire spontaneously, termed dysregulation. When a person consumes something that excites nerves, like MSG or sugar substitutes, nerves and cells in the brain are affected negatively for two reasons: one, they are dysregulated directly from the toxic effects; and two, indirectly by the added toxin's ability to exaggerate the condition that already exists from a hypoglycemic body. The hypoglycemic person (remember our conversation about carbohydrates?) is going to be generally much more susceptible to the toxic effects of food additives and other chemicals. We could look at hypoglycemia as a behaviorally induced chemical sensitivity syndrome: behavioral-induced because most of us could make better choices, but we don't. Keep in mind as mentioned above, that nerves become dysregulated, which leads to cellular death eventually. Dr. Russell Graylock notes that high doses of MSG cause rapid cellular death. Low doses of MSG cause slow cellular death.

Children and Toxins

Children are four times more sensitive to these neuro-irritants than adults. Dr. Graylock notes that the most vulnerable period is the first eight weeks of fetal life. The placenta is only one cell thick, and there is no blood/brain barrier. So a mother's diet high in excitotoxins can begin to damage brain cells before the child is born. Toxicity can permanently distort and misdirect nerve circuits as they develop. This may account for behavioral problems, mood problems, autism, and schizophrenia in child and adolescent years, as well as criminal and violent behavior later in life.

Diet Coke, Anyone?

We find that many of our fibromyalgia patients as children and now as adults regularly consume diet drinks. They admit to having a diet soda habit, thinking that they're doing well because they're not using sugar, but not realizing that sugar substitutes are neurotoxins. Areas of the brain that control hormones, the wake-sleep cycle, hunger, the autonomic nervous system, and the limbic system (emotional centers) are damaged by these toxins. This affects the relationship with the thyroid, adrenals and gonads, the thalamus and amygdala, which has a large responsibility in a person's interpretation and experience of pain. Damaged areas may never repair/recover, encouraging pain and suffering.

Monosodium Glutamate (MSG)

MSG is a substance derived from manipulating proteins. Suffice it to say that any food that is manipulated is no longer in its natural state and is likely to be a toxin. When consumed, MSG inflames, excites, and irritates nerves. It was first suspected of doing neurological damage as far back as 1954. In spite of its well-documented detrimental effects to the nervous system, the strength of lobbyists and an industry whose bottom line depends on the usage of MSG have managed to keep the overwhelming concerns below the radar.

Fibromyalgia sufferers already have overexcited and overly irritated nerves. While I doubt that MSG is the direct cause of fibromyalgia, it certainly could accumulate in concert with other poor habits and subsequently trigger fibromyalgia, if not perpetuate and/or complicate the clinical picture, particularly in people who are genetically more chemically sensitive. It has also been shown that MSG plays a role in chronic fatigue syndrome. For those who are interested in the chemical in MSG that is the most offensive to us, it is called "free glutamate."

Many people suspect that MSG may be in Asian food and look for MSG when checking out food labels. However, MSG hides behind many other names, sometimes called "hydrolyzed vegetable protein." The industry knows that the word "vegetable" makes us feel more comfortable. You will also see additives called textured protein, yeast extract, mono-potassium glutamate, and plant protein. It may be termed as a vegetable protein extract or simply termed "natural flavor enhancers." There's no shortage of ways to manipulate chemicals and perception. Here's the scariest part: as of this writing, the FDA does not insist on labeling MSG in a product unless it is of at least at 99 percent purity. This means that if there is 97 percent or 98 percent pure MSG additive in a product, it could be labeled as No MSG. If you're sensitive to MSG you may ask at a restaurant whether they use MSG. Most of the time you will get the answer, "No, we don't." But again, if it's less than 99 percent MSG, there is no need to admit its use, assuming they even know. They may try their best, yet be fooled by the labeling as much as the public is. Truth be known, I don't believe most people in restaurants or in kitchens know that many of the food additives and flavor enhancers that they use in recipes are MSG or glutamate-rich, or why anyone should be concerned. The best advice for avoiding this neurological toxin is to simply follow the movement started in the '60s with a push to eat natural foods. If it's processed, bagged, boxed, jarred, flavored, or a prepared food, simply stay away from it. It has most likely been compromised in other ways as well that reduce its nutritional value and become a burden to your body and brain chemistry, even if it says "No MSG."

Glutamate-Fibro Connection

Glutamate has been implicated in fibromyalgia and is related to mercury. Glutamate is one of the most common amino acids in the body and acts as a neurotransmitter. This simply means that it helps cells in their communication with one another. Glutamate plays an important role in many brain functions such as learning, memory, neural development, aging, and the proper response to environmental stimuli (Meldrum, 2000; Ozawa, 1998.) However, at high concentrations, it becomes a toxin and can injure or cause death to nerve cells. Glutamate's effect on glial cells is our primary concern with respect to fibromyalgia.

Specialized glial cells known as astrocytes are responsible for keeping the cellular environment healthy and not allowing substances like glutamate to accumulate to toxic levels. We've noted that it is the glutamate in MSG that can cause the glial cells to become so hyperactive that they eventually burn themselves out and literally die. Another possibility when glutamate builds up is swelling, which may cause the glial cells to lose their ability to help modulate pain signals, hence allowing the pain signals to continue firing unimpeded. Mercury and other toxic metals reduce glial cells' efficiency in the brain and central nervous system, which in turn allows glutamate to accumulate and overexcite nerves. When children are overexcited, their behavior becomes exaggerated, sporadic, and uncontrollable (Ascher 2000; Brookes and Kristt 1989; Danbolt 2001). The same thing happens in the nervous system when nerve signals are not being managed well. If glial cells cannot do their job in controlling glutamate, pain signals will be exaggerated, sporadic, and uncontrollable—aka fibromyalgia.

The body does have its own little factory to make an antioxidant in an effort to combat this scenario. The antioxidant is called glutathione. The body's ability to generate adequate supplies of glutathione is dependent on a healthy diet. Dr. Braun references medical studies and doctors who treat fibromyalgia as having found supplements that cause a decrease in glutamate. Ironically, glutamate is essential for the health of glial cells. Yet, when oversupplied, it becomes lethal. So in most patients, continuing to be inoculated by mercury, as well as by other substances such as sugar substitutes, MSG, and grains, will corrupt the balance and pollute glial cells as well as other brain tissue. Wouldn't it be better to eliminate the toxins that allow glutamate to overwhelm the glial cell efficiency, help glial cells to do their job, and create enough glutathione to detoxify and manage cellular communication and help to reduce pain signal perpetuation?

If you must eat processed foods, check the labels; however, anything that you don't clearly understand and wouldn't eat on its own, you can suspect is in the MSG or preservative family. Surprisingly, glutamate is found in barley malt and other things said to be natural flavor modifiers such as food starch, rice syrup and brown rice syrup, and flavorings that you might use in a sauce or soup. Even if it's labeled natural flavoring for chicken, beef, pork, or seafood, any type of seasoning other than natural herbs should raise suspicion. This would include any manufactured or designer types of fats or butter substitutes. Dr. Russell Blaylock MD wrote about this extensively in his book *Excitotoxins*.

A List of a few things that include MSG:

Salad dressings
Steak sauce
Gravy mixes
Chips
Cream sauces/gourmet foods
Flavored nuts
Soybean milk

Miso
Soy sauces
Soups
Chip/crackers
Boxed/bagged foods
Wrapped/prepared foods

Suggested Reading:

Excitotoxins: The Taste That Kills by Dr. Russell Blaylock, MD

The Zone: The Dietary Roadmap by Dr. Barry Sears

Fibro Brain / Brain Fog
There are areas of the brain that control hormones, emotions, movement, and the perception of pain. They regulate hunger and sleep, our biorhythms, and many of the automatic functions and systems during every second of life. Our brain is meant to handle these things flawlessly, on its own, with little to no help from consciousness. The brain has a protective barrier called the blood/brain barrier to protect it, not allowing all substances or molecules to pass. It filters out free radicals that can damage brain cells, as well as toxins that overexcite nerves and cause them to become over-reactive and to fire indiscriminately until they burn themselves out and die. This barrier can be damaged/compromised or simply overwhelmed by substances, allowing them to pass and subsequently build up to toxic levels, wreaking havoc with communication from cell to cell, and from one area of the brain to another. Dr. Blaylock refers to this as "leaks." These leaks in the blood/brain barrier can happen due to physical injury from playing a sport, possibly a stroke, degenerative diseases, infections, or fevers. Leaks are more common in people with low blood sugar (hypoglycemia), those with diabetes, and in people taking medications.

The blood/brain barrier can also be fooled. When something like aspartame (an artificial sweetener) or glutamate comes in contact with it, it is allowed to pass because it thinks it's a neurotransmitter. The blood/brain barrier has no ability to judge how much of any one particular neurotransmitter is enough, too much, or not enough. That's the job of specialized glial cells called astrocytes, internal to the blood/brain barrier. Therefore, when the blood/brain barrier is bombarded with glutamate or aspartame, they are recognized as neurotransmitters, pass through the barrier, and literally overwhelm and overwork astrocytes leading to possible death—not only death to the astrocyte, but they overburden other cells' ability to produce energy (ATP). This is exactly the case of glutamate and aspartame poisoning.

More bad news: there are some areas of the brain that actually do not have any blood/brain barrier, leaving some of the most sensitive parts of the brain that are directly related to fibromyalgia are the least protected. Of particular concern is exposure in utero and in young children; as mentioned earlier, their nervous systems are still forming and the blood/brain barrier is not fully protective.

With free radicals and antioxidants in the news everywhere in the last ten years, you probably would wonder if antioxidants such as vitamin A, vitamins C, E, K, selenium, zinc, chromium, etc., will help. The short answer is yes, they will help. But it's not as simple as that; even a great diet, one rich in antioxidants, cannot combat the dangers and the damage that MSG and artificial sweeteners can cause. The practical answer is to maintain as healthy a diet as possible, eat as natural as possible, and stay as far away from neurotoxins as much as possible. There are, however, supplements and food choices that can greatly help protect; we will cover these shortly.

Environmental Toxins

Many of the everyday plastics and convenience articles like Styrofoam or household products contain toxins. It's probably impractical to think you can eliminate all of these products from your life; however, being aware of them and possibly minimizing them, or choosing other more environmentally safe products, will help to reduce your allostatic/toxic load, lightening up the load on your immune system. The subtlety of how we're exposed to them, and their cumulative effects, can be quite profound over time. Plastics, for instance, can give off benzene, which is toxic to breast tissue, the prostate, and the hormonal system. Different types of creams and wash products that we come into contact with every day are harmful; everything from shampoos to sunscreen can interfere with the endocrine system and upset hormones. Styrofoam cups and bowls will leach into our food and over a period of time, can disrupt the nervous system, causing fatigue, nervousness, insomnia, and can even depress bone marrow, at which point we would call it a carcinogen. There are many rubber and petroleum products that we come in contact with every day whose toxic effects may cause headaches, fatigue, and loss of appetite. Xylene is a solvent found in many products that we use in our homes. Long-term exposure can be similar to mercury poisoning, causing headaches, irritability, depression, fatigue, and impaired concentration.

Detoxifying our systems from these pollutants is difficult; avoidance is the best measure. However, exercise and sweating have been known to help leach some of these toxins from the body; heat saunas and infrared saunas may also help to detoxify a system that has been exposed to heavy metals, plastics, and petroleum-based toxins. There are also other measures taken by some specialists having to do with different forms of chelation. Chelation (pronounced key-LAY-shun) is the use of one chemical substance to bind other substances to it. Once bound, the toxin can be escorted out of the body. Chelation that has been proven to help eliminate toxic excesses was first used in the 1940s by the Navy to treat lead poisoning.

There are many green cleaning/household products on the market. We use SNAP products for house and office. They are green and work great and can be bought through the internet (see appendix for source).

What We Eat

It's no secret that foods can be polluted and toxic. Sometimes this is a result of the way they're grown, using fertilizers, pesticides, or fungicides. The way they're handled or shipped can cause a breeding ground for organisms, mold, and fungus. You can bet that all processing—whether it is growing, handling, shipping, storing, or displaying at the market—is meant first to enhance the bottom line. Many efforts are made to preserve freshness and make things more convenient for us in spite of the health hazards. I remember when you could cut an apple and it would turn brown and shrivel. These days you can cut an apple, have it sit on your counter for a week, and it will still look as crisp and unblemished as the day you cut it. The old adage of "an apple a day keeps the doctor away" may or may not be true, depending on how the apple has been grown, processed, shipped, and stored.

Meats, poultry, and fish have their own set of problems. Fish are frequently toxic; farm- raised are the worst. Wild fish, while more desirable, may have a high level of mercury and other chemicals—sometimes due to natural habitat and other times due to water pollution. Also there are genetically manipulated animals whose meat has high antibiotic and hormone content. Consumer consciousness and demand have driven contemporary farming to raise antibiotic- and hormone-free stock. This by no means cancels out all the toxic considerations; however, it's a start. The safest answer to this dilemma is to try to find local food sources where you have a chance to know the supplier. However, it may be cost-prohibitive to some because most local suppliers are small and production costs are high. Not growing the right stuff (milk, corn, soy, etc.) get all the subsidies/funding because of effective lobbying. A hybrid of locally grown, commercially grown, and a home garden will be the financial and nutritional answer for most. But you can expect to have to invest a little more time.

Good old-fashioned washing and drying will help. Even if you're doing your own growing, a good bath will help to reduce airborne pollutants, fungus, and mold that lives on the skin or in the cracks of the plant or fruit. There are readily available fruit and vegetable cleaners at health food stores or online.

Below find a couple of lists or toxins/poisons to help steer your choices when shopping.

Fish - Mercury Content

Least mercury (Enjoy)	Moderate mercury (Avoid)	Highest mercury (Avoid)
Anchovies	Bass (saltwater, striped, black, Chilean)	King mackerel
Butterfish		Shark
Catfish	Bluefish	Swordfish
Clams	Carp	Tilefish
Cod	Cod (Alaskan)	
Crab (blue, king, snow)	Croaker (white Pacific)	
Crawfish/crayfish	Grouper	
Croaker (Atlantic)	Halibut	
Haddock (Atlantic)	Lobster (N American)	
Hake	Mackerel (Spanish)	
Herring	Marlin	
Jacks melt	Monkfish	
Lobster, spiny	Orange roughly	
Mackerel (N Atlantic, Pacific chub)	Perch (freshwater)	
Mullet	Sablefish	
Oysters	Skate	
Perch (ocean)	Snapper	
Pollock	Tuna (canned albacore)	
Salmon - wild	Tuna (fresh, frozen)	
Sardines	Tuna (yellow fin)	
Scallops	Weakfish (sea trout)	
Shad (American)		
Shrimp		
Squid		
Tilapia		
Trout (freshwater)		
Whitefish		
Whiting		

TOXINS
From the Environmental Protection Agency
(EPA website epa.gov)

Toxic (carcinogen)	Solution
MSG	None
Sugar substitutes	Stevia
Pesticides	Organic
Household cleansers	Lemon juice, baking soda vinegar, cleaners
Airborne	Air filters in house & House plants
Electrical equipment copiers, computers	Filters & exhaust
Smoking cigarettes	Don't
Second-hand smoke	Escape
Drugs OTC and Rx	Replace with foods & natural ingredients or therapeutic efforts
Meat/fish	Eat only grass fed & wild
Heating systems	Change filters & no forced hot air
Barbeque/brown, Slow cook, bake Electric grills, low heat	
Useless "Vitamins"	Natural food
Noise	Ear plugs
H2O	Filters whole & local
Fruit & veggies	Eat organic, wash
Radiation	Lower exposure
Heavy metals	Eliminate & treat

Electromagnetic Radiation

Although we said we were going to stick to toxins/allostatic load due to chemicals, I wanted to add a couple of other important factors to the category of toxins.

In our everyday lives, we are exposed to electromagnetic radiation at every turn. Some of us use electric heating blankets and spend the whole night bathing in an unnatural electromagnetic field. We live near power lines. We are generally exposed day in and day out to low dosages of electromagnetic radiation from our cell phones, appliances, and electronics. These energy fields can wreak havoc with the polarity of cells and damage DNA. Admittedly, there is controversy over how damaging these magnetic fields are. However, I recommend minimizing exposure whenever possible. The precautions that you can take to help reduce the allostatic load of radiation are relatively few unless you want to drop out of society and live off the grid, but even then you'll be exposed to radiation. Consider the following:

1. Try to provide a healthy distance between you and electronic devices, especially for your children (remember our discussion about the sensitivity of the developing brain).
2. Think about the time that you spend with hair dryers, electric shavers, microwaves and electric coffee pots. If you can reduce that exposure, it will be to your benefit. Try more stove and pan cooking.
3. We caution all of our patients not to use an electric blanket or an electric heating pad. The magnetic forces and radiation flowing around the coils will interfere with your polarity, biorhythms and nervous system.
4. Of particular concern is living in too close proximity to high-voltage electric lines or antennas that transmit television, radio, or cell phone signals. Often we will determine that a poor night's sleep can be traced back to a bedroom or to the head of the bed that is close to where electricity comes into the house. Simply try sleeping in another room and see how you do.
5. When using a cell phone, consider a Bluetooth or speakerphone.

Heavy Metal and Plastics Toxicity

We are going to include toxicity from plastic and other petroleum products in our discussion about heavy metals. It's very clear that it's difficult to live without being exposed to plastic or metal. However, in doing so we're exposed to arsenic, cadmium, chromium, cobalt, copper, nickel, and other heavy metals at unnatural levels. These metals are toxic, hence they create free radicals. They stimulate disease processes, speed up the aging process, and reduce our ability to heal and recover from illness. Heavy metals and associated toxicities will sabotage the immune system, affect mood and the nervous system, and cause fatigue and poor concentration. Many people report hair loss as a result of heavy-metal toxicity. We've all heard of lead poisoning due to lead-based paint, which was the only paint produced prior to the 1950s. Lead paint was outlawed in 1976; however, there are still many houses painted with these paints (inside and out) that could pose a threat. Children are the most threatened by contact for two reasons: first, because of hand and mouth contact; and second, their systems are more fragile. Such exposure affects the immune and nervous system in profound ways.

We have already established that the detrimental effects of toxins are insidious and compounded by the cumulative effects of multiple-substance exposure in everyday life. For instance, plastics are convenient, utilitarian and visually pristine; however, there is a disconnect when using them. We have a sense of confidence because we see the food and drink as fresh and protected, giving an extra measure of safety and comfort. Think about how many things we handle that are made of plastic and/or packaged in it. Generally, we can reduce our exposure to the toxins we have discussed by taking into consideration a few things, but keep in mind that the goal would be to do what you can while you can. You're unlikely to eliminate all exposure.

1. Inspect your house for lead-based paint and don't store any old paint around the house.
2. Reduce mercury exposure; see the fish chart above. Discuss with your dentist the difference between what's called amalgam dental fillings and gold or polymer fillings. There are also glass and ceramic fillings available. Not everyone in the dental community agrees that the old amalgam fillings are toxic. I suspect that it's a bit of playing defense due to how many millions of teeth have been filled with this product. I would err on the side of caution and at the very least not get any more amalgam fillings. Some researchers are recommending that the old amalgam fillings be taken out; however, that is an expensive and toxic process in itself. If this is a consideration, it should

be done by a qualified dentist. (See our section on "Good Dentistry or Spin.")

3. Avoid aluminum foil and cooking with aluminum pots and pans. Also, read labels, stay away from cans and containers that have aluminum in them. Aluminum may be in your antiperspirant. This can be absorbed through your skin, as can contact with outdoor furniture, commonly made from aluminum tubing, particularly in the summer when pores are open your body is more susceptible. Wood, painted furniture, or bamboo furniture is a safer choice.

4. Avoid consuming food or drink stored and/or cooked in plastic, such as microwavable foods. While no FDA or officially released government studies have proven current microwaving usage to be harmful, I encourage you not to cook or warm foods in plastic containers.

Detoxification

In addition to attempting to detoxify our exposures and consumptions, we should recognize that the liver has the greatest detoxification responsibilities in our body. The liver has a function of detoxifying fat-soluble and water-soluble substances. Water-soluble substances are much more easily dealt with. Vitamin supplements can be put into the categories of fat-soluble or water-soluble. Water soluble vitamins such as vitamin C are not as worrisome because the liver will manage excesses and eliminate them relatively easily, whereas taking supplements such as vitamin A, D, E, K and F, which are fat-soluble, cause the liver to work harder, hence excesses could build up to toxic levels. The toxic potential in vitamin and herbal supplement dosing is increasing every year due to the abundance of advertising and products pushing their influence on our desire to feel better, live longer and solve problems in the most convenient manner. While we are strong proponents of supplementing nutrition, it calls for a real effort to understand supplementation and foods. Most people don't have the time; they are too busy earning a living and taking care of their families to study. It's our recommendation that everyone should have a health coach—a doctor or another person he or she can turn to who has the proper education, experience, and attitude to coach a person through balancing nutrition and understanding the intricacies as well as possible interaction with medication.

The message is that indiscriminately taking supplements can be harmful. However, the same holds true for medications. Whether prescribed or over-the-counter; medications are toxic—if not in and of themselves, then when combined with other medications that add to the allostatic load of everyday stress and exposure. There is a federal mandate for all doctors to have electronic medical records by 2015. This will enable any and all of our doctors and pharmacists to see what medications we are taking, and their dosages. This is being done to provide a safer and more efficient medical system. In the *Journal of the American Medical Association (JAMA)*, July 26, 2000; 284 (4): 483-5, an article by Dr. Barbara Starfield of Johns Hopkins School of Hygiene and Public Health reports that iatrogenic death is the third leading cause of hospital deaths in United States; after heart disease and cancer. Every year it kills over 225,000 people who would not otherwise have died if not for being in the hospital. Over 112,000 of these deaths are directly related to medication errors and reactions. She notes that these statistics are for deaths only and do not take into account the negative effects that are associated with invisible disability, illness or discomfort due to iatrogenics. Invisible disability includes conditions such as fibromyalgia and chronic fatigue, which are not included in the statistics. Imagine including the 6,000,000 fibro cases to the iatrogenic statistics. It raises the question for fibromyalgia sufferers as to whether they are suffering any toxic effects of drugs exposed to or consumed.

There are liver tests that can gauge the level of toxicity in the liver and are a great starting point. Check with your doctor.

Mercury
There are two looming concerns in reference to mercury toxicity. One is the usage of high-fructose corn syrup (HFCS) containing mercury. The second is the massive number of dental fillings using amalgam, which leach mercury.

In a study published by the *Journal of Environmental Health* 2005, Dr. David Walling reported that mercury was found in nearly 50 percent of sampled commercial high-fructose corn syrup. It is used in prepared foods such as breads, cereals, beverages, nutrition bars, luncheon meats, soups, condiments, yogurt, etc. According to the Institute for Agricultural Cultural and Trade Policy, the average American eats about twelve teaspoons of HFCS per day. Some of the brands tested were Quaker, Hershey, Kraft and Smuckers. However, consumers should be wary of all processed and prepared foods. Remember the no bagged, boxed, jarred or prepared food rule.

How does this happen? *The Journal of Environmental Health* went on to explain that for decades, HFCS has been made by using mercury-grade caustic soda (hydrogen peroxide) produced in so-called "chlor-alkali" or industrial chloride plants that use mercury cells. The caustic soda, which can thus contain traces of mercury, is used to separate the cornstarch that goes into making the syrup from the kernel. When we add these reports to the concern about genetically modified corn, overconsumption of calories, hypoglycemia, diabetes, etc., the best advice is to avoid consuming any products that contain high-fructose corn syrup. If you start reading labels, you'll discover that it's nearly impossible to find products that you're used to stocking that don't have high-fructose corn syrup. Eat natural real foods; take the time to pick them out and prepare them yourself. This includes preparing your own condiments, sauces and dressings. See Chapter 13 for more important information about HFCS; this is "you need to know" stuff.

Dental Fillings

Amalgam/Mercury Fillings Controversy: *Good Dentistry or Spin?*

Think back to the 1990s when the tobacco company scandals took place. There were lawsuits, class actions, government involvement, penalties, and payouts that tobacco companies had to deal with in the tens of billions of dollars; I'm betting it's not over yet. Can you imagine what would happen if we reached that same level of concern, societal outrage, and scientific clarity regarding amalgam fillings, aka mercury fillings? Tens of millions of people on every continent, particularly Baby Boomers, have their mouths full of mercury fillings. Mercury has been implicated in millions of dollars of health-care costs, with untold consequences believed to contribute to degenerative diseases and functional diseases, everything from Alzheimer's to fibromyalgia, rheumatoid arthritis to lupus.

Amalgam filling material is comprised of approximately 50 percent mercury. This mercury can and will begin to break down while it is in your mouth. As it is processed through your digestive system, it will be further broken down into methyl-mercury, which is one step more toxic than mercury. The pituitary gland, thyroid gland, and brain/neurological tissues are the primary targets for the toxic effects of the mercury.

The dental community's long-standing claim has been that while mercury is in fact toxic, fillings pose no risk because the amalgam is sealed once it is applied to the tooth. In making such a claim, they obviously hope to assuage the public's fear with regard to their placing potentially poisonous material in their patients' mouths. I have not unearthed any credible scientific evidence that supports their claim.

How a person tolerates toxins is dependent on several factors: the health and well-being of the immune system, genetics, the body's detoxification efficiency, susceptibility and the seemingly innocuous effects of cumulative toxins (diet and environment) will all play a role as they increase the allostatic load. The variability means a person may develop toxic levels even if he is exposed to very low levels of toxin, or it may lead to an otherwise healthy person with no genetic predispositions who breaks down over time due to increased levels or chronic exposure. When mercury makes its way into a person's system, it attacks the brain, pituitary gland, hypothalamus, thyroid, and adrenal glands. It may upset the balance among the hypothalamus, pituitary, and adrenal glands (HPA axis). It has also been known to cause fatigue, musculoskeletal pain, sleep disturbances, gastrointestinal problems, as well as neurological problems like MS and Alzheimer's. In reference to Fibros, I'm concerned with glial cells in the brain and their short- and long-term reaction to exposure, which dysregulates brain activity.

Dr. Braun cites a study of 86 patients with chronic fatigue syndrome. Seventy-eight percent of participants within a short period of time reported significant health improvements after replacing amalgam fillings. Additionally, a special immune reactivity test ("Melisa") showed a significant reduction in white blood cells compared to before the removal, meaning that the patient's immune system was not working as hard. This in turn would be expected to help symptoms of fibromyalgia, neurological disorders, autoimmune problems, and chronic fatigue.

There's a division of the Centers of Disease Control called the Agency for Toxic Substances and Disease Registry. A representative of the ATSDR, Susan Castile, reported that 4 to 19 micrograms per day of mercury can leach out of amalgam fillings, causing central nervous system disturbances, tingling, tremors and fatigue, and memory, mood, and behavior problems. She went on to say that elderly people with respiratory problems, pregnant women, and children are at the greatest risk to be affected by mercury. It would seem to me that the amount of amalgam fillings in a person's mouth could drive the cumulative leaching parameters of 4 to 19 micrograms per day sky-high. Let's consider a woman 55 years old who had the sum of six fillings by age 35. Now let's add the following list as a very real-life backdrop:

1. She has had one or two pregnancies
2. Her diet is high in carbohydrates, primarily grains
3. She's exposed to MSG through restaurant and prepared foods
4. She uses sugar substitutes
5. She's exposed to her share of pollutants and carcinogens
6. She's predisposed to fibromyalgia, or at the very least she is chemically sensitive
7. She has a fairly typical lifestyle deprived of sleep on top of a good dose of domestic and financial stress

It's not hard to believe that a mouth full of amalgam could tip the scales and, as we discussed, inspire everything from autoimmune diseases such as lupus and rheumatoid arthritis to chronic fatigue and fibromyalgia, as well as central-nervous-system degenerative conditions such as Parkinson's, Alzheimer's and ALS. With ever-improving technology, surely specialized materials have been designed that can be used without compromising patient health, restoration, longevity, and profit margins. The rationale for amalgam fillings seems to have passed. Why challenge our physiology when it's unnecessary?

What Should We Do About Those Old Fillings?

The bad news is that there may not be anything that has a good risk/reward ratio for those who already have amalgam fillings in their mouths in terms of having them removed, as it is possible that removing them may prove more harmful than simply leaving them in. If removal is something that you consider, you should consult the American Academy of Environmental Medicine and research biological dentists. The cost for removal (as of this writing) is also fairly prohibitive. But let's talk about it a little more.

Amalgam Removal

The question of whether to remove amalgam fillings is difficult to answer. There are toxic risks in doing so. If we are talking about fibromyalgia specifically, and possibly chronic fatigue, it would seem prudent to at least look at the data and consider personal chemical sensitivities before plunging into removal.

When considering removal, it is important to weigh risk/reward. The first step would be to get tests done to establish the baseline of mercury toxicity as well as other heavy metals. If it is determined that your body has been handling toxicity well and there is a low level of risk in removing the amalgam filling, consider looking into biological dentistry.

An internet search can find articles that will equate biological dentistry with biological "quackery." It's important to keep in mind that while the internet is a useful tool, there is no regulation in terms of what people are allowed to publish on it. While researching, keep in mind the bias that certain people/organizations will bring to the table for financial gain or to protect themselves.

One of the organizations I recommend consulting is The International Academy of Oral Medicine and Toxicology (AIAOMT). Their advisory board is made up of PhDs from the United States, Sweden and Canada. They have chapters in 14 countries, and their motto is "Show Me the Science." The AIAOMT is two decades old and reports that they've chronicled the research that proves beyond a reasonable doubt that dental amalgam is a source of significant mercury exposure and is a hazard to health. They have taken the lead in educating dentists and allied professionals in the methods of safely dealing with amalgam fillings as well as disposing of the waste. They are in the process of developing more biocompatible approaches in other areas of dentistry including endodontics, periodontics, and disease prevention. By labeling themselves biological dentists, they are not attempting to create a new dental specialty; rather, biological dentistry "describes an attitude that can apply to all facets of dental practice and to health care in general. To always seek the least toxic way to accomplish the mission of treatment, and to do it while treading as cautiously as possible on a patient's biological terrain." Their website is www.AIAOMT.org.

While the American Dental Association (ADA) may be looked at as having a conflict of interest, it would still be wise to search their data for information as well that of non-biological dentists. Another source that we strongly believe you should look into is The International Academy of Biological Dentistry and Medicine.

It's important to note that it is not our belief that amalgam fillings on their own are the sole source for problems such as Alzheimer's or Parkinson's, nor is it our opinion that amalgam fillings alone will exacerbate or perpetuate fibromyalgia and chronic fatigue. However, they are one more toxic load for the body, and one there is no need for, despite conventional wisdom giving the okay for it. Of course, this is the very same conventional wisdom that signs off on MSG and sugar substitutes in our food supply, so you may wish to consider the source.

Everyone can at least become more conscious of and reduce additional exposure. Eliminating or reducing the intake of MSG, chemical sugar substitutes and processed/manufactured foods will go a long way toward improving overall health. Also, you can improve diet and help support the body's innate detoxification system, in particular making sure that there are adequate live foods rich in minerals and enzymes.

Heavy Metal Testing

Mercury and heavy-metal toxins hide in the brain, organs, and tissue. Therefore, conventional testing methods such as blood tests, or urine or hair samples, may not be depended on. The most reliable method for testing for mercury is called a "provoked urine challenge." This method introduces a chelating agent that helps to pull toxins like mercury out of the tissue, after which it is excreted through urine. The urine is collected and analyzed by a special laboratory. You'll want to make sure that your medical doctor, dentist, and/or naturopath are very familiar with these procedures, because there are some contraindications.

Just for perspective, I have included a printout of the results of the toxic elements screening. The test evaluates urinary excretion and looks at a diverse spectrum of toxic elements and excessive levels for a total of 20 potential toxic elements. This example was supplied by Genova Diagnostics of Asheville, North Carolina. Doing this test may help with a decision as to whether to remove filings or not and give you a baseline perspective of your toxic load/environment exposure.

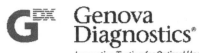

Genova
Diagnostics®
Innovative Testing for Optimal Health

Order Number:

Completed: September 09, 2005

Received: July 20, 2005

Collected: July 20, 2005

Toxic Elements			
Results in µg/g creatinine			
Element	Reference Range	TMPL	Reference Range
Lead	0.4		<= 1.4
Mercury	0.86		<= 2.19
Aluminum	1.2		<= 22.3
Antimony	0.012		<= 0.149
Arsenic	0		<= 50
Barium	0.1		<= 6.7
Bismuth	0.19		<= 0.76
Cadmium	0.05		<= 0.64
Cesium	0.0		<= 10.5
Gadolinium		0.821	<= 0.019
Gallium		0.413	<= 0.028
Nickel	0.45		<= 3.88
Niobium	0.082		<= 0.084
Platinum		0.078	<= 0.033
Rubidium	0		<= 2,263
Thallium	0.133		<= 0.298
Thorium	0.083		<= 0.124
Tin	0.78		<= 2.04
Tungsten	0.094		<= 0.211
Uranium		0.046	<= 0.026

You may find the following helpful if you continue to be concerned about amalgam fillings.

The following was taken directly from www.mercurypoisoning. com, accessed December 2013. I thought it was helpful, with additional resources noted. Hopefully, it will help you in sorting out and understanding considerations in mercury-filling removal. This is Marie's story, and, as Marie would say:

"This story is simply offered as-is for educational purposes only, and does not replace a personal consultation with the health-care professional of your choice."

Should I Remove My Amalgam?
How Do I Choose a Doctor and Dentist?
How Many Fillings Do I Remove at One Time?
Marie Flowers
Updated November 2006

If your dentist wants to replace some amalgam because it is old and cracked, you could become ill if you allow him to do it. Will he use precautions while removing it? Not if he is a regular dentist, or even a mercury-free dentist. Now is the time to seek a biological/holistic dentist who will protect you from mercury vapor and will be more knowledgeable about replacing the amalgam with a safer material. Your regular dentist might take out the amalgam and put back more amalgam! If a filling needs to be replaced in your lower left side, a biological dentist could redo all the amalgam fillings on the lower left side at the same time if not too many need replacing.

Dr. Hal Huggins recommends seeing a medical doctor first. See a medical ACAM doctor who understands mercury toxicity (www.acam.org or 1-800-LEADOUT) and he will give you supplements (multivitamin/minerals) to build up your immune system before the dentist starts removing the mercury. He will also give you mercury-removing supplements (such as high doses of Kyrolic garlic, vitamin C, and some like Dr. Mercola recommend chlorella) to take so you will be prepared for your dental revision. This will reduce your chances of being further poisoned or becoming poisoned.

Other doctors who treat mercury toxic patients include doctors from The American Academy of Environmental Medicine (www.aaem.com). Another organization I just heard about from Dr. Rebecca Painter, an ACAM physician who testified at recent FDA hearings on dental amalgam, is The American Board of the Clinical Metal Toxicology (www.abcmt.org). There is a doctor listed with this organization in Greensboro, NC for you folks in my area of Virginia. I don't know her and have not been to her.

One good way to find a good alternative health doctor who understands mercury toxicity is to call the biological dentists' offices and ask them who they recommend. Good and experienced biological dentists work with these doctors and know who to refer their patients to.

If you are sick, or want to avoid being so, you definitely need to look into biocompatibility testing of dental materials, before you start removing the mercury fillings. Go to the discussion on bio-compatibility testing, and check with your biological dentist to see if he has this kit in his office.

If you are not sick, but yet you want your amalgam replaced, you could replace it slowly and safely over a course of time, using safety precautions recommended by the IAOMT. See www.saveteeth.org for the IAOMT protocol. Also check out the IAOMT.org web site for a story with picture of how fillings should be removed safely. It would also be easier on the pocketbook to pay for one quadrant at a time.

They will have to be replaced one day anyway, because they don't last forever. Get yourself educated so you won't become poisoned when a tooth with an amalgam filling breaks or you have an emergency situation.

Knowledgeable people, such as chiropractors and alternative health doctors who know about mercury's toxicity, may choose to do a complete removal of amalgam in their own mouths as a preventative measure. If I had cancer I would remove my fillings so my immune system would have the best chance of fighting the cancer. Dr. Vincent Speckhart, alternative cancer specialist of Norfolk, VA, now retired as of 2002, required his patients to remove mercury and other toxic materials from their mouths in order to take stress off the immune system. If I was having many of the symptoms of chronic mercury toxicity, I would start removing mercury fillings. If I had a neurological disease, I would start removing mercury fillings.

If you choose to do a complete dental revision, then the whole mouth is revised using precautions and under the care of both a biological dentist and a medical doctor. The holistic/alternative doctor will supply supplements to strengthen the immune system, and mercury-removing drugs or supplements.

DAMS recommend that you do not take the drugs like DMSA or DMPS until after you remove your fillings. There is so much mercury already stirred up when you are poisoned; you don't want to stir up any more with mercury fillings still in your mouth. The idea is to pull out only a little mercury at a time and excrete it. You don't want to pull out great amounts; your body will not able to excrete it and then it will redistribute back into your body. In fact, DAMS is very cautious when it comes to chemical chelators, and recommends other chelators that don't involve chemicals.

I have had mercury settle in my back muscles after doing a glutathione push that was too much for me. A push is a syringe that is inserted into a vein over a short 10-15 minute period. I felt like I had been poisoned all over again. It wasn't the doctor's fault. I didn't tell him I had been taking DMSA also. The combination of the DMSA and the glutathione together just pulled more mercury out of my body than I could excrete.

I had ten fillings removed over a period of five office visits to the biological dentist within a month's time. If you are suffering from MS or other serious illness, some suggest waiting for longer periods of time between mercury removals. DAMS recommends removing only two fillings per session or staying in the chair no longer than two hours. On the DAMS web site (amalgam.org), they recommend that you schedule your appointments a month apart.

Some of the dentists want to get in your mouth and take out lots of fillings in one visit. You have to judge your health and what your body can stand. If I had three fillings in one quadrant and that quadrant was numb, then I would consider having all three fillings removed at one time since the area was already numb. Once again, it depends on how sick you are and what your body can stand. I know one woman who was so poisoned that the dentist feared for her life if she didn't get them all out as soon as possible. This happened to a lady in Wales whose brain was on fire from mercury in her brain.

Another thing you need to consider in choosing a biological dentist is not just whether he is safe, but is he also competent in replacing your fillings with other materials? Will the bite be right? Will the restorations look good and fit without leaks? I have had some people contact me whose dentists messed up their bites so badly that they couldn't get their teeth together. Some were traditional dentists and some were biological. So if you do only a few teeth in the first visit, you can judge the quality of the dentist's work. Then he won't be redoing half your mouth and leaving you in a mess. That is why it is good to have recommendations as to a dentist's safety and skill in restorative work.

It is also time to visit a biological dentist when your regular dentist wants to place a crown. My regular dentist placed a crown in my mouth that chemically and electrically interacted with the mercury filling and caused a "galvanic" reaction between the different metals in my mouth. Placing these metals together caused me to become sick to my stomach, as the mercury was leaking out of the crowned tooth. I felt like I was dying and spent several nights without sleep.

This is what my regular dentist did when he placed a crown:

He knew that I had been taking prednisone one month previous to my dental visit with him. Prednisone, a steroid drug, makes a person more susceptible to contracting diseases. You should not have mercury removed when your immune system is compromised due to medications or illness unless under a doctor's orders.

But most dentists do not take this into consideration. My dentist only partially drilled out the mercury filling and exposed me to the mercury vapor while doing so. He did nothing to build up the tooth in order to strengthen the tooth before placing the crown. He placed a crown containing metals over top of the mercury filling that interacted with the mercury filling, thus making me physically sick. This crown had to be later replaced during my complete dental revision. Cost of the crown with my regular dentist: $550 (back in 2001) and I still had a mercury-filled tooth underneath!

This is what a biological dentist will do to place a crown:

He will not want to do mercury removal unless you are on immune-enhancing supplements. He will safely remove all of the mercury filling in that tooth and not expose you to vapor while doing so. He will build up the tooth with a porcelain inlay to strengthen the tooth. He will place a crown that does not contain metals to make you sick. Cost $850 to $1000 plus and that will now be a mercury-free tooth. Some of the dentists have a Cerec machine in their offices where they can make the crown or inlay on the spot and you don't have but one office visit for that tooth.

So amalgam can be removed gradually or in a shorter period of time, depending on your health situation. There is a direct correlation between the number of amalgam fillings in your mouth and your toxic exposure to mercury vapor over a lifetime. Check out other sites such as Bernie Windham's at www.dams. cc. He can give you the references.

In fairness to my local dentist, he was not the only one to cause oral galvanism in my mouth. The dentist that I had seen in TN when my tooth first broke off had placed a "patch" on my tooth at my request. The dentist in TN should not have placed dissimilar metals in my mouth. He should not have put a "patch" on that tooth. I didn't know that dissimilar metals were dangerous in the mouth. That was when I first started tasting metal. So the poisoning started with that tooth in the dentist's office in TN.

But my dentist did not tell me the truth when I asked him why I tasted metal in my mouth. If my dentist had not been "gagged" by the ADA and the VA state dental board, maybe he would have felt that he could have honestly explained to me what was happening. However, since dentists are "gagged" because of fear of losing their licenses if they tell the truth about mercury, patients have mercury-poisoning symptoms and don't even know what is happening to them. My dentist did tell me that maybe I was tasting metal because I was grinding my teeth. That is half the truth. Patients who grind their teeth do have more mercury released from their mercury dental fillings. However, he could plainly see the dissimilar metal that had been placed on the tooth by the dentist in TN. (The dentist in TN didn't look at the tooth; his assistant did the patching.)

This is what should happen in order for patients to receive proper care from dentists.

Even if the federal bill HR 4011 to ban mercury fillings is passed, people with existing mercury in their mouths will not be protected. People will not know that dentists should be using a special protocol to remove mercury fillings. They will also not know that dentists should not be placing dissimilar metals in the mouth in the form of braces, crowns, partial plates, and bridgework in conjunction with mercury fillings. For patients to be protected, dentists in VA need legislation from Richmond that would allow them to freely discuss dentistry with their patients without fear of reprisal. Hometown dentists need to be able to say,

"I don't have the equipment in my office to properly remove mercury fillings from your mouth. But I am going to refer you to a special biological dentist who uses a special protocol to start removing mercury from this quadrant of your mouth. Then you can come back to me as your general dentist and we can resume our patient/dentist relationship. In the future I will be placing only non-mercury fillings in my patients' mouths. If you need dental fillings replaced in another quadrant of your mouth or if you need a crown, I advise you to go back to the biological dentist and have the mercury also taken out of that quadrant of your mouth. If you are having health problems that a medical doctor is thinking is related to mercury fillings, I would advise you to have a complete dental revision and remove all the mercury fillings."

The state needs to write legislation so that dentists are "ungagged," and so they would be allowed to advertise that they use a special protocol to remove mercury fillings. They would not be allowed to advertise this now, as the VA state dental board will not allow it. Many mercury- free dentists are afraid to even advertise that they are mercury-free. The VA state dental board doesn't want you to know that your "silver" fillings are 50% mercury. They don't want *you removing mercury fillings and they don't want you to know there is a safe protocol for the removal of mercury fillings.*

The state dental board believes what the state dental school teaches dentists about amalgam is "scientific" and that silver amalgam mercury dental fillings are not harmful. The favorite ADA line is "only 100 people have ever had an 'allergic' reaction to silver fillings."(I guess my brain was having an "allergic" reaction when it was burning and on fire, vibrating inside my skull and causing me to have L'hermette's sign--electrical charges shooting from the brain stem throughout my body.

As of 2006, the ADA can't say that any more. If your dentist tells you that only 100 people have ever had an allergic reaction, ask him, "Well what about that group of over 2000 people who sent stories to the FDA in the fall of 2006 that had been poisoned from their fillings? That is a little more than 100, isn't it?" Tell your dentist to get on my website and read victims' testimonies and see their pictures and read the transcripts from the FDA web site where the FDA Advisory Panel REJECTED a report of the FDA saying the fillings were safe.

I wish I had been reading an article like this before I went to my dentist in August 2001. I did not have the knowledge I am giving you. It would have been much cheaper for me to have found a biological dentist, traveled some distance to go to the appointments, and paid a little more to have the crown placed correctly without exposing me to mercury vapor. I could have avoided all this pain and suffering, the cost of DMSA to remove the mercury from my body, the cost of hormones to keep me thinking straight, and the cost of many supplements to keep me going.

Here are some notes from back in 2002: Each 200-mg DMSA pill I take to remove mercury from my body costs me $1.04. Insurance has already paid for more than half of the cost of the pill, but I still have to pay $1.04. Vitamins/ minerals cost me $50 or more a month and hormones cost me $45 a month out of pocket after the insurance pays its share. When I was first poisoned and received help from my ACAM doctor, I was also taking yeast-removing drugs that cost more than $300, and the insurance company didn't want to pay for some of them. I also took enzymes, olive leaf extract, licorice, and other supplements that were recommended by my ACAM doctor. So it hasn't been inexpensive, being mercury poisoned.

Also, ACAM doctors are usually not participating members of your insurance company, so the office visits also cost more. However, it is cheaper to go to one good ACAM doctor than to go to six MDs who know nothing about mercury poisoning.

Fillings don't last forever, including amalgam mercury fillings. So it is not a question of "Should I remove my amalgam?" but of how and when they will be removed. Under what conditions will you choose to have them removed? It is your mouth. You are in charge of your own dental health. Be wise, and do it right when they need to be replaced. Gradually over a period of time you can become mercury-free!

Your bumper sticker should read "Mercury-Free and Healthy!"

December 29, 2003 update:

After talking to many people who have contacted me by phone or by e-mail, I am adding to this discussion of "Should I have my amalgam removed?" If you are sick with poisoning symptoms, don't make the mistake of waiting too long to have the dental work done. Some people keep postponing the work because they think they can't afford it. As they wait, they get sicker. If you get sick enough, you may have to quit your job completely--and some I have talked to have gone on disability in their thirties. If you wait until you get so sick that you can't work and then have to retire, it is likely that you will have even less money for the dental work.

I think some postpone this work because they are not convinced yet that the problem is their fillings. So get convinced. Do the research, before you get too sick. Don't just keep avoiding the issue. As you read more and more and you see your symptoms in the medical research, and in the personal stories, you will then be able to make an educated decision. And don't let a low score for mercury on a heavy metals test keep you from the dental revision. It is very hard to rely on heavy metals testing for mercury. I am so glad my physician understood the symptoms and treated me for mercury even though my test scores were not very high.

My husband just retired this past summer due to complications from a war injury. But before he retired, he had all the mercury removed from his teeth. I am so glad he got this work done while he was still employed.

Elmer Cranton (www.drcranton.com). It is less expensive for the patient, because he doesn't have to go in for three-hour IVs of EDTA chelation (www. drcranton.com).

www.flcv.com/dams.html

toxicteeth.org

amalgam.org

IAOMT.org

Back to the top

Back to Mercury Poisoned main page

Disclaimer:

This information is provided for educational purposes only, and does not replace a personal consultation with the health care professional of your choice.

(c) 2002 by Marie Flowers.

***

When I checked out some of the links to doctors' offices who treated heavy metals, some mentioned only EDTA chelation. This is not the drug of choice for mercury toxicity. EDTA attaches to other heavy metals before it attaches to mercury. If using chemical chelators, DMSA (an oral pill) is a better choice, according to Dr. Elmer Cranton (www. drcaanton.com)

Total Plasma Thiol Test

Earlier we spoke of plasma thiol testing to help measure our health status and estimate our DNA's ability to repair damage from toxic exposures. The test is an extension of established thiol testing for cells' protective antioxidants in the glutathione family. The implications of the test are for immune competency and general health status. In other words, how is a person holding up under the stresses and toxicities of life? Additionally, it measures how resilient/protected people's physiology may or may not be as they age.

Biogerontolgists suggest that pharmaceutical therapy, social, behavioral, physical activities, and diet can be resourceful in improving thiol levels. This information of course is common knowledge: improve diet, exercise regularly, control social and behavioral stresses, and possibly take vitamins; immune competency and general health status will rise. However, up until 2005 the only intervention proven to raise thiol levels was nutraceuticals. In February 2005 the *Journal of Vertebral Subluxation Research* (JVSR), reported a study demonstrating that as little as three years of regular chiropractic wellness-care will help to optimize human health status and raise serum thiol levels. It's hoped that with further study, insurance companies will realize financial savings for their shareholders and incorporate long-term chiropractic wellness-care into policy coverage. Consumers, of course, just want to improve health and not have to suffer the health problems that they've seen older generations endure. For a Fibro, reducing pain and increasing energy will do just fine. Raising thiol levels is clearly a way to help. Proper supplementation and regular chiropractic wellness-care checkups will be the pivotal additions to your lifestyle.

Biomedical Diagnostic Research, Inc.
P.O. Box 3638
Goodyear, Arizona 85338

Patient: First E Last Patient ID Number 3070 Doctor:	Date Collected: 2-Aug -13 Date Received: 2- Aug -13 Date Completed: 2- Aug -13

Serum Thiol vs Risk of Active Disease

Mean ± SD Controls
indicated;
p< 0.05 compared in all
Diseases categories

Serum Protein Thiols (nmoles/0.76mL/0.2 ml serum)

■ Serum protein thiol ■ Your Results

Kidney Dis – Kidney Disease, CV Dis – Cardio-Vascular Disease, Cancer – All Cancers, Meta Dis – Metabolic Disorders, Neuro Dis – Neurological Diseases, Diabetes – All forms of Diabetes, Blood Dis – Blood Disorders, Inf/ Inflam – Infection and Inflammation Diseases, Thyroid Dis – Thyroid Diseases, All Dis – All Diseased Categories combined for analysis.

This serum protein thiol test is NOT a diagnostic tool, but a measure of health status. The mean depicted in the graph (120) is subject to some variance over time. Presently, a value of 90 or less would indicate reduced DNA repair capacity and immune competence since the standard deviation (2) is 28 away from the average ."All disease" means the average value of all the results for subjects with known disease diagnoses. This was first observed in a published study on 306 individuals with classifications as shown above. Your value, if below the mean, doesn't diagnose a disease. For example a result of 91 does not mean you have thyroid disease. Values of 61 and below do indicate that a medical assessment would be recommended, in the absence of a known diagnosis. Values above the mean have been shown to correlate with good cellular aging and longevity, and is a good health category with a 5% risk of active disease.

Serum Protein Thiol Test Result: 138

Prof. Joseph Cummins
Technical Director

Arthur F. Rossi, Ph.D.
Laboratory Director

CLIA ID Number: 36D1005069

Vaccinations

The Centers for Disease Control reported that, according to the Arthritis Foundation, there is no known link between vaccines and fibromyalgia—and further, that the rise in fibromyalgia statistics is not alarming. They feel that the increase may simply be because of an aging population. Further, they suggest that fibromyalgia is a type of Baby Boomers' disease. But only in the last ten years or so has there been an increase in physicians' willingness to accept fibromyalgia as a diagnosis. Therefore it's impossible to know whether or not the increase in cases represents a true increase in fibromyalgia incidents, or an improvement in acceptance and reporting.

The cynical side of me wants to point out that once the pharmaceutical industry finds a way to make money, invisibly disabling diseases such as fibromyalgia will be brought to the foreground of public consciousness for shareholder profitability. We are seeing it with millions being pumped into advertising for Lyrica. Pharmaceutical companies would capitalize on the need of physicians who for the most part don't know what to do with fibro patients. I was at a conference with internists/PCP physicians where, in conversation, several docs said that if prescription medicine was not available, medical doctors would be out of business because they would have no idea what to do to help people. I guess I never thought of MDs that way before.

Pharmaceutical companies work hard to prove to the FDA that there is a therapeutic value to their products and, in spite of the side effects and inconsistent benefits, voilà, these drugs makes it to market. This has already happened with Cymbalta, Lyrica, and Savella, to name a few. They are palliative medications at best. They help to manage or reduce symptoms—and I'm not saying that this is bad thing—but they offer no hope of changing the outcome of fibromyalgia. We'll talk more about these medications in later chapters.

Republican or Democrat?

Controversy over whether or not to vaccinate our children is a never-ending debate. While there is much to discuss about vaccinations, my concern in this writing is how vaccinations affect fibromyalgia. Considering the vulnerability of the developing child's brain, it's scientifically valid to judge that additional exposure to toxic substances challenge the immune system, disturb brain growth and neurological connections, and subsequently encourage and set the stage for fibromyalgia to be triggered. If a person is already genetically predisposed to fibromyalgia, this becomes more of a concern. With the current vaccination schedule of our children, receiving multiple injections before they even leave the hospital, many antigens and significant amounts of toxins are injected into newborns' bloodstreams. This regimen continues for up to five years. Chemicals and heavy metals that we all know to be toxic are used in vaccine preparations. It amazes me how many pediatricians advocate vaccines at birth, and in the same breath point out that babies are not ready to eat cereal until they are six months old due to an immature digestive system. I get it; the digestive system just hasn't matured to handle cereals well yet. It seems it would make sense to apply that same protective principle to vaccinations; babies' physiology and immune system, in particular the brain and central nervous system development, are every bit as immature. The differences, in my mind, are embarrassing. We humans respond to observable "cause and effect" phenomena. What I mean is that the closer the observable effect is to a cause, the easier it is and clearer it is for our judgment to correlate the two with conviction.

Vaccines vs. Cereal

Vaccines vs. cereal is a case in point. Administering vaccines that may undermine and challenge brain and immune integrity involves an insidious, silent, and painless process, taking its toll over decades. Cause-and-effect consciousness doesn't exist in a time frame that correlates with human "cause and effect" barometers. However, it eventually may express itself as neurological problems such as fibromyalgia, reflex sympathetic dystrophy, MS, etc., at a time frame far removed from the "shot." There is also immune stress from vaccines at a vulnerable time in childhood development. Subsequently maturing to adulthood, childhood immune weakening may reveal itself as rheumatoid arthritis, lupus, or general multisystem breakdown as seen in Gulf War syndrome, chronic fatigue syndrome, and fibromyalgia. Sadly, because of the protraction of time between cause and effect, the correlation between what we expose our newborns to and conditions we suffer from in later life is hardly even questioned. Cereal, on the other hand, has a cause and effect that is very real to us—it's "now." The cause and effect is immediate and messy. We have a much easier time emotionally and intellectually accepting and reacting to a baby's sensitivity to cereal and the mess on our shoulder. I won't get into any of the specific chemicals such as mercury and aluminum or other contaminants in vaccinations in this chapter.

Gulf War Syndrome

There have been various associations described between vaccinations and multisystem breakdown conditions such as fibromyalgia, chronic fatigue, and Gulf War syndrome. Gulf War syndrome is characterized by chronic fatigue, malaise, brain fog, depression, difficulty sleeping, digestive problems, multiple chemical sensitivities, and general musculoskeletal aches and pains, very much like what we see with fibromyalgia. Out of respect and to add perspective, Gulf War syndrome can be considered synonymous with post-traumatic stress disorder that we've seen in other deployments—such as World War II, Bosnia, and Iraq, among others. In any event, the pattern and relationship of vaccinations and the subsequent physical and emotional trauma helps to tie these concepts together. In the case of vaccinations, there are several theories that propose vaccinations at the very least being co-triggers for the development of multi-system disorders.

Cytokines

We will be discussing cytokines in more depth soon. Suffice it to say here that cytokines are communication proteins in our bodies. Cytokines turn on, turn off, increase, and decrease pain and inflammatory responses. Frequently we speak of cytokines in reference to local neurological synaptic responses. However, cytokines are ubiquitous and work in unison, managing our immune system and just about every defensive and protective response of the body. But this doesn't mean the system is perfect. Wallace (1999 to 2001), reports that cytokines have been shown to cause a reduction in a person's pain threshold as well as possibly being responsible for brain fog and sleep disorders, leading to fatigue. He also found specific abnormalities directly related to fibromyalgia. So cytokines are involved in defense, repair, and communication processes. Dr. Alan Leon Chaitow reports that Monro (2001) found that the normal cycles of cytokines are capable of being disrupted by multiple vaccinations, as discussed above.

German Measles

German measles, aka rubella, is a virus named after a German physician. There are reports (Leon, Alan, 1988) of the rubella immunization having significantly elevated antibodies in patients against rubella in fibromyalgia patients. This in itself is not so surprising. But, Alan further noted that a new rubella vaccine in 1979 caused an upsurge of reported cases of chronic fatigue and fibromyalgia.

This section is not meant to be a comprehensive dissertation on, nor a vote for or against immunization. Rather, it is intended to bring to light additional hypotheses. Vaccinations inherently are meant to challenge the nervous system and the immune system for a greater good. The challenge to the immune system helps to put into perspective another avenue of understanding how fibromyalgia can be triggered or develop over time. Also it raises the question as to how much consideration we should give to further immunizations as adults, and what the impact of shots for flu, whooping cough, shingles, and influenza has on us unknowingly. What is the greater gamble health wise, to get them or not? Once again, these are questions to pose to your health team. To be fair and consistent, let's remember your doctors' and health team's advice means medical as well as non-medical practitioners. Then you can make a more balanced/informed decision for yourself and your children. Depending on medical advice alone means you will not have a balanced perspective.

Vaccine Alternatives

Frequently the question will come up as to whether there are alternatives to vaccination. Living as healthy a life as possible, and developing a strong immune system naturally, would begin with long-term breast-feeding. This subject in itself is huge and daunting, but only to those who find reasons to not breast-feed. Overwhelming evidence and opinion by the medical and non-medical community agree that breast-feeding is immunologically, physiologically, and emotionally superior. That's not to say that in and of itself breast-feeding is "the vaccine alternative," but simply that it should be a starting point for consideration. The question of whether to breast-feed, is of course, personal, and all considerations should be given appropriate weight.

Vaccinate by State

I found an interesting resource: National Vaccine Information Center (NVIC).

NVIC details each state's exemption criteria in regard to vaccination. The center outlines the reasons why someone may not have to vaccinate a child. Vaccination requirements are most likely to come into play for children and their families when they first attempt to enter school (daycare, public education, or private education). Each state has established its own vaccination requirements and allowances. Vaccination exemptions appear to fall into three categories: medical exemptions, philosophical exemptions, and religious exemptions. For further information, refer to the National Vaccine Information Center.

Introduction to Inflammation

There's no shortage of hypotheses and opinions as to the cause of fibromyalgia, triggers leading up to a fibromyalgia diagnosis, and/or the perpetuating factors. For research purposes, it's all interesting. For practical purposes, it would seem that the perpetuating factors are all that matter right now if a person has already been diagnosed. We do find, however, that very often the trigger or the triggers bringing fibromyalgia to clinical expression are the same factors that perpetuate the condition. Genetics, of course, would apply, and stress in its various forms: physical, chemical, and emotional. And then there are allergies, infections, inflammatory conditions, obesity, and malnutrition as well as peripheral and central neurological sensitization. Certainly discerning one or more of these components that make up the present clinical picture would be resourceful.

Inflammation is part of the immune system's protective vigilance, attempting to manage anything that threatens the body's ability to maintain homeostasis. Our first thoughts or indication of inflammation is usually redness, heat, or soreness around the area that is insulted in some way. However, inflammation exists throughout the body 24/7 without our conscious awareness, managing all kinds of toxins, imbalances, and insults that are simply a result of the physiology of life. Whether acute or chronic, observed, suspected, or simply covert, management of inflammation calls for changes in the vascular system to deliver plasma and white blood cells to the area. Chemical mediators/neurotransmitters are delivered to heighten cellular awareness and sensitivity as well as communicating with all other functions of the body, especially keeping the brain in constant neurological awareness and control.

Understanding inflammation is one of the keys to begin putting into perspective how we can reduce the burden that a fibromyalgia patient is under when dealing with everyday stressors. By reducing inflammation, we can support the immune system and other bodily defenses to fight the all-important neurological toxicity issues that plague fibromyalgia sufferers.

When inflammation exists systemically, it tends to linger just below the radar. Over time it can raise havoc and cause breakdown of cells, tissues, and organs. Inflammation can show up as psoriasis or eczema; or bowel problems such as Crohn's disease or colitis. Alzheimer's, multiple sclerosis, heart disease, Parkinson's, and chronic pain due to central sensitivity syndrome have been linked to chronic central nervous system inflammation. We also see the effects of inflammation demonstrated in rheumatoid arthritis, allergies, arthrosclerosis, diabetes, and cancer.

To control inflammation and prevent it from becoming chronic, we want to first look at diet, lifestyle, nutrition, and everyday emotional stress. When chronic or systemic inflammation is suspected, lab tests can be done to evaluate the level of inflammation. A common lab test that will demonstrate inflammation in the body is called C-reactive protein (CRP). This is a chemical produced by the liver that elevates in any condition that threatens health. It's stimulated to be produced by the release of inflammatory chemicals in an area that's been injured or is being attacked by toxins or bacteria. The liver can also be triggered to produce CRP from emotional stress.

Hopefully we'll help you to gain a perspective on inflammation and not have to wait until lab tests have to be conducted. We can be relatively assured that most people have lifestyles that cause their bodies to generate more inflammation than is healthy. You'll see the term pro-inflammatory, referring to the state of body chemistry encouraging inflammation more than it should. The term pro-inflammatory can also be used to define a substance's or activity's impact on the body. Examples are sugar, carbohydrates, and bad fats in our diet. Emotional stress is pro-inflammatory as well.

Inflammation
Every moment, the body is trying to process waste products and toxins and deal with invasive and threatening organisms, as well as preventing illness. However, when things get out of hand, inflammation itself becomes a problem. Approximately 90 percent of all the cells in the body are not even human cells. They are cells that we live with—hopefully synergistically—cells such as bacteria that we have in our digestive system to break down food. Some of them actually produce vitamins and nutrients that we depend on. Others are foreign and destructive, having their own agenda contrary to ours. Regardless of whether we categorize cells as friend or foe, there are toxic byproducts/consequences that the body's physiology must deal with.

Many companies have created anti-inflammatory products that include herbs, different vitamins and minerals, and antioxidants to combat toxins and reduce inflammation. Some of the herbs that are useful in fighting inflammation are turmeric, bioflavonoids, plant enzymes, boswellia, and botanicals such as Chinese skullcap, ginger, devil's claw, and cat's claw.

There are plant enzymes such as pineapple enzymes, bromelain, papaya enzymes, and papain, as well as some animal enzymes such as trypsin and chymotrypsin. These plant and animal enzymes have been found to be very effective for sports injuries, arthritis, and chronic inflammation such as arthritic conditions, strains, sprains, and even cancer treatment. Many studies have been done with bromelain, which has not only been found to be safe and effective but more potent than many current available drugs to reduce inflammation.

Diet

The body's main tool in controlling inflammation is diet. There are foods that can cause inflammation and there are foods that can reduce inflammation. Diet (how we eat) tends to be overlooked by most people as a therapeutic/health necessity. Rather, diet is dismissed as old news relating primarily to how we look and what size belt we wear.

We are very aware of preservatives and chemicals in manufactured and manipulated foods as being toxic and pro-inflammatory. The worst and most common offenders are manipulated/bad fats and carbohydrates.

We find that many substances and their detrimental effect relate to their ability to cause the body to become more acidic. When the body is too acidic, it becomes more pro-inflammatory. Foods such as red meat, soybeans, and sugar create acidic body chemistry. On the other end of the spectrum we have green leafy vegetables, sweet potatoes, and asparagus to help to alkalize the body and combat an inflammatory lifestyle.

Toxins

Toxins are a recurrent theme in this writing. I don't think we can hear often enough that practices like smoking or consuming preservatives, flavor enhancers, or highly acidic foods are destructive to our health and subsequently will raise CPR/inflammation and threatened disease. Retail companies that produce products with substances to hook us on flavors and convenience will spend millions of dollars day after day to appeal to our senses. They not only make us comfortable with consuming these products, but convince us that we are smart to consume them and that we're healthier for it. Because they convince us of that, we're actually willing to pay more money for their products than for something natural. Consider salad dressing: You can spend $2.00 - $6.00 on a bottle of salad dressing full of chemicals and mostly bad fats, but you could probably make it yourself for $.75 to $1.50 with zero chemicals and good fats--and it will taste every bit as good, if not better.

Special Diets

There are thousands of diets and recommended eating strategies. They all seem to work for some people, but don't work for all people.

They tend not to do the job our physiology/chemistry needs, or they lack the emotional and lifestyle balance that allows long enough participation to succeed. I've noticed one diet that has a high potential of meeting a productive balance between body chemistry, emotional/ social balance, and lifestyle factors: namely, a Mediterranean diet. A Mediterranean diet has been shown to reduce CPR by 20 percent when practiced regularly. It is relatively higher in the consumption of cold-water fatty fish, olive oil, and red wine, all of which have been shown to decrease inflammation. Examples of cold-water fish are salmon and sardines. And, as aforementioned, reducing inflammation and CRP will help to reduce and control cardiovascular disease, rheumatoid arthritis, inflammation, inflammatory bowel conditions, fibromyalgia, components of chronic fatigue syndrome, and even inflammation due to myofascial trigger points.

In our clinic, due to the difficulty of always getting fresh fish in large enough quantities, we supplement patients' diets with essential fatty acid complexes. Interestingly enough, when compared to buying fresh cold-water wild-caught fish, supplementation of marine oils to increase Omega-3s is little to no more expensive, and tends to be more convenient. Further, considering that the rest of the average person's diet is still too high in pro-inflammatory foods, it's easier to try to combat it by adding Omega-3 oils than it is to give up a favorite cereal or sandwich. I'm not saying that supplementation is better than eating natural foods; I think with this issue as well as many other discussions in this book, a level of practicality is resourceful. It's a rare person who's going to be a purist about any diet or take the time to delve into the chemistry of foods enough to manage everything on his own. (As a disclaimer, I would have to admit that ethnic background and the region in which someone lives will play a role in the effectiveness of any eating strategy. So although I've mentioned the Mediterranean diet, by no means is it the diet for everyone; it is mentioned only to provoke further investigation.)

We would all be wise to adapt an anti-inflammatory and natural eating strategy. Taking time to learn and adjust your lifestyle is okay, but time marches on, as will inflammation, undermining health and brain function. Many people wait until there is a health crisis/obvious threat to life before seriously working at it. Fibros are already in crisis, so they need to be serious and work at it right now. Fibros can't afford cellular energy depletion or destruction of brain neurons and glial cells, so don't be confused or reject the recommendation due to reading that fibromyalgia is not considered an inflammatory condition. I don't know of a fibro case that doesn't have coexisting conditions with inflammatory components. Eat wisely and continue to do better.

As Dr. Russell Jaffe puts it, "Absence of evidence is not evidence of absence." Assume exposure, even if something feels good. Toxins are stored primarily in fat, muscles, and bones. When understanding that lifestyle and environmental toxins contribute to neuromuscular and skeletal destruction, it becomes imperative to reduce exposures where possible and to optimize the body's defenses. Defenses are generally through nutrition (diet and supplementation) and functional adaptation.

CHAPTER 13

Surprise Toxins

Chapter Topics:
> *Sugar and Tobacco*
> *Artificial Sweeteners*
> *Gluten Toxicity*
> *Alcohol*
> *Body Fat*
> *Weather Changes*

Sugar and Tobacco

A colleague of mine reviewed this manuscript and was surprised that I didn't cover the toxic effects of sugar and tobacco. I told him that I thought these two toxins have been proven over and over again to be health hazards. With a touch of sarcasm I have included this short paragraph. Sugar and tobacco have been written about and the dangers have been known and preached for decades. I didn't feel I could bring any new light or motivation to the subjects. I simply hope that everyone will heed the warning. Sugar—eliminate it. Tobacco/tobacco smoke—stay away. Its products and byproducts can do nothing but challenge every physiological component of your being.

High-Fructose Corn Syrup (HFCS)

HFCS is a culprit of its own. We pointed out some concerns in the last chapter. But here is the rest of the story. We have a natural attraction to sweetness. Fructose tastes very sweet. Interestingly enough, in spite of its sweetness, it does not trigger the production of insulin, thereby being a great marketing tool for diabetics and people trying to lose weight.

White table sugar is part glucose (no sweetness) and part fructose (very sweet). In 1971, the Japanese found a way to economically produce fructose from corn, and it is sweeter than sugar. Its utilization increases sweetness in foods, which creates more cravings and an increase in pleasure centers within the brain. Hence more consumption, plus it is cheaper to produce than regular sugar, yielding more profit.

HFCS is in just about any commercial food that isn't in its natural state. The important thing to understand is that HFCS is metabolized differently than sugar. Instead of being broken down for energy, it's transported to the liver almost completely intact, where it is converted to triglycerides. Triglycerides change the way insulin receptors on cell membranes act. This causes the cell to become insulin resistant. (Insulin resistance=increased inflammation, pain, and loss of energy.) The triglycerides cannot get into the cell, so they go to fat cells for storage rather than being burned to produce energy. Under some conditions these particular stored-fat calories cannot be processed out of the fat cell to be used as energy even when we need them for exercise, or when restricting calories hoping to burn fat. The more HFCS consumed, the more fat is stored and the person continues to feel hungry, eats more, and yet loses energy.

The reason that HFCS is appropriate for this chapter is that it is an unsuspected toxic chain of events causing insulin resistance, fat storage, and loss of energy—a Fibro's nightmare.

Artificial Sweeteners

Artificial sweeteners are of concern for everyone, but especially for Fibros. Artificial sweeteners carry with them confirmed toxic influences on the nervous system and blood sugar management. On the other hand, they are regularly recommended by doctors for controlling dental cavities and the management of diabetes. The FDA has rated most artificial sweeteners as GRS, meaning "generally recognized as safe." Yet all artificial sweeteners have been shown to produce serious health hazards, particularly in the way they affect neurological tissues. That means the brain, just as we discussed above. The worse offender appears to be aspartame; it's as dangerous as MSG. Artificial sweeteners are considered excitotoxins, and when consumed in a typical diet that includes MSG, the nervous system is in great danger as neurotoxins accumulate and multiply their detrimental effects.

Aspartame

Aspartame has been around since 1969 under the trade name NutraSweet. Aspartame, like other sugar substitutes, is many times sweeter than sugar and has a tendency to lose its sweetness when heated. It's created from aspartic acid and phenylalanine, which are two amino acids. Some people are hypersensitive to phenylalanine and have the disorder phenylketonuria (PKU). When the levels of phenylalanine get too high, a person with this condition may suffer brain damage and mental retardation. It's so important that newborns in the United States are screened for PKU. People with this condition need to have a low-protein diet. For this reason, products that have phenylalanine are required by the FDA to be labeled as such. Other research has shown that aspartame can affect other amino acids and neurotransmitters negatively in the brain, influencing serotonin levels. These toxic effects were reported in *The Journal of Pharmacology and Toxicity* in 1991. The last thing that a fibromyalgia patient needs is to challenge neurotransmitters and consume anything that would be considered an additional stimulant/irritant to already overly stimulated pain nerves.

Some foods are clearly labeled as having aspartame additives. Other times you'll see it as NutraSweet. Keep in mind the power of lobbyists, political pressures, and questionable decisions by the FDA. After 1969 studies showed aspartame created tumors in test animals, somehow it still got through and was approved by the FDA. It's scary to think that substances like aspartame and MSG are creating tumors in test animals.

When we restrict artificial sweeteners, patients report decreases in headaches and fibro fog, while memory improves. We've had reports of improved balance and fewer aches and pains. Patients report sleeping better and we've noted that restless legs improve if not resolve.

There have been many conditions and reactions reported to the FDA. Most all of them revolve around how aspartame affects brain cells, causing conditions such as fatigue, depression, insomnia, vision problems, anxiety, slurred speech, memory problems, and loss of taste, among others. It's interesting that the FDA very carefully regulates a substance called methyl alcohol. When methyl alcohol is consumed, it is converted into formaldehyde and formic acid. When aspartame is consumed, it breaks down into methyl alcohol and formic acid. So we are effectively consuming formaldehyde. Formaldehyde is used as an embalming fluid and is clearly a carcinogen. The other component, formic acid, as Dr. Graylock has reported, is the poison that fire ants secrete, causing intense pain.

Imagine combining these substances with water, adding some flavorings, maybe some flavor enhancers (MSG) and sticking them in an aluminum can (which is toxic as well) and we have a tasty drink that could be marketed as a soft drink…go figure. Let's add that the company producing this drink has millions of dollars to spend on advertising to you and your children, making it impossible to not see, read, or hear about it every day of your life, and you can buy it for less than the cost of one apple.

These drinks are part of our culture, so common that they are taken for granted; they are bought and consumed without thinking. In the meantime, we're destroying cells. Alzheimer's and other neurological disorders such as Parkinson's, MS, and Huntington's disease are on the rise, as well as fibromyalgia/chronic pain.

Dr. Russell Blaylock, MD, in his book *Health and Nutrient Secrets That Can Save Your Life* notes that diabetics who drink large amounts of aspartame-sweetened drinks are more likely to go blind. He poses the question, "If these excitotoxins (poisons) have such strong evidence of their damaging effects, why is it that the American Diabetic Association and thousands of doctors encourage their diabetic patients to use artificial sweeteners—in particular aspartame?" The answer seems to be that one of the FDA's largest financial contributions comes from Monsanto Company, the makers of NutraSweet, aka aspartame.

Carol Simontacchi, in her book *The Crazy Makers,* reports that aspartame breaks down at 86 degrees Fahrenheit. Transportation and storage temperatures will routinely go higher than 86 degrees, so when it's a drink in a can it has already broken down before we even pop the tab, which means we are consuming straight methyl alcohol. The Aspartame Consumer Safety Network reports that the most well-known problems with methyl alcohol poisoning are vision problems, retinal damage, and blindness.

Some might say, "Well, I don't drink any soda at all, or hardly any." But aspartame is used in everything from breakfast cereals to cocoa, gelatin, chocolates, desserts, and it is even found in vitamin pills and salad dressings. The list is endless. At the end of any given day the average American could have consumed enough aspartame to encourage fibromyalgia. It can certainly increase susceptibility to blindness, degenerative diseases, and an array of central sensitization issues, sensory disturbances (idiopathic pain/fibromyalgia) and functional deficits. An article in *The Annals of Pharmacotherapy, 2002,* noted that removing aspartame from the diet for four consecutive months could eliminate chronic pain symptoms.

Saccharin
You'll see saccharin labeled as Sweet 'n' Low, or possibly Sugar Twin. It was initially felt that saccharin was linked to cancers. However

in 2000 the warning label was removed from saccharin and it seems that the FDA, The World Health Organization, and the scientific community of the European Unions as well as the US Congress are all satisfied that it's safe. While it very well may be safe by their standards in extremely small dosages, most people consume artificial sweeteners in excess of nerve cell capacity to tolerate. We advise our patients not to use saccharin. Plus I don't trust that the government's standard of safe is safe.

Sucralose

Sucralose is commonly named Splenda. There is a website that I'd like to quote-- www.FAQS.org. I thought the way they put sucralose into perspective, whether approved by the FDA or not, raises questions of compromising and trying to fool human physiology. From FAQS. org: *"Splenda is 600 times sweeter than sugar. Sucralose is not absorbed from the digestive tract, so it adds no calories to consumer food. It is made from rearranged sugar molecules that substitute three atoms of chlorine for three hydroxyl groups on the sugar molecule. Sucralose has been tested in more than 100 studies."* By the way, most of these sugar substitutes will have a similar story of engineering and altering molecular structure to fool the senses and the nervous system—in other words, the brain.

Sugar Alcohols

Sugar alcohols you would recognize by the names sorbitol, xylitol, lactitol, mannitol, isomalt, or maltitol. While these substances are generally accepted as safe, they are not technically considered artificial sweeteners. However, you'll frequently see them in sugar-free foods on the diabetic shelves of your grocery store. They do have calories, but fewer calories than sugar, and do not cause a sudden spike in blood sugar. The reason for this is that the bloodstream does not readily absorb them. Products utilizing sugar alcohols are required to carry a warning label. The warning is *"Excessive consumption may have a laxative effect."* The reason is that the digestive tract cannot fully absorb them; ultimately they act as an irritant, causing the body to want to dilute the irritant/poison, producing watery, loose stools. Further, these substances can upset the balance between good and bad bacteria in the intestines. Once the balance of the intestinal flora has been upset, it opens the door to a variety of toxic events and conditions. Not the least of concerns is that the intestinal walls may become compromised. These conditions can cause toxicity, encouraging irritable bowel syndrome (IBS) and causing leakage of toxins out of the intestines and back into the system due to intestinal wall permeability (leaking gut syndrome). Actually, leaky gut syndrome is not a bona fide diagnosis that MDs learn in medical school, so there is controversy about its existence not so dissimilar to the attitude some hold about fibromyalgia. Diagnosis or no diagnosis, considering that the gut is the largest organ contributing to immune function, loss of integrity is a problem that burdens physiology.

Stevia

Stevia is the only sweetener that we recommend. Stevia comes from a South American shrub called the yerba dulce. And while the FDA does not presently regard it as safe, and The World Health Organization has determined that the data is insufficient to label it as a sweetener, our research tells us that it is the safest sweetener when used in moderation. It's natural and it hasn't been molecularly altered. There have been studies by the FDA with animals suggesting that it could reduce sperm count and possibly cause infertility in rodents. On the other hand, there are studies showing that in humans there are health benefits, such as lowering blood pressure, helping to control blood sugar, increasing energy, and reducing cravings for alcohol and tobacco. It may also contribute to reducing bacterial count in the mouth.

The stevia shrub is in the sunflower family and brings with it some political and economic implications. The United States banned stevia in the early '90s and allowed it to be labeled only as a dietary supplement. The United States in 2008 approved Rebaudioside, meaning "sweet leaf," which is the sweet leaf of the Stevia plant.

Stevia, as with all sweeteners, has a little bit of a different taste. You may need some adaptive time to enjoy it. When you're used to sugar, any change may taste strange or bitter until your palate adjusts. Stevia is no different. It's sensitive to heat, so if you put it into a beverage that's hot, you could use quite a bit of Stevia and get surprisingly low sweetness. As the beverage cools the sweetness intensifies. Our advice is to experiment, and if you must use sweetener, use the least amount possible.

Having reviewed sugar substitutes, we hope that you'll put them into perspective and generally accept that they're all a bad idea for fibromyalgia patients, if not for all people. Stevia is the least offensive and the least toxic. However, to reduce toxicity, improve metabolism, and improve neurologic function, as well as reduce cravings for sweeteners in the first place, "lose the sweet tooth." See nutritional advice, below.

Miscellaneous Toxic Sugar Substitutes

I'm including different sugar substitutes only to give you conviction and perspective when someone tries to sell you a product explaining that the "special" sugar substitute that they use is safe and has all kinds of benefits as opposed to using another substitute or good old-fashioned sugar, honey, maple syrup, molasses, etc.

Maltodextrin

Maltodextrin is usually highly processed from a starch. In the United States it is derived mostly from GMO corn; in Europe, from wheat. The majority of the proteins in the wheat have been removed, so there is a tendency to look at maltodextrin as gluten-free. It would, however, be wise not to rely on the safety of any product that claims to have had all the gluten removed. Refined from corn or potato starch, maltodextrin in recent years has been used in sports drinks as well as meal replacement bars. It's said to have a beneficial effect on muscle recovery for athletes. It also has been known to improve taste and texture, help to provide someone with a fuller feeling, reduce blood sugar swings, and reduce cravings. Anyway, that is what many of the reports profess. We believe it should be considered a sugar and should not be considered a sugar substitute. Whether it's considered a sugar or non-sugar, it should be avoided.

Federal Drug Administration (FDA)

Most of us look for food substances to have the FDA stamp of approval on them, giving us a sense of security, quality and safety. I'm afraid that may not be a valid assumption. An article in *The Star Tribune* of Minneapolis, MN, by Jim Spencer, March 7, 2012, had the headline "FDA Survey Uncovers Concern over Influence." The FDA is politically motivated, generally overburdened and carries with it all the human frailties and possibility of errors that any other organization or government body would have. FDA approval should not be ignored, but it might not tell the full story.

Spin and Deceit

There are millions of dollars spent each day to study and understand the psychology of communication and how words and concepts can be used to influence, guide, and direct our attention and often fool, deceive, and mislead us into consuming products that will kill us (slowly). In a great article written by Mike Adams, we see how he extracted information from grocery warnings about artificial sweeteners. He noticed that Monsanto, the original creator of NutraSweet (also sold under the name of Equal and Spoonful) has their own so-called spin doctors. Their spokesman, a man by the name of Farrell, described NutraSweet as an artificial sweetener. He said that the term "artificial" was distasteful because to many people it conjured up ideas of cancer, headaches, rat laboratory studies, allergies, and epilepsy. Consequently, the description "artificial" was not very appetizing. So from that point on they decided to call it a sugar "substitute." They then found that psychologically people didn't like that either because they didn't want something to sound like it replaced the beloved sugar they grew up with. Apparently Farrell said, "Memories of sugar take them back to their childhood, a simpler time when there was less to worry about, and sugar was a sweet treat. Our own words were defining our product and words that created thoughts being unnatural, unsafe, un-sweet were negative." The name NutraSweet hit the mark, suggesting that something nutritional and sweet was better than the most beloved product in history. So after studying human psychology, Monsanto found that the most appealing words were NutraSweet.

Psychologists have found that Americans love and admire discoveries and innovations gained through hard work and that words such as substitute, artificial, chemical, laboratory, and scientific were removed from any advertising or labeling of aspartame and replaced by words that were appealing to the public such as discovered, choice, variety, unique, different, and new taste. They knew exactly how to appeal to us when our busy lives don't allow us the time to think about every purchase and every ingredient in the foods we buy. Unless we have unlimited time and an abiding desire to pick all the labels apart and understand them, our safest choice is simply to eliminate foods from our diet that are processed, manufactured, bagged, boxed, prepared, or tampered with in any way. Remember, artificial sweeteners/ sugar replacements are considered "excitotoxins." As we stated earlier, excitotoxins, aspartame, and most artificial sweeteners fool/sneak by the blood-brain barrier as a neurotransmitter and then sabotage cells and nerves inside the brain. They overwhelm and cause poisoning by free radicals in the brain—your brain. As a fibromyalgia sufferer, you can't afford to lose any more brain cells.

Weight Loss

It has been documented through the Centers for Disease Control that using artificial sweeteners has been found to help people gain weight rather than lose weight. Because of this, the FDA has changed its mind and no longer allows manufacturers to label drinks and foods as weight-loss products. They can however still say that a product is a diet drink or a diet food.

Nutritional Advice

I believe that the first piece of advice we've already exhausted: avoid—better yet, eliminate—MSG and sugar substitutes. However, there are many other neurotoxins we should stay away from as well: processed, preserved, engineered, and pre-prepared foods. And don't forget the consumption of chemicals orally (dental products), through the skin (cosmetics and cleaning products); and through the air (cleaning products and environmental pollutants). Choose these products wisely. We have focused on MSG and sugar substitutes simply because they seem to be the most common unsuspected dietary faults, along with the abuse of glutens and sugar.

We find that while people are adjusting to a healthier lifestyle, eliminating toxins and modifying their behavior to control blood sugar, supplementation is helpful. In a perfect world, it's best to get all our nutrients from whole, fresh foods. There are live foods rich in vitamins, minerals, and enzymes. However, at least in the early stages, supplementation will help. There are high-quality proprietary formulations to accomplish this. Remember that all supplements are not created equal, and you get what you pay for. Two of our favorite companies to work with are Moss Nutrition from Hadley, Massachusetts, vand nutraMetrix/Isotonix from Enfield, Connecticut. nutraMetrix/Isotonic formulations have a unique delivery system, assuring optimal absorption. They add their flagship product, POC-3, to many of their formulas specifically for its antioxidant qualities in managing toxicities, helping to reduce pain while increasing energy. Additionally, supplementing with fish oil will help manage blood sugar and serve to limit the effect of toxins and repair cellular damage. See our appendix for contact information.

I don't believe it is wise to eliminate all carbohydrates. However, unless you have special needs, you can get all the carbs you need from vegetables and fruit. I've tried to ease into the idea that even complex carbs, especially grains, can have serious insulin/body chemistry drawbacks. Fruits have been reasonably acceptable carbohydrates, but recently have come into question due to having been manipulated genetically for more sweetness, higher production, shelf life, and visual appeal, so go easy on them. Fruit juice is a simple carb. Even if you juice it yourself, it will still lack fiber. You'll be better off eating the whole fruit. Eating quality proteins, and eating four or five regularly planned mini-meals throughout the day, are recommended. I'm frequently asked about portion size. An example of how to judge proportions and the type of feeding that works best would be a fresh raw vegetable salad—include some avocado with a variety of greens, and four to six ounces of a lean protein—preferably organic protein such as free-range chicken, beef, eggs, seeds, nuts, or wild fish. The visual proportions and allocations, when putting together a feeding, might look like the drawing below. A homemade dressing of cold-pressed virgin olive oil and freshly-squeezed lemon or unfiltered organic cider vinegar is recommended. This food combination has a balance of vitamins, minerals, enzymes, live foods, lean proteins, quality essential fatty acids, and antioxidants, and it strikes a healthy balance between acid and alkaline foods. This visual also strikes a good balance between alkaline-forming foods and acidic-forming foods. At any given meal, if we remember that our diet is best to follow the 60/40 rule; about 60 percent alkaline and 40 percent acid, then we will want to try to at least mimic that with a meal. Sources will differ on their recommendation of alkaline/acid-forming foods. There is a range that's healthy, depending on the person. However, keep in mind that good fats, while being relative acid producers, have anti-inflammatory advantages that net a systemic advantage. Therefore there is no need for most people to shy away from consuming them. Plus they add taste and satisfy the hypothalamus, reducing the urge to eat carbohydrates.

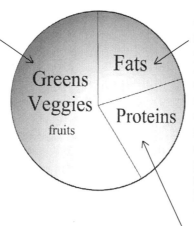

Allocate about 100grams/day of carbohydrate from vegetables to maintain weight. Go easy on the starchy ones as well as fruit. No corn or soy.

Allocation: about 10 grams/day from fish oil, coconut and olive. Raw nuts; macadamia, and walnuts also hemp and chia seeds as well as avocados. Note: no other fats are wise except from healthy protein sources, see Eveyln Tribole M.S.R.D's book; *The Ultimate O-3 Diet*

Protein allocation: 50% of body weight in grams/day.

Gluten Toxicity or "The Staff of Life"

It's doubtful that the biblical staff of life exists any longer. In the 1960s and '70s, genetic engineering transformed wheat and other grains into poorly nutritional but more profitable products. Engineered grains have challenged physiology and general health. The culprit appears to be glutens. Gluten is a generic term in that all grains have glutens that are made up of subsets of proteins. Different grains have different proteins in different concentrations. One type of protein in wheat gluten is called gliadin, which makes up about 69 percent of the total protein in wheat. It is the most-studied protein, as it appears to be the major culprit in celiac disease. Celiac patients are classically defined by and warned of sensitivity to wheat, rye, oats, and barley. However, all grains have glutens. So, depending on the person, there can also be sensitivity to corn, millet, rice, etc., as they have irritating proteins within the gluten other than gliadin. This is a cautionary lesson in that if a person has celiac, gluten allergies, or is generally intolerant, he or she may still have trouble with all types of grains, even if the product is labeled "gluten-free." Before we go any further, let's pin down definitions for gluten allergy, gluten intolerance, and gluten sensitivity, and how this applies to Fibros who don't have Celiac.

Gluten Allergy: This is when the body sees a substance (in this context glutens) as a threat or foreign and mounts an autoimmune response to eliminate it and protect the body, hence causing an allergic reaction.

Gluten Intolerance: This is when the body just doesn't like it or has a difficult time digesting it, and in general the person simply doesn't like the way she feels after consuming it.

Gluten Sensitivity: This category is seen as the causative condition of celiac disease; in other words, celiac is a manifestation of gluten sensitivity. Gluten sensitivity in itself is not a disease; rather, it's the state of being or a genetic condition and is systemically/physiologically detrimental.

My advice is to stay away from all grains if:

- You've been diagnosed with or suspect any of the above.
- You notice symptoms such as digestive disturbance, bloating, brain fog, fatigue—generally any of the symptoms that are common to fibromyalgia or chronic fatigue syndrome. This probably includes 99 percent of our readers.
- You have been diagnosed with any gut disease or digestive problem and need time to heal. As mentioned above, don't

trust labels or any grain to be safe until you're healed and feel confident in reintroducing one grain at a time. (Don't start with wheat.)

Dr. William Davis, author of *Wheat Belly*, notes that gliadins are degraded in the intestinal tract. They break down into exorphins that absorb/leak into the system and are capable of crossing the blood/brain barrier and binding to opiate receptors in the brain. This may induce changes in appetite, possibly accounting for hundreds of calories more than normal to be consumed each day, adding to the challenge of managing blood sugar—which, as we know, is of prime importance to the management of pain and energy.

Dr. Davis also notes that the covert consequence of children eating genetically altered grains can be recognized in behavioral changes such as ADHD and autism, social detachment, schizophrenia, and bipolar disorder. More directly related to fibromyalgia, if you recall, opiate receptors must be available for natural endorphins and other neurotransmitters to be innately effective in managing pain. Eating grains, particularly for someone with sensitivities, keeps the nerve circuits clogged and disallows the brain's ability to manage pain innately. This means exaggeration and perpetuation of pain signals.

The bottom line for Fibros and chronic pain and fatigue sufferers is to consider grains categorically toxic until proven otherwise. There are lab tests to determine sensitivities/allergies; however, there is a high percentage of false negatives and benign positives. It is prudent to run the tests, but regardless of the results, we recommend initially stopping all grains, allowing the body time to detox and begin to heal. This is particularly revealing when a person at any age has no medical problems that account for symptoms as noted above. Most people will be happy with the results and the way they feel within 30 days; however, stretching it to at least 90 days is best. Then a choice can be made to continue a grain-free lifestyle or selectively introduce one grain at a time and judge tolerance of it.

Alcohol

Here is just a quick comment about alcohol consumption. As of this writing the medical community has jumped on the bandwagon, touting that a glass or two of red wine has beneficial effects, claiming that it can actually decrease stress and decrease inflammation. Assuming that a person has no other conditions or sensitivities that need to be dealt with, or weaknesses that would cause overindulgence,

I would agree with the two-glass-of-wine limit. Note that not all alcohol is okay, only wine, primarily red wine. However, don't think that you are getting enough resveratrol and flavonoids or anti-aging phenols in a couple of glasses of wine to make a real difference in the antioxidant department. The primary value is the relaxing and social aspects of sipping the wine. Alcohol in general is considered a detriment to the nervous system and inspires chronic pain and inflammation—not a good idea for Fibros. Further, for you men out there, alcohol is a testosterone downer. A person who is controlling weight, improving diet, and basically trying to live an anti-inflammatory life will be able to take more liberties socially and get away with it. But the bottom line for fibromyalgia sufferers is to stick to a one-glass-of wine rule. For those who see the wisdom in supplementing their wine diet, I recommend an Oligomeric Proantho-Cyanidin formulation by nutraMetrix-(OPC-3). See appendix.

Usually the first feedback I get from patients beginning OPC-3 is that within 48 hours they feel more energy. Yet they are calm, not rattled from energy like coffee.

Body Fat
The more body fat a person has, the higher the C-Reactive Protein (CRP) seems to be. The location of body fat will be a factor as well. For instance, having abdominal and visceral fat (fat around the organs) tends to create more inflammation than fat storage in other areas of the body. This is why television personality Dr. Oz harps on about reducing belly fat—to reduce inflammation and lower the risk of degenerative diseases, cancer, arthritis, and neurological disorders as well as heart disease. Notice he says "neurological disorders"; that's fibromyalgia.

So how can you know if abdominal fat is at an unhealthy point for you? One of the most common ways is Body Mass Index measurement (BMI). BMI relates a person's height-to- weight ratio. However, a more valuable measurement is a ratio of *waist to height*. This ratio will help to assess lifestyle risk of developing inflammatory diseases and in general quickly put into perspective your general health. The measurement is simple: measure your height in inches and divided by your waist measurement in inches. A healthy result would be a waistline approximately 50 percent of horizontal height. As an example, a 6-foot individual (72 inches) should have no more than a 36-inch waist. Don't be too disappointed when you make this calculation; use it as a motivator. I had always thought I was doing pretty well staying in shape, but after the first time I made this calculation, I got back on the treadmill.[45, 10.]

Interestingly enough, the body actually has built-in mechanisms to control inflammation. But for most of us, lifestyle, diet, and stress levels override the built-in mechanisms. A by-product of exercise physiology is that we produce waste products, toxins, and inflammation. At the same time, muscles have the ability to produce chemicals called cytokines that help to manage the waste products and inflammation produced. Cytokines, along with stimulating endorphins during exercise, is part of the reason why exercise is at least transiently beneficial to Fibros. One of the reasons the upswing in spirit, energy, and comfort does not last, however, is due to other toxins circulating that are not managed as well. However, there is a way to gain ground and over time increase exercise and lengthen the phase of improvement.

An exciting study came out in Pub-Med in February 2014. The study showed for the first time that systemic inflammation could be reduced in adults with Type II diabetes by participating in progressive resistance exercises (lifting weights). Everyone could benefit in the same way. Why wait until hypoglycemia or diabetes has been diagnosed? By increasing skeletal muscle mass there was a reduction in CRP as the ratio between fat/muscle shifted. Cellular energy (ATP) will increase as well, supporting all the goals of a fibro recovery effort. Therefore, to optimize an anti-inflammatory lifestyle and increase energy, lifting weights should be incorporated along with an improved dietary plan.

Generally, I think you would be safe to cross train, meaning participating in resistance as well as aerobic exercise, mild to moderate, on a regular basis—and at the same time varying the activities within those two categories. For instance, vary aerobic exercise by doing some walking, rowing, swimming, or get on an elliptical machine. With resistance exercises, you may want to start off with a program of circuit machines or resistance bands and eventually graduate to free weights. But, as the study reported above, resistance exercise should be progressive. This means lifting the same 10-pound weight over and over, week after week, won't work. Try to lift a weight that allows you to complete only about eight repetitions. Consult your doctor first and begin by working with a trainer to learn proper form and warm-ups. We will go over more exercise strategies in Chapter 21.

Weather Changes

Most patients will report that changes in the weather cause fibromyalgia symptoms to flare up. Whether it be fatigue, headaches and muscle pain, or poor sleep, the physical, energetic and emotional symptoms become more obvious. In spite of the fact that classic fibromyalgia is not recognized as an inflammatory disease, most patients react almost exactly as a patient would with an inflammatory disease such as arthritis. So if you react this way, you're not wacky. It turns out that all fluid bodies respond to changes in barometric pressure. Ask any sailor how barometric pressure affects tides. Considering that our bodies are made up of about 70 percent fluid, we can expect that barometric pressure changes will force the fluids in our body to adjust. When they adjust, we will know it.

To put this concept into perspective, imagine a balloon or an empty plastic bottle. Its shape in large part is dictated by having an equal amount of pressure on the outside and the inside. If the barometric pressure goes up, there would be more pressure on the outside, putting pressure on the walls, collapsing the plastic bottle and shrinking the balloon. If the barometric pressure goes down as a storm front moves into the area, the pressure inside pushes the sides outward and the plastic bottle and balloon expands. Any area of the body (most notably joints or muscles) that has extra fluid/inflammation is already challenged and has your attention. With the increased pressure from the inside out as the barometric pressure goes down, muscles and joints will become more achy/painful. Keep in mind that this scenario is not isolated to those with a defined inflammatory disease. It can simply be an area of neurological hypersensitivity, as in fibromyalgia, hence flare-up symptoms.

Let's assume for a minute that you don't have arthritis, injuries, or infections; you have fibromyalgia. Might there be other factors complicating your fibromyalgia, in turn allowing the barometer/weather changes to affect you so radically? One of the most common reasons has to do with toxicity and fluid retention. The most common cause of general fluid retention is sensitivity to foods such as gluten. A great experiment would be to restrict sweets, starches, and, in particular, gluten (primarily wheat as discussed above) from your diet. Continue for 90 days; then pray for a rainstorm to come into the area so you can test out the theory. My guess is that you'll feel better and possibly lose a little weight while you wait for that rainstorm. As the storm approaches, you can decide whether your fibromyalgia is reacting to barometric pressure or the barometric pressure is being blamed for an overly toxic lifestyle.

Be patient with yourself when changing lifestyle and mindset. The changes you make will benefit you and your family for a lifetime. Plan at least a three-month process of reading labels and considering alternatives: autopilot won't do. Transitioning home supplies, shopping habits, and the family's taste buds will take some creativity. Eating out and social events will require consciousness to make better choices. Plan, plan, plan; prepare, prepare, prepare.

CHAPTER 14

Genetics, Family and You

Chapter Topics:

Genetics	*Dopamine*
Alcohol	*Family*
Serotonin	*Children*
Catecholamines	

Genetics: Is Fibromyalgia Contagious?

The short answer is yes, fibromyalgia is contagious; however, it's not contagious like you catch a cold or virus. Fibro is contagious in the genetic sense as an inheritance. There are no physicians or therapists who work with fibromyalgia patients who would disagree as to whether there is a genetic or familial relationship to how or why a person might have fibromyalgia. The theory is that fibromyalgia is passed along due to a genetic mutation that takes place in a person's chromosomes due to damaged DNA.

Some people might ask: "If I have my mother's habits, attitudes, behaviors and posture; couldn't my aches and pains and poor energy be learned somehow?" This seems like a logical question, and I guess in some ways it's true. The key understanding is that learned behaviors are known to trigger expressions of a genetic predisposition to a disease; however, only infrequently are they considered to be the cause. Diabetes, heart disease, obesity, fibromyalgia, and many other conditions may just be hibernating; encoded in our genes, waiting to express themselves if challenged by unhealthy behavior, disease, or injury.

There are many behavioral and environmental factors to be considered. We won't discuss all of them in this section. However, I thought I would include one of the most common practices in our society proven to affect gene expression—namely, alcohol. With this discussion, you will gain a better understand of neurology and neurotransmitters (cellular communicators). These are crucial concepts as we go on to build a vocabulary and refine our perspective on fibromyalgia. I've purposely included it right at the beginning of this section for its practical value in everyday life. And subsequently we will delve deeper into more scientific research covering inheritance and genetic predisposition. In this section we will also cover how you might've "caught" fibromyalgia and what blood tests will tell us.

Alcohol Exposure

Alcohol is a common contributor to triggering fibromyalgia when genetic predisposition exists. The developing fetal brain is very sensitive to alcohol. National surveys show that about six out of every ten women of childbearing age (18 to 44 years old) use alcohol. Slightly less than one-third of the women in this age group who drink alcohol are binge drinkers. The Centers for Disease Control and Prevention reports that 7.2 percent of pregnant women use alcohol, which increases the chances of fetal alcohol syndrome.

It's no secret that alcohol use can disrupt menstrual cycles and increase the risk of infertility, miscarriages, stillbirths, and premature delivery, and make menopause more difficult. Many reports suggest that one or two glasses of wine are healthy. However, in the context of fibromyalgia, I believe that zero alcohol use is the only acceptable level during pregnancy, considering we have no way of confirming how susceptible any one person's gene pool happens to be. Additionally, a suspicion of susceptibility to developing fibromyalgia may not even surface until after a formal diagnosis has been had—only then do questions begin to surface about Grandma's rheumatism, and Mom's irritability or fatigue. Why should one gamble when there is only one shot at doing a great job before delivery?

Specific to fibromyalgia is the effect that alcohol has on the development of the fetal brain. Alcohol literally poisons neurons and glial cells. Neurons, as you know, are the communication channels (nerves). Glial cells are cells that surround, support, detoxify, and modulate; they orchestrate and help nerves learn to keep up with adaptive demands. Nerves in the brain are practically helpless without healthy and effective glial cells. What this means is that the brain is not just nerves; it's nerves and glial cells. The mass of glial cells in the brain is called white matter. White matter makes up approximately 80 percent of the total brain mass. In the fetal brain, white matter forms a matrix to help guide the development and nerve projections, which are pathways from one area of the brain to the other—therefore in large part it will be responsible for the health and efficiency of our brain. Glial cells manage chemicals (neurotransmitters) that help ensure the passage of signals along nerve fibers as well as hold back signals when they get out of control. Control can be lost due to too much nerve stimulation (hypersensitivity), which allows normal signals to be exaggerated or amplified. An example, as we have gone over in the past, would be the way a light touch on the leg is perceived to be painful by a fibromyalgia sufferer.

Exposure to alcohol does not mean that a mother must be completely intoxicated in order for damage to occur. Minimal exposure can do its damage on the sensitive and developing brain matter. The damage that occurs during this stage of development can be permanent. In fetal alcohol syndrome, the damage can show up as mental retardation.[31] The worst time for a fetal brain to be exposed to alcohol is during the third trimester when the brain is going through a growth spurt. Neurons, as well as glial cells, are dividing rapidly at this stage. Alcohol exposure may stunt development and may be irreversible. Neurons and glial cells of the hippocampus and cerebellum are particularly susceptible at this stage. The hippocampus is part of the limbic system, which includes the amygdala, anterior thalamic nuclei, septum, limbic cortex, and fornix. We will discuss some of these brain structures in other areas of the book; for now, know that many of these structures of the brain manage emotions, behavior, motivation, and long-term memory. Compromise of these structures can cause the brain to interpret signals that we then experience as loss of energy, brain fog, loss of coordination, fatigue, and generally the aches and pains of fibromyalgia.

The cerebellum is important for memory and physical coordination. When physical coordination is impaired, it opens the door for a host of musculoskeletal imbalances that can show up as stiffness and a lack of coordination, and may generate pain for no apparent reason. Clearly even minimal exposure to alcohol will add an unnecessary challenge to a developing nervous system and questionable genetics.

In the last chapter we touched on the toxic effect of alcohol. However, since we have brought up the discussion of glial cells and neurons making up the brain, I thought I would add a little more perspective before moving on. Remember we said that glial cells manage chemicals (neurotransmitters) that help ensure the passage of signals along nerve fibers, as well as holding back signals when they get out of control (inhibition). Signals can get out of control due to too much stimulation (hypersensitivity), which in turn allows normal signals to be exaggerated and amplified. As a nerve signal moves along a nerve, it must jump from one nerve to the next over little junction spaces called synapses (we've discussed this earlier). To jump over this space, nerve A disperses a chemical neurotransmitter into the synapse, which is then picked up by nerve B.

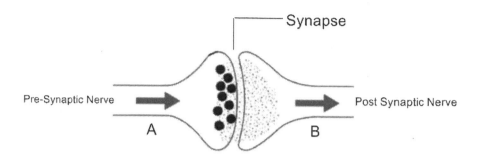

When chemicals jump across a synapse, they look to dock on special receptor sites on nerve B. The goal is to continue the path of communication toward the brain. Ideally, at this same site, attempts are made to control the pain signal by completely short-circuiting or just dampening it. What's interesting is that the receptors where docking takes place to control signals/pain are the same receptors where alcohol--as well as other chemicals, such as Valium and barbiturates--are welcome to take up residence. In and of itself this doesn't seem so bad, because we could use Valium, barbiturates, or alcohol to control the pain, and that is exactly what many of us do. The problem with this scenario is that with chronic use of alcohol or drugs, receptors effectively become immune and reduce their ability to receive the inhibitory neurotransmitters that the body naturally produces. This increases the chances that overstimulated and hypersensitive nerves will continue sending pain signals unimpeded and possibly all on their own for no apparent reason. Subsequently, in order to accomplish the same amount of inhibition that used to work naturally or with a certain amount of alcohol or drugs, there needs to be an increase in dosage and/or frequency. This is one of the ways we become alcohol or drug-dependent. You can see how undesirable this would be for a fibromyalgia sufferer. Alcohol has similar effects on other receptor sites, causing neurotransmitters such as dopamine and serotonin to be less effective. Dopamine and serotonin are involved in regulating our mood and outlook on life—here again encouraging alcohol dependency in order to boost spirit /mood.[31]

Alcohol can also contribute to impaired memory, dehydration, oxidative stress, vitamin deficiencies, and can increase fatigue; it may also conflict with medication, all of which is particularly egregious to Fibros. The scary thing is that most fibromyalgia sufferers already have all or most of these symptoms. There is an additional subconscious threat with moderate and social drinking not being perceived to have any negative effects. The person continues to drink, causing more damage and dependency, without thinking that he or she is contributing to their own problems.

The bottom line is that alcohol consumption poses too many risks and complications for mom and child.

Genetic Predisposition
Genetic predisposition means coding of DNA molecules that render an individual more susceptible to expressing a particular trait or disease. In our conversation, the disease is fibromyalgia. The disease could ultimately be expressed—or we might say triggered—hence, fibromyalgia is expressed. The trigger could be simply the lapse of time, as in aging—aka adult onset, with symptoms of fibromyalgia showing up in our 50s or 60s. This is not so uncommon; we can point a finger at aging for many diseases. When we are genetically predisposed, other environmental factors can be a trigger, such as another disease, infection, or possibly receiving a vaccination. Some types of overwhelming stress or environmental exposure could be triggers, as well as alcohol or even a wheat allergy that causes stress to the system. The list of stressors is endless.

How Did I Catch That Fibromyalgia Gene?
Well, as I mentioned, you don't really catch it; you inherit it. It's handed down similar to the way genetics help to determine the color of one's eyes or hair. This is termed polygenetic, meaning the product of two or more genes. These traits are inherited, but they're not necessarily consistent, and they don't show up in any predictable way or time frame. Having the gene could skip one child but predispose another, or skip a generation. Other polygenetic traits are autism, cancer, Alzheimer's, obesity, even migraines, along with numerous other conditions. The adult-onset version might be something more like diabetes, epilepsy, hypertension and psoriasis, or thyroid disease.

There are many hypotheses as to the primary cause of fibromyalgia, and with each hypothesis genetic predisposition plays a role. But to get further into the genetic relationship is beyond this writing, and unnecessary. Suffice it to say that one could possess a genetic predisposition. But here's what's interesting: the predisposition may not specifically be for fibromyalgia, yet it may set the stage to develop fibro. The predisposition may be for thyroid abnormalities or central nervous system disturbance, possibly for abnormal muscle physiology or a predisposition for hypersensitivity to pain. With hypersensitivity to pain, a person could develop neuropathic pain, meaning pain of unknown origin. Sometimes termed "idiopathic pain," this is when we define pain as a disease in and of itself (possibly from a known or unknown origin). Whether the pain is coming from the central nervous system or peripheral nervous system, hypersensitivity of nerves is not the major question.

The major question in the study of genetics is: "Is there a specific documentable fibromyalgia gene variation that will allow a person to develop specific tests to diagnose, or possibly even protect or prevent adults and children from developing fibromyalgia?" This is the question that has yet to be answered. There is much research underway, so we won't go into every possibility, but we will discuss a few interesting thoughts for diagnostic specificity.

Blood

Dr. Leon Chaitow in his book *Fibromyalgia Syndrome* reports blood testing as a possible diagnostic tool to understand stressors that would influence genetic expression. However, there is no test as of yet that has arisen to the degree of diagnostic specificity. There are however some revealing blood findings that may possibly help in managing fibro.

Phosphorus has been looked at by Dr. St. Amand as a genetic glitch. He finds that fibro patients' kidneys mismanage phosphorus. The kidneys fail to eliminate phosphorus efficiently, causing it to back up into the bloodstream. When phosphorus is too high in the blood, the body, in an attempt to normalize the blood, will store phosphorus in bones, muscles, and other tissues. Even though phosphorus is an important element for creating energy, at some point cells become overburdened and energy generation begins to lag. St. Amand's theory goes on to explain how calcium, sodium, and chloride try to balance and dilute phosphorus. He states: "Those cellular visitors (calcium, sodium, and chloride) cause swelling and produce the lumps and bumps of fibromyalgia. In turn, that squeezes nerves and sends distress signals to the brain. There, the problem is interpreted to express the symptoms of fibromyalgia: pain, burning, crawling, tingling, and numbness. The brain itself isn't immune to the process, so add fatigue and cognitive impairment."

To mention a few common findings, vitamin D is commonly low in tests. Malic acid may be low as well. It helps to deter pain and participates in the generation of ATP if low cellular energy goes down. The balance between Omega-6 essential fatty acids (EFA) and Omega-3 EFA is important in the body's ability to manage pain as well as inflammation and blood sugar. This is a very important issue; we will explain in Chapter 22 how you can be tested. Magnesium levels were shown to be low in fibro patients as well, which causes loss of energy, low ATP in muscles, and spasms. With treatment of as little as 300mg/day, tender points improve. But still none of these tests can be considered to be diagnostically specific.

Genetic Mutation

The Buckman Research Institute, along with Dr. St. Amand, published a paper in the *Journal of Experimental Biology and Medicine* (2008).[66] The study involved testing blood from fibromyalgia and non-fibromyalgia patients. Their studies pointed to genetic mutations as a possible cause for fibromyalgia. In particular, they studied the activity of cytokines. Cytokines are communication molecules; some of them work in very close proximity and others are more ubiquitous, affecting the whole body, similar to a hormone. They have the ability to up-regulate or down-regulate gene activity. They also help manage metabolism, immune reactions, pain, and inflammation.

The study helps explain how a fibromyalgia patient could have pain without inflammation, simply suggesting that cytokines can malfunction; they can overreact or underreact. When there's insult to an area, cytokines help trigger inflammation and pain. In the case of fibromyalgia, it has been shown time and time again that areas of pain have no evidence of inflammation. The study suggests that pain cytokines are turned on and inflammatory cytokines have been turned off. The pain then causes the body to develop tender nodules that can be detected on palpation of muscles, tendons, and ligaments—but, as aforementioned, without inflammation at the site. While still unproven, it seems that Dr. St. Amand's guaifenesin therapy not only affects tissue phosphorus, but influences cytokines to do a better job.

Healthy Perspective

A healthy perspective in reference to a genetic link would be to understand the predictability value genetics hold for fibromyalgia sufferers. I'm sure the future will bring the possibility of manipulating genes and reducing or eliminating many diseases, including fibromyalgia. For now, genetics can at least give us some insight to susceptibilities, hence providing motivation to improve behavior and environmental factors, with a goal to mitigate genetic predisposition. Consider implementing as many as possible of the self-help recommendations made throughout this book; they will empower you to "do what you can while you can," everything from diet to posture and exercise to attitude. You can also help yourself and your children by simply being aware of detrimental behavior learned from your parents or grandparents.[47]

It's clear that genetics play a role in fibromyalgia. Exactly how the inheritance takes place is not known for sure. Some gene theories relate serotonin, dopamine, and catecholamines as complicating, perpetuating, and possibly causative in fibromyalgia. I'm going to make a brief comment about each of these, if for no other reason than that you will find the terms in other chapters or research that you read.

Serotonin

Serotonin is a neurotransmitter—aka neural communication molecule. It plays an important role in our general perspective of life, well-being, and happiness. It affects mood and appetite. Serotonin affects our wake/sleep cycle, memory, learning, and clarity of thinking or lack thereof (brain fog). It's interesting to note that most serotonin (90 percent) is produced in the gut. Serotonin plays a large role in the health and the mobility of the gut, as well as absorption of nutrients. It has been reported that too much serotonin production could cause irritable bowel syndrome (IBS); the reverse may be true as well. IBS will upset serotonin balances, altering mood, and set the stage for food allergies and other gut problems. Too little serotonin could cause constipation. For these reasons, along with the fact that the gut houses its own enteric nervous system and is in constant communication with the brain, some people have called the gut "the other brain." This explains at least one of the links between fibro, IBS, and depression.

Low serotonin as well as gut malfunction can be related to low back problems. The nerves of the low back help to control the gut. When nerves are irritated due to poor posture, injury, or subluxation, a cascade of neurological mismanagement and inflammation can occur, directly affecting gut physiology, serotonin, and consequently mood, energy, toxicity, and allergies.

Catecholamines

Catecholamines are a broad category of chemical communicators that include dopamine. Other catecholamines related to fibromyalgia are adrenaline and norepinephrine. Both are produced by the adrenal glands as part of the fight-or-flight response (stress response) that we hear so much about. Stress--any stress, good or bad--calls upon the adrenal glands to produce these special catecholamines. This is normal and welcome. They cause an increase in blood pressure, the tightening of muscles, mental sharpness, and a sensitized nervous system so our readiness for response becomes more acute: hence the term "fight-or-flight." When someone is under chronic and daily stress, adrenal glands don't have a chance to recover. Consequently, they stay in this heightened state of adaptive readiness. This heightened condition is due to the catecholamines' effect on the sympathetic nervous system. When the stress is chronic, the sympathetic nervous system believes it needs to dominate bodily systems. This is termed "sympathetic dominance." In this state, most of us will notice tightness between the shoulders going up into the neck and head. Fibros are no strangers to these feelings, especially when stress and responsibility increase during the workday or as the stress of a hectic family life with financial and/or health challenges mounts.

Under normal conditions (or should I say controlled conditions) when stress abates, the production of these chemicals stops and the gland has a chance to recover, stopping catecholamine production. Chronic stress and sympathetic dominance relentlessly calling upon the adrenals to produce catecholamines eventually fatigue the adrenal glands.

A body can literally lock itself into this fight-or-flight condition; complicating, perpetuating, and possibly even triggering the expression of fibromyalgia. So we see that controlling stress is synonymous with controlling the physical or chemical body. This is why we have discussed life management concepts so often, whether that be through, diet, nutrition, exercise, avoiding overwhelm, or simply gaining control by self-directing recovery, aka self-advocacy. I will cover similar complications when we explain the relationship between the hypothalamus, pituitary, and adrenal glands, termed the hypothalamic-pituitary-adrenal axis.

Dopamine

Dopamine is a neurotransmitter in the catecholamine family that plays a role in learning, motivation, and pleasure. For instance, when you receive a present, the good feeling is stimulated by dopamine. What is interesting is that the person giving the present releases more dopamine than the person receiving the present. This might account for the saying, "It is better to give than to receive." Many of the rewarding feelings that people get from using alcohol, cocaine, and methamphetamines come from directly stimulating dopamine. This understanding may have some application in drug rehab. Incorporating deeds and service to other people will stimulate dopamine and other feel-good chemicals. Dale Carnegie, in his book *How to Win Friends and Influence People,* wrote at length about this concept. It helps to manage emotions and bring purpose to a person's life. It's not such a far-fetched strategy to consider repurposing oneself in service to others to avoid overwhelm and to stimulate feel-good chemicals, particularly in the early stages of managing fibromyalgia when attempting to stimulate endorphins through exercise may actually hamper recovery.

Family and Relationships

Ninety-five degrees and humid was the forecast for the day, and it was ripe for a change. It was, after all, summer in New England. Philip and Sarah sat in front of me for their first consultation. The humidity was really getting to Sarah. She had been diagnosed with fibromyalgia nine years before. As she shared with me what she had been going through, I noticed that Phil's body language and expression mirrored hers. When Sarah paused, I turned to Phil and asked, "What's it been like for you, going through this with Sarah?"

"Well, all I know is that I've lost my best friend," he said. "We were married seven years when all this began. Sarah had always been the life of the party. We used to go dancing and take weekend trips with friends." He gazed over at Sarah as he said she used to love to hike and bike ride. They stared at each other and both kind of shook their heads as if to say, "Yeah, I remember." There was an uncomfortable pause. Phil, continuing to stare at Sarah, and nodding his head ever so slightly, said, "We took tennis lessons once but we were both horrible, so neither one of us misses that." They each cracked a smile as he turned back to me and said, "I'm afraid we'll never get our lives back. And I don't know how to help her."

While there was sadness in this conversation, optimism prevailed. The fact that Philip even came to the appointment was a major plus. It told me he cared and was likely not to be part of the problem in the privacy of their home. Significant others frequently don't understand what a fibromyalgia patient is going through. The patient may have to go home and hide, fake, deny, or defend everything she feels and her behavior. Philip, on the other hand, was open to learning and helping in any way he could. Open communication is the first key. Men generally are plagued with this stuff called "testosterone" and, you know, "ego." To men, when their relationship changes and their wives become incapacitated to some degree, there's a sense of having an unfulfilled promise in the relationship--a sense of loss, possibly resentment or anger, particularly if they feel sexually neglected. Admittedly, this is a generalization, but men's first instinct is ego- and testosterone-driven. They want to fix it! Fix it means they fix it themselves, and they're frustrated when they can't. To men, fix it does not mean talk about it. Women, on the other hand, need to talk about it. They need to know they've been heard; their feelings need to be validated. Men need to understand that this is a large part of the fix. The fibro family will smooth out when men understand that they simply need to hit the communication, validation and "I hear you" mark.

I'm kind of a do-it-yourselfer. Even though counseling can be resourceful, I've found that nothing can replace a couple's willingness to team up and agree to learn and grow in the communication area on their own. My background doesn't necessarily give me the ability to explain why men have such a tough time sinking their teeth into these types of efforts. It's probably the testosterone, ego-caveman thing, and the same reasons that men hate to stop and ask for directions. While I am sure that there are many choices and many avenues, books and courses that could be helpful, I recommend reading the "Letter to Normals" at the beginning of this book and/or any other chapter you feel would be particularly helpful in your relationship. Also, take a look at Gary Smalley's information (http://smalley.cc/) and consider reading: John Gray's *Men Are From Mars, Women Are From Venus.*

I'm obviously singling out men here; however, the same challenges can be seen with female partners as well as adolescent children. So we're really talking about "the other person or persons" in your life. Remember that the other people in your life are at least as confused as you. And you in some ways have an advantage, because at least you have the physical feelings that explain and help put into perspective how you function and think—whereas the other people, when observing how you function, and your emotions and attitudes, will make up stories and excuses in their own minds to try to cope. I think the communication skills that Gary Smalley and John Gray offer are good basic communication skills, no matter the gender or the ages in the relationship.

Children
Although it seems that communication with children poses a whole other set of problems, basic communication skills always apply.

Whether you're a single parent or couple parenting, the resources as we've described above will be useful. Single parents will hopefully have a relative as part of their team who is close enough to effectively co-parent youngsters. In either case, the significant other/co-parent should put each other first, not the children. Together, with communication and understanding, they would then put the children first in their lives.

Whether we're playing a game by choice or necessity, we need to know the rules of the game and have a game plan. If you have fibromyalgia, that is a family game-changer, especially if you have children, just like pregnancy is a game-changer. So after you've come to terms with fibromyalgia yourself, and then with your spouse, open and honest communication will be the key with your children. Depending on their maturity, you could have them read the "Letter to Normals" or read it to them. In the meantime I am going suggest a list of things that children need to know—the rules and kind of a game plan. By no means is this list complete or necessarily in order of importance. You may decide to explore counseling resources at your child's school, religious affiliation, or support groups as well.

- Fibromyalgia is a medical condition.
- It's not something that I am likely to get over, like a cold or the flu.
- It's not contagious like a cold or flu either.
- Like having a cold or flu, I feel achy and tired all the time.
- I have some pretty good days and some really bad days.
- I really don't know how I'm going to feel from day to day.
- I could feel good in the morning and bad in the afternoon.
- Whatever I feel, it will be a surprise to me and to you.
- When I'm not feeling good, I could get crabby.
- When I am a fibro-crab, you can tell me that I'm being crabby.
- TVs and music bother me, but we can get you head phones if you want.
- I want you to ask questions any time you want.
- Tell me what's important to you and I'll tell you what's important to me.
- (Dad, significant other, co-parent) may get tired and crabby too.
- Nobody caused it.
- Would you be willing to help me with (XYZ)?

- What do you think about e-mailing each other once in a while?
- This is a family matter. I won't put anything on Facebook if you don't—agreed?

I'm sure there are many more things that need to be communicated and parameters to be put on family life. You will accumulate them as necessary during your process. You won't want to make your child feel like he or she is responsible for taking care of you. Yet children are no different from adults; they become more centered and fulfilled when they feel they have purpose/worth, and are happy to be helpful and contribute. An appropriate amount of responsibility helps emotionally, and balances humanness. With sufficient praise, appreciation, and the family working together, children will usually rise to the challenge and be proud to help.

I mentioned e-mails above. The more avenues of communication you can open up, the better off you'll be. You will want to default to whichever type of communication your children are comfortable with and emotionally open to, whether that is through e-mail, in person, letters, cards, or through a third party. Special talk time routines are empowering and comforting too. Try one-on-one chats first thing in the morning, when they get home from school and want to share their day with you, during your evening meal, or a few quiet moments before they go to bed. Let it be their choice and something that they can count on— you must never be the one to break the commitment. Those of you with teenagers might be saying to yourselves, "That ain't gonna happen." But you just might be surprised. Of course it would be a help if this pattern of communication was already established pre-fibromyalgia.

The last thing I'll mention is that befriending other families who have a Fibro is extremely helpful in maintaining normalcy. This provides a built-in support system for not only the child, but significant others and co-parents. Outings and get-togethers can be fun and therapeutic.

> It has been said that an apple doesn't fall too far from the tree. Genetic predisposition does not mean genetic expression. At least 70 percent of genetic expression can be controlled by lifestyle.

CHAPTER 15

Perpetuating Factors

Chapter Topics:

Hydrogenated Fats	*Cholesterol*	*Magnesium*
Trans Fats	*Niacin/B3*	*Malic Acid*
Statins	*Vitamin D3*	*Insomnia*

The following are some factors known to confound, complicate and possible perpetuate the fibromyalgia picture. When addressed, they may greatly improve symptoms, if not resolve them.

Partially Hydrogenated/Trans Fats

During an annual physical, it is likely that your doctor will conduct a blood test for C-reactive protein. C-reactive protein (CRP) is produced by the liver in response to inflammation. The test can't determine where inflammation is in the body or why it exists, but the test is useful in determining whether there is an acute or chronic inflammatory condition. It helps to include or exclude other conditions that could account for symptoms that need to be addressed. CRP may be indicative of an acute transient process, such as immediately after surgery, in which case we know what the body is doing and that the inflammation should subside in approximately three days; if not, we would suspect an infection. It's also seen in chronic inflammatory conditions such as lupus, rheumatoid arthritis and inflammatory bowel disease. Chronic inflammation contributes to diseases such as heart disease and Alzheimer's.

Another way of assessing subclinical chronic inflammation is to evaluate essential fatty acid (Omega 3, 6, and 9) balance. A discrepancy in the balance is liable to signal inflammation long before C-reactive protein is positive. Unfortunately, routine blood work does not usually include this assessment. Even if you were to request the tests, it is unlikely that your MD would understand the implications and the relative balance among fatty acids. This is another case that necessitates an opinion beyond your family doctor (PCP). Your best bet would be to consult a naturopath (ND), chiropractor (DC), or medical doctor (MD) who specializes in functional medicine. The

American College for Advancement in Medicine (www.acam.org) would be a great place to start investigating practitioners to uncover more subtle inflammatory conditions. These specialized practitioners will not only run these tests routinely, but will be well-versed in interpretation and treatment options. We use Lipid Labs out of Minnesota. (see appendix). They have an in-home blood spot test to determine the ratio of Omega-3 to Omega-6 fatty acids. While there is some controversy as to the healthiest ratio, it is generally accepted that as the percentage of 6s in the blood goes up, surpassing 3s, inflammation goes up--and with it, the risk of disease. This data is crucial if we are to control diet, inflammation, and pain, and to preserve brain function. With this information in hand, appropriate dietary changes can be instituted, working toward better numbers, and avoiding or weaning off statins. Approximately every four months we would retest and continue to steer recovery.

Most of us are aware that there are various types of fats; some of them are good, and many are not. One of the major problems with trying to take in only good fats, or trying to avoid the bad fats, is the labeling of products. If you are a person who spends time in the grocery store reviewing labels before you purchase, you may think that you are making an informed decision about what you are putting into your body.

Due to the FDA's rules with regard to labeling, when you purchase a product that states that it has zero trans-fats in it, or that there are no hydrogenated fats/oils, there still may be. The Nutrition Facts Label can state zero grams of trans-fat if the food product contains less than 0.5 grams per serving. Thus if a product contains partially hydrogenated oils, then it might contain small amounts of trans-fat even if the label says zero grams of trans-fat.[19] However, in late 2013, the Federal Drug Administration declared that partially hydrogenated oils are not recognized as safe any longer. Rules have been proposed to make these types of fats illegal; this of course will take some time as food producers make the transition to zero tolerance. For now, continue to watch the labels—even a small amount of trans-fat per food item can add up and accumulate over time and cause inflammation.

Even if you choose to make your own food at home, you need to be wary of how you cook and what you cook with. The goal should be to avoid any foodstuff that contains either partially hydrogenated oils or trans-fats, and avoid heating all oils to their breakdown temperature. When you're cooking at a high heat, you want to use oils that are stable and don't oxidize or go rancid easily, forming free radicals. A higher content of saturated fats in the oil are the most stable. My best suggestion is to use coconut oil or real butter. Coconut oil has 92 percent saturated fat allowing relatively safer cooking at high temperatures; butter comes in second at 68 percent. Still, check the label to see temperature tolerance. Than make sure you stay below that temperature.

Statins

Have you ever noticed that your muscles and joints ache or have pain on movement? How about your legs? Do they cramp or feel restless? Maybe you feel all of these things in addition to being so tiered that some days you don't think you can make it through. Well, one of the first things I would ask you in a consultation is if you're on any statin medication. The most common ones are Lipitor, Crestor, Vytorin, and Lovastatin.

Statins lower the cholesterol that the liver produces. The liver produces about 75 percent of our total cholesterol, and the other 25 percent we get from our diet. Wouldn't you think that if the liver produces cholesterol, it does it for a reason--and a good reason, at that? One of the great lies traditional medicine has perpetrated upon itself and the public in the last 30 years is that cholesterol and fats in general are bad—and further, that high cholesterol causes heart disease, and statins are the answer. Yet pharmaceutical companies report a 99 percent statin failure rate. This fact did not diminish statin sales. JAMA reported in 1994 that hyper-cholesterolemia posed no important risk factors in heart disease. In 1995 the *Journal of Physicians and Surgeons* reported that tightly controlled clinical trials have never concluded that lowering LDL can prevent cardiovascular disease. As recently as 2007, JAMA reported being baffled by findings that lower cholesterol levels were not linked to reduced risk of stroke.

We have been told there is good cholesterol and bad cholesterol, but like any other substance that's necessary for a healthy, functioning body, there must be balance. So when people talk about good cholesterol HDL (high-density lipoprotein) or so-called bad cholesterol LDL (low-density lipoprotein) the goal is to strike a healthy balance. To do this we need a certain amount of fat and cholesterol in our diet. However, we've been told for several decades that "fat is bad" and "cholesterol will kill you." These are scientifically naïve and worse yet, possibly blatantly manipulated warnings. They can be found to be true under certain circumstances, but are generally lies that have brought stumbling blocks to our general health and are of great concern for people who are tired, in pain, or overweight. I will tie in the relationship of cholesterol, statins and fibromyalgia in a moment. But first let me put into perspective how the no fat/no cholesterol warnings have affected general health.

For the fibromyalgia sufferer, inflammation and pain are of great concern. One of cholesterol's jobs is to help control inflammation. If you consume a lot of carbohydrates, and most of us do, as well as restrict fats—in particular, cholesterol, as we've been told to do—the body, desperate to control inflammation, causes specialized hormones to activate an enzyme in your liver to produce cholesterol from glucose. The trouble is, when this enzyme (called HMG Co-A reductase) is cranking and putting out needed cholesterol, the medical community judges the extra circulating cholesterol as too high. With statin prescriptions, inflammation is allowed to escalate, as demonstrated by aches and pains.

The next step is to counteract the symptoms with anti-inflammatories. This is not a healthy cycle, but a profit machine for pharmaceutical companies; they make money on the statins to lower the cholesterol, in turn making money on anti-inflammatories to lower the inflammation due to the lack of cholesterol. Good deal, for them. We will talk more about statin medication shortly.

Statin Myopathy: Statins may cause muscle pain and tenderness (statin myopathy). In severe cases, muscle cells can break down and release a protein called myoglobulin into the bloodstream. Myoglobulin can impair kidney function and lead to kidney failure. Certain drugs when taken with statins can increase the risk of myopathy. These include gemfibrozil, erythromycin (Erythrocin), antifungal medications, nefazodone (Serzone), cyclosporine, and niacin. If you take statins and have new muscle aches or tenderness, consult your doctor.

Statin Neuropathy: Neuropathies or peripheral neuropathies are characterized by weakness, tingling and pain that most often occur in the hands or feet. However, fibromyalgia patients will frequently report tingling in all areas of their body. Mary Enig, PhD, reports research from Denmark where nine percent of a 500,000 population sample taking statins was likely to develop a neuropathy. Subsequently she found that taking statins for one year actually increased the risk of nerve damage by about 15 percent. For patients who took statins for two years or more, the risk of nerve damage rose by 26 percent. Is has also been noted that for people taking statins over a long period of time, the nerve damage may be irreversible.

Dizziness: Dr. Beatrice Gold MD, PhD notes that dizziness is a common adverse effect of statin therapy, believed to be due to a drop in blood pressure. Fibro sufferers would not welcome dizziness on top of the brain fog that they already experience.

Avoiding Statins

It is a little peculiar that between non-medical and medical doctors, it is the non-medical doctors who are labeled as "alternative," given the way each separate branch chooses to primarily care for their patients. Non-medical doctors seek to provide therapeutic solutions and health enhancement while utilizing the least amount of engineered pharmacology that they can. Medical doctors, on the other hand, almost always operate under the exact opposite paradigm, looking to drugs of all kinds to assist their patients in controlling symptoms. This dichotomy is in spite of both types of doctors working with the same science.

Long gone are the television advertisements that simply told you to go to your MD and get a prescription for a statin drug. The new adverts clearly state that statins may be of assistance "when diet and exercise aren't enough." This is a profound change in the pharmaceutical companies' thought process, and we can hope that it will trickle down to many MDs as well. Their new ad campaign may be nothing more than their attempt to hedge their bets as more research continues to reveal that cholesterol in and of itself is not a cause of heart disease. There may still be medical professionals, as well as pharmaceutical people, who are stuck on cholesterol as the "bad guy" in the heart disease battle, and for those who are, I highly recommend Gary Taubes' book *Good Calories, Bad Calories*.

I'll further discuss fats in short order, but for the moment, let's focus on the fact that 75 percent of the cholesterol in the body is produced naturally by the liver. There are certain ethnic groups, such as those of Mediterranean heritage, that tend to produce higher levels of cholesterol than "normal." Even with a great exercise regimen and a proper diet, there may be little that can be done to lower their cholesterol number. If there is an actual need to lower cholesterol level, and your medical professional starts talking about prescribing statins, you may wish to discuss the following options that are more natural.

Niacin (Vitamin B3)

The Archives of Internal Medicine, in 1994, reported that niacin outperformed statin drugs in controlling cholesterol. Additionally, niacin was found to reduce other risk factors with regard to heart disease and also helped lower LDL (bad cholesterol) as well. In 1988, the *British Journal of Clinical Practice* reported that niacin was effective in treating intermittent claudication, a condition that involves heaviness, achiness, burning, and cramping in the legs that is frequently experienced while walking. Intermittent claudication is known to be a result of poor blood flow. Niacin helps simply by improving blood flow. Niacin also assists with cellular respiration and energy production (ATP), which is of great value to fibromyalgia sufferers directly and indirectly. However, as in all health decisions, consult your health team before changing your strategies.

Consider the following recommendations taken from Dr. Michael Dobbins, 2012, "The Fats of Life." Discuss them with your medical team as an alternative to statins for management of cholesterol and inflammation, or at least to help your body mitigate some of the consequences of taking statins.

- Antioxidants: vitamin C, E, selenium, lipophilic acid and CoQ10. (I would add a healthy dose of a Proantho Cyanidin formulation by NutraMetrix-OPC-3; see appendix).
- Essential fatty acids are high in Omega-3. Remember that while there has been much emphasis on low-fat diets, the most credible research and studies show that low-fat diets actually increase LDL. It may be more important to include more fats in your diet, the exception being the elimination of all trans-fats and partially hydrogenated fatty acids, and replacing them with polyunsaturated and monounsaturated fats.
- Diet: consume more garlic, ginger, onions, chromium, folic acid, B6, B12 and betaine.
- Increase fiber, especially water-soluble fiber, fruits, vegetables, and vegetarian sources of protein.
- Carnitine: This is important in fatty-acid metabolism found to be depleted in cardiac muscle during acute infarctions.
- Avoid trans-fats, which are known to contribute to inflammation.
- Avoid refined sugars, sugar substitutes, and carbohydrates.

- Consider taking evening primrose, borage, or black currant oil; all are sources of
- GLA, which the body uses to make anti-inflammatory prostaglandins.
- Eat high-quality saturated fats such as coconut oil, which is known to have an antibacterial and antiviral quality that protects against inflammation of the arteries and intestines.

Vitamin D and Cholesterol

Cholesterol is an important precursor to vitamin D production. Vitamin D is a necessary nutrient not only for metabolizing calcium in supporting bone health, but also to help modulate inflammation, insulin sensitivity, and immune function, joints, muscles, hormones, and the health of the skin. Further, it helps to support the pancreas and stomach, and maintains a healthy blood pressure along with helping the entire cardiovascular system to run smoothly; it protects the brain and reproductive organs and has anti-aging properties to boot. However, without the proper levels of cholesterol, our bodies do not produce sufficient vitamin D, which can lead to deficiency. This helps account for the epidemic proportion of vitamin D deficiency in the United States as of this writing. Before we go any further, I should note that in spite of the accepted term "vitamin," vitamin D is really a hormone that the body produces under the right conditions.

Vitamin D comes from diet, supplementation, and from being exposed to ultraviolet rays of sunlight—hence the nickname "the sunshine vitamin." D2 is the D found in fortified foods like milk, juices, or cereals; and D3 is the form that is synthesized by the skin when it's exposed to the sun. Ten to fifteen minutes of exposure (without sunscreen) is recommended three to four times a week. Obviously, this synthesis takes place through the skin. However, without adequate cholesterol in the skin, D production doesn't happen. If the diet is low in or void of fats or a malabsorption syndrome exists, D production will plummet regardless of whether there has been enough sun exposure. This is yet another symptom of conventional wisdom's insistence on reducing or eliminating fat from the diet, hence the epidemic need for D supplementation. When non-medical doctors spoke about the relationship between D and fats decades ago, it was considered quackery.

Peer-reviewed clinical research documents that D deficiencies are linked to chronic musculoskeletal pain. Additionally, such deficiencies are linked more specifically to muscle weakness, fatigue, fibromyalgia, arthritis, headaches, migraines, various mood disturbances, fatigue, and seasonal affective disorders.

Cholesterol and Hormones

Cholesterol is a basic building block of sex hormones (testosterone, estrogen, and progesterone) as well as cortisol and aldosterone, which are produced by the adrenal glands. Adrenal health is crucial for the regulation of blood pressure, managing the body's response to stress and stabilizing the immune system. It is crucial to the relationship within the hypothalamic-pituitary-adrenal axis. The thyroid is also helped by cholesterol to maintain its relationship with the hypothalamus and pituitary. Imbalance in any one of these systems can help trigger, perpetuate, and/or complicate fibromyalgia.

Cholesterol and the Liver

We often read that the liver is a filter system. This is true, but it's only part of the story. The liver decides what substances should be eliminated and what substances should be recirculated or combined to reorganize and construct other substances that are useful for the body.

The liver removes toxins. The two primary toxins designated for removal are urea and bile. Urea is a byproduct of amino acid (protein) metabolism and is excreted in urine. Bile is made up of a combination of cholesterol and waste products. Bile is used to assist in the excretion of waste products from the bowel, but it also helps in the digestion of fats. The liver is constantly producing bile, and then it shuttles the bile over to the gallbladder for storage. After eating, bile is excreted from the gallbladder, helping to emulsify fats into smaller particles so they can be absorbed. And, at the same time, it helps breaks down food for removal in the intestines.

What's interesting is that the metabolic pathway in the liver that produces cholesterol also produces CoQ10, which is a powerful antioxidant.[19] It is crucial to all cells if they are to produce adequate amounts of ATP (energy). We know that low levels of CoQ10 cause muscle damage, leading to muscular aches and pains, leg cramps, fatigue, restless leg syndrome, and chronic fatigue. Does any of this sound familiar? Most medical recommendations, in spite of the error in insisting on reducing cholesterol, realize that statins reduce CoQ10 at the same time. If you are/have been on statins, hopefully you were told to supplement with CoQ10.

Magnesium

Magnesium deficiency exaggerates fibromyalgia symptoms due to its reducing the cells' ability to create energy/ATP. Muscles become hypertonic and cramp; a person can suffer from anxiety, headaches, poor sleep, numbness, and increased pain sensitivity, aka hyperalgesia. We also frequently find that Fibros suffer from constipation with poor intestinal peristalsis due to magnesium deficiency. Modern societies' dietary habits are common co-conspirators in degrading health, with poorly mineralized water and a low intake of leafy green vegetables. Additionally, dietary habits encourage metabolic acidosis, which increases the loss of magnesium by urination. Deficiencies are also seen in conjunction with vitamin D deficiencies, malabsorption, and chronic stress. There was a study done by Selda Bagis, MD, that showed that 300 mg of magnesium combined with 10 mg of amitriptyline (an antidepressant) proved to improve more fibro symptoms than either one alone. This makes sense considering our previous discussions on how resourceful antidepressants are in the management of fibromyalgia. So if you're already taking an antidepressant, you may find improved results from the addition of as little as 300 mg of magnesium. If you're not on antidepressants, I recommend starting with about 600 mg and monitor results.

Malic Acid

Malic acid is the organic compound found in tart fruits such as Granny Smith apples, cranberries, and certain grapes.

Malic acid, like magnesium, helps cells to generate energy/ATP. In fibromyalgia, it is felt that malic acid may prevent hypoxia (loss of oxygen) to the muscle tissues, and hence improve ATP production. The *Journal of Rheumatology,* in 1995, reported that a study done with 24 fibromyalgia patients taking three tablets twice a day of a product called "super malic" (a combination of malic acid 200mg and magnesium 50mg) showed an Improvement in muscle strength, endurance, and reduced pain. There is a little lack of clarity as to whether it's the magnesium or the malic acid that's the most effective of the combination. You'll find most companies combine the two when targeting fibromyalgia.

Cold-pressed unfiltered virgin apple cider vinegar will supply malic acid naturally. The nice thing about supporting malic acid naturally with apple cider vinegar is that the vinegar helps to alkalize body chemistry, which in itself reduces inflammation and pain and improves muscle energy.

Note to Physicians

If you are not already trained in functional medicine or are not well-versed in nutrition but are looking for a system of pulling together your years of education and experience, take a look at Functional Medicine University http://www.functionalmedicineuniversity.com/.

This educational step will help you practice with more cost-effective diagnostics in understanding multidimensional functional/physiological impairment as seen with fibromyalgia, chronic fatigue, diabetes, idiopathic pain, heart problems, etc. Naturopathic physicians' education inherently accomplishes this. Chiropractors' education is heavy in nutrition and integrative sciences, but could benefit from postgraduate studies. However, medical doctors have virtually no education in nutrition. They have no choice but to seek postgraduate integration of academics and the human condition. Functional Medicine University may be a good starting point in this effort. Another great resource would to contact Dr. Jeffrey Moss from Moss Nutrition of Hadley, Massachusetts. He will be able to point you in the right direction.

Insomnia

I chose to include insomnia as a perpetuating factor. Some feel that it is a cause of fibro; others noted it as a co-existing condition. What we do know is that it's always part of the constellation of fibromyalgia symptoms. Insomnia tends to run in families and is more common in women.

One night of sleep deprivation is enough to cause generalized hyperalgesia (pain) as well as encourage anxiety, which supports further sleep deprivation. Even one episode of transient insomnia will alter circadian rhythms. A person may begin to have anxiety and associate bedtime/rest with the struggle. This encourages more sleep deprivation; the pattern repeats itself with more anxiety, hence establishing a chronic pattern.

People with insomnia may show low levels of melatonin. Some studies have reported consistently high levels of the stress hormone cortisol. Both may cause reduction in REM sleep. Depending on the person, high levels of cortisol may cause poor sleep, while poor sleep may cause high levels of cortisol in others. Growth hormone (HGH) has also been implicated. Growth hormone is normally secreted at night by the pituitary gland; it's associated with growth and repairs as well as deep sleep. As a person ages, the growth hormone naturally declines.

A percentage of insomnia cases are related to some type of substance abuse, especially alcohol, social drugs, and sedatives. We also find that shift work causes circadian rhythms to be inconsistent with normal/healthy day/night cycles and is of great concern in fibromyalgia cases and insomnia. In my experience, shift workers are unlikely to make progress with fibro until they change back to regular dayshift hours.

Medication may be helpful with both duloxetine (Cymbalta) and milnacipran (Savella) approved by the FDA for sleep and fibro. Additionally, these drugs help either directly or indirectly with musculoskeletal pain. For non-drug options, we start patients on a combination of calcium and magnesium with melatonin, and incorporate a growth hormone secretagogue to help modulate sleep, control stress hormones, and repair muscles and nerves. A secretagogue is a substance that encourages another substance to be secreted--in this case, growth hormone from the pituitary gland (see appendix for sources).

Some patients find that taking an adrenal support will help to control cortisol/stress hormones through the sleep cycle. Hypoglycemia through the overnight hours can be of concern as well; some patients' sleep improves simply by including a snack before bed, which helps with blood sugar, hence cortisol. Try a slice of apple with walnut butter on it.

> Any condition or abuse, suspected or unsuspected, can perpetuate symptoms and frustrate case management. However, the perpetuating factors that are promoted or prescribed by people with the authority of white coats and stethoscopes worry me the most. This is another reason to be sure that your health team has a diverse representation of medical and non-medical health care professionals. If you depend on only one type of doctor, you are liable not to get the complete story--or, worse yet, to get the wrong story.

INSIGHT # 4

AWARENESS AND COVERT CHALLENGES

Trying to find the right path…is being on the right path itself.
—Siddharth Astir

CHAPTER 16

Find the Right Doctor

Chapter Topics:
    Believers   *Non-medical*
    Non-believers   *The Interview*
    Medical

Finding the Right Doctor

Forget it! The chances of finding "the right doctor" are pretty remote. First, I know that's not what people want to hear. Second, most probably don't believe me. The reason I say forget it is that "the right doctor" suggests that there is one doctor who can do it all and save you from fibromyalgia. There is not. There are, however, doctors who believe that fibromyalgia exists and at the same time have the interest and ability to work with you. There are doctors who will have an open mind and an understanding of other disciplines, doctors and therapists likely to be key participants in recovery; however, they can be hard to find.

Without your determination to complete this book and become your own advocate (in spite of the fact that it may be uncomfortable and confusing at times) you are unlikely even to know when "the right doctor" is in front of you. Most sufferers get caught up in their need to feel better and trust in their doctor's "power as an authority," causing them either to put too much unfounded trust in the doctor, or too much trust in their own personal research, perceptions, beliefs, and commitments regarding what fibromyalgia is and is not, and what they should do on their own.

Reality Check

Before we get into some of the things to look for as well as the dos and don'ts of doctor/ patient fibrology (the study of fibromyalgia), let's take a reality check about doctors.

As we develop an understanding of doctors, how they think, and how they may best serve us—as well as how we can best serve ourselves in finding the right doctor—let's agree: there is no question as to whether fibromyalgia exists; it's very real. The only question is whether you'll find the doctor who not only believes this, but will believe in you—one who is willing to work with you. The American College of Rheumatology, The World Health Organization, The American Chiropractic Association, The National Institute of Health, and The American Medical Association all accept fibromyalgia as a real medical diagnosis: standard AMA diagnostic code ICD-9=729.1 (myalgia and myositis). Revised and more specific coding to standardize diagnostic codes across all of health care is termed ICD-10. Under the new coding, fibromyalgia has a specific diagnostic code of its own, M79.7. So don't waste your time with any doctor or therapist who has any question as to the veracity of fibromyalgia as a disease to be dealt with.

This chapter will possibly be the most important one to set the stage and perspective for your success; at the same time, it is liable to be the hardest chapter to read. You may feel that I'm shaking the only stability you have and challenging your relationship with "your doctor," the one you have trusted up until now.

Doctors, therapists, and paraprofessionals reading this chapter are liable to be offended, see it as arrogant, and adopt an attitude that diminishes the value and perspective of this entire book. My job is to prep the fibromyalgia sufferer with the best vantage point to critically evaluate doctors and the possibilities that they offer for an improved outcome. Doctors are just people with different educations. They have all the prejudiced opinions and hang-ups, etc., that everyone else has. They're not gods; they don't know it all. We all just want to believe that each of them does. Have you ever had friends tell you that they are lucky to be going to a fair-to- average doctor? No, it's always "My doctor is the best in the state [or country or world]." People are compelled to support/reinforce their own decisions and affirm their confidence in their doctor regardless of his/her qualification or how things have been going. I might add that it is no coincidence that every doctor has a list of affiliations and certificates, plaques, and degrees. Doctoring is a business, and accolades sell. The point is, don't be taken in by appearances. It's what is not hanging on the wall that tells the story.

Most fibro sufferers are adults and have already established relationships with doctors. They have a certain amount of confidence in them and also have beliefs about other types of doctors. People have a tendency to hold on to their beliefs and their perspectives and remain committed/loyal, sometimes to a fault. I hear patients say things like: "I don't believe diet has anything to do with fibromyalgia," "I don't believe in taking medication," "I don't believe in chiropractic," and "I don't believe a rheumatologist could do anything more than my family doctor is doing." Most of these beliefs and opinions are unfounded, uneducated, and are likely to just have been handed down through someone in the family.

We're going to spend a lot of time on this topic, as it's crucial for a patient's success. You may have to loosen your grip on everything you've believed up until now in order to open your mind to a solution or two that might surprise you. I believe that without the right team of doctors and caregivers you will stall, complicate, and possibly sabotage your progress but never know it. Further, any other value that you get out of this book having to do with the science, possibilities, and clinical factors will be minimized or completely lost if you don't have the right people to join with you, and/or if you refuse to play the role as your own advocate.

Coach

Being your own advocate is like being the head coach of your own team. The coach is the leader who sets the tone and the attitude of all that takes place. A coach teaches and trains, looks to everyone else on the team to know their job, and is responsible for the understanding and integration possibilities—the big picture of how to win. Further, the coach should demand that everyone on the team respect each other and communicate accordingly.

The coach has a play-by-play feeling for how things are going. He organizes all the players involved and coordinates a team that has an understanding of each person's job in light of the challenges. The coach needs to appoint a captain, the coach's right hand. It's the captain of your team who will be the initial pivotal person--a doctor, in your case, to help you negotiate the weeks and months ahead.

The Doctor

Good News / Bad News

I always like the bad news first. The bad news is that doctors are human. I know most of us don't want a human for a doctor; we want a superhuman, someone to cure us on the spot. Most doctors cringe at the thought that they might not possess these superhuman abilities that are expected of them. After all, they are doctors. Nevertheless, doctors have all the frailties, ego, prejudices, and misconceptions that patients have, and are compelled for the most part by the science and paradigm of their education and chosen specialty.

The Good News

The good news is that along with human frailties, doctors have a driving thirst for knowledge and an extraordinary dedication to remove suffering and improve the human condition. They are every bit as worried about you as you are. When you don't mend quickly, they share your frustration. They have all the compassion and concern that you hope they will have.

Believers / Non-believers

There are some special categories that I've put doctors into in reference to fibromyalgia. There are the believers and the non-believers. Each of these categories has three subcategories. You will recognize and be familiar with some of them. After we discuss them, we'll break them down into finer detail.

As a side note, let's acknowledge that when we speak of prescriptions, we're referring to prescribed treatment—whether it is a medication or a non-drug treatment like exercise, massage, or acupuncture. For instance, you could be working with a chiropractic physician, a naturopathic doctor, or an osteopathic doctor. A prescription may not necessarily be a type of pharmaceutical but may be some type of physical medicine, or may be self-help treatment such as vitamins, diet, exercise, or yoga.

My intent in this section is to discuss with you general attitudes of doctors, what to look for, and what/whom to possibly stay away from.

We said the first category was believers. I break believers down into three subcategories: 1. Enthusiasts, 2. Neutrals, 3. Buts.

Believers

These doctors generally "get it." They know that fibromyalgia is real and they understand what you're going through. These doctors know that the science of "cause" and the art of "cure" are evolving on a daily basis. You will feel in these doctors a sense of compassion and understanding and a genuine interest in what you're going through; they listen to what you have to say.

Believer Enthusiast

This type of a believer is enthusiastically engaged in understanding your special situation. An enthusiast tends to specialize in fibromyalgia and fibromyalgia-like conditions. An enthusiast loves working with fibromyalgia and fibromyalgia-like conditions and has a lot of contact hours with them. They understand the complications and the coexisting conditions that confuse and frustrate you as well as the pain, stiffness, fatigue, and depression you feel. This doctor will tend to be relatively open-minded and a good captain for your health team. He/she knows you need extra time to be heard and is willing to give it to you.

Believer Neutral

The neutral believer knows that your condition is real and does all he or she can to help. However, this doctor, at best, has only general knowledge about the condition. You're very likely to know more than your doctor—especially if you finish reading this book. The neutral will be very busy with other interests or conditions he is treating. He doesn't really have the time for or the interest in fibromyalgia patients. As we mentioned earlier, with the science of fibromyalgia evolving daily, this neutral doctor may also be too busy to keep up with fibro research and literature. Most neutral doctors tend to be nonassertive and non-confrontational; they are distracted with pressures from managed-care insurance organizations and the pressures of being part of a physician's group, HMO, or PPO, as well as the rules and regulations that take up time and add paperwork. This means that your care is possibly based on your insurance coverage (we all know the insurance companies hold the purse strings). Nonetheless this doctor does want to help you, so he may run some tests and be quick to prescribe the most common types of medication targeting your worst symptoms, frequently defaulting to sleep or mood medication as well as some type of anti-inflammatory. The effort, of course, is to help you, as well as stay within the parameters of your insurance policy. This is definitely not the worst-case scenario, but it's not good enough.

Believer Buts

"But" doctors are believers; "buts" are relatively frank with you as well as themselves in that they don't want anything to do with fibromyalgia patients. This doctor either feels inadequate concerning your condition and is up front about it, or simply doesn't want to take the time to deal with it. This doctor is more than happy to refer you to an enthusiastic colleague who specializes in fibromyalgia or

245

fibromyalgia-like conditions. The referral will most likely be to a physician within their discipline/group; MDs refer to MDs, meaning that if a medical doctor is the captain of the team, you will be referred to another medical doctor. That's not a bad thing, but it too is not good enough.

Non-believers

Non-believers come in the same three varieties: enthusiasts, neutrals, and buts.

Non-believers generally do not believe that fibromyalgia exists. They simply see someone's symptoms as a bunch of separate issues. Non-believers are becoming fewer as time goes on and information is more readily available about the science and cause of fibromyalgia. But know that the non-believers are likely to feel annoyed with you and your presentation. These guys aren't hard to recognize, but you may have to go home for a good cry after an appointment with one.

Enthusiasts

Non-believer enthusiasts are enthusiastic about convincing you, the patient, that fibromyalgia does *not* exist. You won't see even a spark of empathy in them, and you will receive little to no validation from this type of doctor. You'll be able to recognize a mile away the few who are out there. They can't hide it; the enthusiastic non-believer is too arrogant even to try.

Neutral

The non-believing neutral doctor will mirror the believer-neutral doctor in the area of trying to help you with the symptoms you present. The difference between the two is the that the non-believer will, in a sense, patronize you, never really believing that all of your symptoms are real or relating to you in any way, but never really letting you know that he is a non-believer. This doctor will not come across as being arrogant. Like the believer neutral, the non-believer neutral is also a non-assertive person, avoiding confrontation with you or the insurance company. This doctor, too, will prescribe for you the most common medications—again, all the while staying within the parameters of managed care. Hopefully, as in the case with the believer neutral, this doctor's efforts will at least help.

Buts

The non-believing buts will listen politely, but they will be thinking, "She's one of those." This type of doctor will be a little bit short with you; he will acknowledge your concerns, but may make the effort to talk you out of believing that fibro is real, leaving you feeling insulted. Based on the fact that this doctor will not believe what you're saying, he may refer you to a rheumatologist, chiropractor, or psychiatrist to get rid of you. His goal would be to rid himself of you as soon as possible. To save face, he may have you leave with a non-refillable prescription but no future appointment.

As you can see, the doctors who are enthusiastic about fibromyalgia and the but doctors are likely to be your best friends in the sense that they are perfectly clear where they stand. You can team up with them, take their referral, or simply move on.

Neutrals, on the other hand, although they have good intentions, may work with you for months or years, but you will end up with little to no results. They are dangerous and will waste precious time.

If I haven't made it clear yet, when I talk about doctors I'm talking about all doctors—all types of doctors, whether medical, osteopathic, chiropractic, or naturopathic.

Every once in a while there will be a report—an article or something on the internet—that a doctor professes a "cure" for fibromyalgia because he has had good results with a few patients. What's interesting is that in all doctor categories, the neutral doctor tends to be the quickest to report these types of successes. It has been quoted too often but it does seem to hold true that "If something sounds too good to be true, then it is too good to be true." The doctors who profess a so-called "cure" are likely to misjudge their clinical results for one of two reasons:

Reason number one: The patient has learned to cope with self-help methods, along with just enough relief from the doctor to be convincing. After suffering for months or years, patients will naturally begin to develop and discover self-help coping skills. They will learn these skills to help tolerate the pain, tenderness, aching, and fatigue. Other patients find ways to compensate for the poor sleep and daily fatigue. Still others will evolve past emotional stress issues, thus improving symptoms. They feel like they are, in a way, cured. So the doctor believes he has succeeded and will attempt to capitalize on it.

Reason number two: The patient never had fibromyalgia in the first place. For example, a patient consults a chiropractic physician and begins to receive treatment. Some weeks later, the patient feels 100 percent better. Or maybe the patient is under medical management, taking prescriptions for inflammatory symptoms, and then she is all better. These two sample patients were most likely misdiagnosed initially, or had come up with their own diagnosis originally and the doctors they were working with chose not to confirm it. So please consider the source of your diagnosis. Fibromyalgia labels are not always true or classic fibromyalgia; many are fibromyalgia-like conditions.

Attitude

When acknowledging the human side of doctors, it's not hard to imagine them feeling that they should or could be all things to all people. After all, that's what their academic education strives to instill: confidence. But some come across as self-absorbed and arrogant. I say this not because most doctors are this way—it just seems like fibro patients run across these doctors more frequently than the general population of patients do. This poses an added challenge to Fibros. As a Fibro, the last thing you need is another challenge. If you have a suspicion that your doctor—or anyone else that you're working with— has a closed mind, has misunderstandings or misconceptions about fibromyalgia, or restricts your possibilities to the arrogance of their education, it may be time to find another doctor.

Remember, as you develop your vocabulary and your understanding, it will be your job as your own head coach to put together the "right team." There's absolutely no room for attitude. Later we'll go over some effective interviewing techniques to weed out some of these different types of doctors and attitudes.

It's clear that a multidisciplinary approach to fibromyalgia is the best hope. This approach utilizes the best of medical science and non-medical science, taking advantage of each of their arts, paradigms, knowledge, and understanding to expand possibilities for you. It's up to you to maintain the attitude of a coach and make a decision about who will be on your medical and non-medical health team.

Medical and Non-medical Doctors

For now, let's acknowledge that there are two broad groups of doctors.

Medical doctors: Medical connotes medicine--"of or relating to the science of medicine or to the treatment of patients by drugs and or surgery."

Non-medical doctors: "Of or relating to the science of treatment disease without the use of drugs or surgery, emphasizing prevention and robust health."

Regardless of specialties or subspecialties, doctors put many years into studying their science and their art. While their art and paradigm may differ, their intent is the same: to improve the human condition. It's unfortunate that many doctors don't understand disciplines/specialties outside their own "doctor culture."

The science of pain management and wellness care is evolving rapidly. New drugs, nuclear medicine, arthroscopic surgery, robotics, and nanotechnology have revolutionized the practice of medicine. There's also telemedicine with patient–doctor and doctor-doctor management via phone, e-mail, and internet. Your medical doctor (MD) is no longer the pill-and-potion-pusher your great-grandparents remember. By the same token, the largest body of non-medical physicians, at least in the United States and Canada, is chiropractors. Chiropractic has evolved to the subtleties of neuromuscular and neurobiological imbalances, as has the science of nutrition and laser therapy for noninvasive pain management. This has revolutionized the practice of chiropractic. Your chiropractor (DC) is no longer the back-cracker your grandparents remember.

Philosophy
All doctors are working with the same science, anatomy, and physiology. The difference is in the approach—the art and paradigm. We see similar challenges when contrasting Eastern medicine with Western medicine: same science but different approach, art, and paradigm. This understanding can greatly influence your decisions and your course of treatment, as well as the type of team you put together. Remember, you're looking for open-minded doctors who are educated and aware enough to help you negotiate the maze of possibilities, and not just within the confines of their office or group. If you're currently working with a Non-medical doctor, possibly a chiropractor, you'll want to decipher three things as quickly as possible. First, does he/she believe in fibromyalgia and understand what you're going through? Second, does he/she understand the need for medical co-management? You don't want to work with a doctor who has an attitude toward medicine. Third, the chiropractor or naturopath must not attempt to restrict your efforts or your care to non-medical means.

By the same token, if you are currently working with an MD, you must pose the same questions. Does he believe in fibromyalgia and understand what you're going through? Does he understand that chiropractic, neurobiological medicine, and functional medicine are necessary in fibromyalgia management, or does he have an attitude reminiscent of 40 years ago? Lastly, does he want to restrict your treatment to medicines? By the way, this is not theoretical information. You absolutely must have medical and non-medical doctors in place if you are to help the progress of your body's potential.

Good News and Bad News

Once again, here's the bad news first. The job of being a good patient and a good student of fibromyalgia can be overwhelming, especially when discovering things that you don't feel you should have to have the responsibility to deal with. You've been taught all along that we should put our trust in doctors. Many years ago, I met a great man from Algeria. His name was Hakim. Hakim was a devoted spiritual man. He told me of a saying in his religion: "Trust in God, but tie up your camel." As your own advocate, as the coach of your health team, tying up your camel means doing the best you can to know more than your doctor knows. I don't mean the academics, biology, neurology, etc., or how to interpret blood tests—but the basics, the lay of the land, the multidisciplinary possibilities in health care delivery. By doing so, you can at least guide and set the tone and attitude of your team. You will be able to ask better questions—important questions that can make all the difference in the world to you and your family.

The Good News

The good news is that you've now begun to build a solid foundation of awareness and realistic perspective about doctors and fibromyalgia. You're developing a broader vocabulary that will serve you well. As we've mentioned earlier, when the learning and discovery process gets to be uncomfortable, you're quite possibly closer to discovering some piece of information that have been missing—a seemingly little piece of information that will help you discover something that's been holding you back from getting better. It could be a piece of information that will resonate in your heart, and stimulate your mind, letting you know that you are on the right track, possibly a new track with the right doctor/doctors. Be patient with yourself. Don't forget you're human, too. Remember, in this game you are the coach.

Perspective

We're going to take another look into the perspective of medical and non-medical care. To do this we need to discuss Eastern medicine vs. Western medicine.

Your judgment and your ability to put your personal health team in place will necessitate a perspective of Eastern and Western medicine. The distinction will clarify doctors and caregivers that you seek out, as well as knowing if you have found the medical doctor (a believer, and an enthusiastic believer) who can offer you not only good medical advice but possibly serve to co-coach and be a teammate all at the same time.

It may feel that I'm being condescending to medicine/medical care. However, it's quite the contrary. I believe that "the right doctor," primarily a medical doctor, should be in the foreground of the diagnostic process. This pivotal doctor must be open-minded and have understanding and enthusiasm to co-manage your condition with other disciplines. I am intentionally being disparaging and condescending. It's done to acknowledge the disparity of information, power, and influence that the medical and pharmaceutical industries exert on our society—on you, me and the media.

Eastern Medicine vs. Western Medicine

Consider the fact that doctors, both medical and non-medical, will see the fibromyalgia patient through the eyes of their education, beliefs, paradigms, and the mentorship of their predecessors, all of which colors their perspective and their reality. As it is for all people, perspective and reality is dynamic, ever-changing. What's real and valid today is not only different from year to year, day to day, and patient to patient, but is different from discipline to discipline, doctor to doctor, from Eastern medicine to Western medicine. This mindset of what's real will dictate the types of questions that a doctor is able to pose intellectually on the path to diagnosing and treating each patient.

Different doctors and different disciplines pose different questions. That's why they get different answers. When we ask better questions, we get better answers. When we ask more diverse disciplinary questions, we not only get better answers, we get multidimensional answers, the likes of which may change the course of someone's suffering and life. Obviously we're focusing on fibromyalgia, but all patients and human conditions stand to benefit. Doctors, like everyone else, have patterns of thinking and questioning, as well as anecdotes that recycle in their brains, like a menu that their brains default to. When the main menu is accessed, it reinforces itself as accurate and true information. However, it's likely to stifle creativity in the art of doctoring. This goes back to why there is *no* one doctor who's the right doctor. Let me give you an example.

Example: An Eastern medical doctor inherently has an Eastern medical philosophy and therefore is likely not to ask the question, "Should I prescribe Synthroid or Armor Thyroid for my patient diagnosed with hypothyroidism?"

This doctor would ask the question, "Should I prescribe a food high in iodine such as kelp, wild-caught fish, or possibly iodized salt to help support my patient's thyroid weakness?"

What does this mean to a fibromyalgia sufferer?

It helps to put doctoring into a finer perspective. As we look more closely at Eastern and Western approaches, I think you'll see how it will help you and direct your care in integrating medical care with non-medical care.

Eastern Medicine

Eastern medicine refers primarily to medicine of Chinese origin. In 1985, I studied at the Nanjing College of Traditional Chinese Medicine on mainland China. I studied acupuncture, herbal medicine, Qigong, energy medicine and, an ancient art called Tui Na. Tui Na is a combination of what we know in the West as orthopedics, physical therapy, chiropractic, and massage. All are intended to help the body heal itself. Let's acknowledge that the body is an amazing machine that has the ability to heal itself, if not interfered with. The ability to heal is primarily under the control of the master control system, namely the brain and nervous system. When you cut yourself, the doctor takes credit for the stitches, but the healing comes from the inside out, beginning with the brain's ability to interpret, manage, and orchestrate healing at the site. This is a pivotal concept acknowledged by East and West, medical and non-medical. However, in everyday practice, particularly in the West, it's overlooked. Or maybe it's taken for granted; nevertheless, it makes a difference as to how a doctor practices.

My studies in China helped me to reinforce the reality, relationship, and exchange that flow between living tissues. I realized that the lines are blurred, with no distinct separation between time, space, motion, rest, sickness, or health. Rather, there is only a gradient of relative distinction, and the balance between health and disease is fragile. There is no right, there is no wrong, and our perspective, philosophy, and beliefs are determined by the eyes that we see through.

The physical is not distinct from the human spirit; nor is one more valuable or corruptible than the other. Neither should be left out of the clinical picture when diagnosing and treating. Admittedly, this might be too philosophical, but nevertheless it holds some valuable lessons of how and why traditional Western medicine has failed the Fibro community.

Western Medicine

Western medicine historically has adopted a paradigm that separates humans into parts and systems. This is applied to academics as well as in a clinical setting. It has seen us as physically distinct from our spirit, energy, essence, or life force which ironically is ultimately responsible for life and healing. This paradigm was originally adopted in an effort to afford structure for learning as well as developing theories—called "scientific theories." It brought control, power, and lines of demarcation with religion. This formed an elite "club" if you will; which agreed to be committed only to those things that could be repeated and that everyone could agree on. Western medicine therefore viewed the body as basically a machine of parts to be dealt with as if only to have physical connections—and no medically relevant connections to other people or to nature.

I don't believe that our medical forefathers really believed the simplicity of these principles but never the less believed "medicine" and "science" would be served. What's unfortunate is that the mindset became cemented in with a consciousness that pushed energetic relationships within the body to the fringes of critical thinking. It has in many ways stalled progress. Contemporarily; instead of all principles conforming to the scientific theory, medicine has begun to judge risk and reward balances which allows for convenient and profitable compromise of the "parts and systems" version of scientific principles. This has been an unspoken shift in recognizing its incompleteness when considering the human condition.

If these concepts interest you, consider reading:
Power and Force by David Hawkins, MD
Between Heaven and Earth by Harriett Beinfield and Efrem Korngold
Energy Medicine by Dr. James Oschman

Fibromyalgia and Integrative Options

Most countries now have a dichotomy in health care, categorizing doctors, as aforementioned, as medical or non-medical. I've listed the doctors that are most important to consider for a Fibro health team. All of the doctors listed below are considered to be physicians by the

US Health Education and Welfare and are licensed accordingly, except for acupuncturists.

Doctors, Medical:

Primary Care Physician
Rheumatologist
Neurologist
Orthopedist
Endocrinologist
Psychologist
Osteopath

Doctors, Non-medical:

Chiropractor
Naturopath
Acupuncturist

I don't want to insult any other professions, therapists, or caregivers. Clearly there are other disciplines such as APRNs, physical therapists, massage therapists, and those with advanced degrees in nutrition who could very effectively round out your health team. The medical community will continue their intensity with diagnostic and surgical technology, and pharmaceutical superiority--and frankly, I wouldn't have it any other way. Who would want to live somewhere that doesn't have great medical care? But we're here to talk about fibromyalgia, and as strange as it may sound, comprehensive "medical care" is just not enough; comprehensive "health care" is the answer The nonmedical categories may need a little more explanation; however, we will start off with medical.

Medical Doctors

Whether PCPs (general practitioners, internists), rheumatologists, neurologists, or osteopaths, they will all have the same basic paradigm. Each of them, however, may have special interests. You'll find that a great place to start would be with your PCP. Also, the way many insurance policies work these days, your PCP may be a necessary place to start for your best advantage to access insurance benefits. Your insurance company may look at this doctor as a type of gatekeeper. Insurance companies will feel that they have the most control over costs by insisting that your health care efforts begin here. More costly insurance products will give you more flexibility and freedom of choice. But generally, benefits are shrinking and premiums rising; a fibromyalgia patient can expect to carry the financial load.

Rheumatologists

Rheumatologists are medical doctors with advanced and specialized training, mostly concerned with inflammatory, autoimmune, and soft-tissue conditions involving pain, such as arthritis, rheumatoid arthritis, gout, lupus, and tendinitis, as well as fibromyalgia, to name a few. Rheumatologists are generally classified as musculoskeletal specialists, although it's not that cut and dried.

Primary Care Physician (PCP)

PCPs are the family doctor or general practitioner that our parents remember. They will usually be your first contact for health problems, as well as ongoing medical wellness care. Lately, urgent care and walk-in care are centers are popping up. They take the place of a family doctor and seem to be a little more efficient, but lack establishing a more traditional relationship. However they serve immediacy, convenience, and cost control. These practitioners are diverse and well-rounded within the medical paradigm. PCPs make a relatively high percentage of referrals to other medical doctors. Once fibromyalgia is suspected, there is likely to be a referral to a rheumatologist or neurologist for an opinion/diagnosis. If fibromyalgia is confirmed first, medical effort would consist of medications such as Lyrica, antidepressants, or sleep aids.

Functional Medicine

There are chiropractors, naturopaths, and medical doctors who practice "functional medicine." However, this section is about medical doctors. Whoever it is that's practicing functional medicine will generally take a more subtle integrative approach to the relationship between physiological systems and lifestyle. The medical doctors who practice functional medicine tend to specialize, due to the fact that they don't receive the training in medical school. They will incorporate some of the so-called "natural" approaches that chiropractors, naturopaths, and osteopaths have respected for 100 years. Non-medical doctors head the charge toward health care by default, while the brilliance of traditional medicine keeps us alive in spite of life-threatening illnesses and injuries. Medical doctors who have matriculate into a functional medical practice are wonderful additions to a system that has traditionally been focused on illness.

Osteopaths

Osteopaths (DO) have a historical philosophy, art, and education, as chiropractic physicians do, with the addition of minor surgery. They also prescribe pharmaceutical treatments. So, at present, while they function as medical doctors, they are not technically considered allopathic physicians, as medical doctors are. Osteopathic philosophy and practice focus on a more holistic approach, the way functional specialists like chiropractors or naturopaths would. They acknowledge that all bodily systems are interconnected and that the musculoskeletal system is especially important, as it affects all other conditions and systems of the body. Some DOs play the role of the PCP, particularly in more rural areas of the country.

Chiropractic Doctors

I'll talk a little more about chiropractic simply because it's the largest non-drug, non-surgical health-care profession in the United States and Canada. Chiropractors and chiropractic specialize in neurobiological systems. Chiropractic's paradigm and portal of entry to influence neurological and biological systems of the body is through the neurology of movement and structure, sometimes termed physical medicine. Chiropractic's adjunct focus is on lifestyle and nutrition. Unfortunately, in spite of the need for comprehensive health care, chiropractic has been in the shadows due to the lack of publicity and funding from the big money of pharmaceutical and technology companies that the medical community has prospered from. The simple reason is that pharmaceutical companies and big technology have not found a way to make money off the chiropractic profession.

Chiropractic awareness has inspired more and more people to demand less medication and fewer surgeries. Pharmaceutical companies are taking note of a possible opportunity to expand their drug market. It has been proposed that chiropractors shift their philosophy and paradigm to include prescribing anti-inflammatories and pain medication. I believe there's a pharmaceutical experiment taking place as I write, encouraging chiropractors in New Mexico to prescribe drugs. Many multidimensional facilities are springing up throughout the country, which include MDs, chiropractors, naturopaths, and physical therapists. Many hospitals are staffing chiropractors in their "integrative health" departments.

I won't get into the philosophy of why chiropractic has not wanted to participate in prescribing medicine; suffice it to say that chiropractic is not about the practice of medicine. It's different. If the New Mexico experiment proves profitable, big pharma will push for chiropractors in all states to prescribe and will subsequently infuse money into the profession. This scenario worries me, as it would blur the line between medical and non-medical doctors, similar to the lack of clarity between medical and osteopathic. Although it would help more people to be aware of the opportunities that chiropractic holds for them, I see it as a long-term negative for societal health. We already have great medical doctors serving up more prescriptions than any other country in the world. What Fibros need is a better balance, more choices, and diverse opportunities—not more doctors prescribing. The best of medicine from medical doctors, and the best of non-medicine health care via non-medical specialists, will serve best. For now, awareness and education will help bring the patient to confident self-advocacy and a healthy balance between the two.

Fibromyalgia protocols, as well as the diagnosis, treatment, and management of other chronic pain conditions, are evolving rapidly. The medical community has developed new drugs, nuclear medicine, arthroscopic surgery, robotics, and specialized imagery that have revolutionized the practice of medicine. Chiropractic has evolved to the subtleties of neurobiological imbalances and their relationship to the structural/dynamic influences of the spine and central nervous system.

Naturopathic Doctors

Naturopathic medicine is based on the belief that the human body has an innate healing ability. Naturopathic doctors (NDs) teach their patients to use diet, exercise, lifestyle changes, and natural therapies to enhance the body's ability to ward off and combat disease. Naturopathic physicians craft comprehensive treatment plans that blend the best of modern medical science and traditional natural medical approaches to treat disease and to restore health.

The past 30 years have seen an extraordinary increase in consumer demand for safe, effective, and cost-effective natural health care, along with chiropractic. Naturopathic medicine has emerged as the health care profession best suited to meet this demand. Although naturopathy almost disappeared in the mid-twentieth century because of the popularity of drugs and surgery, naturopathic medicine has resurfaced and now offers safe, effective natural therapies as a vital part of the health-care systems of North America.

Acupuncturists

While most acupuncturists are not licensed as doctors in the United States, I've included them in this category due to their increasing popularity. There are also physicians—medical and chiropractic—who have taken certification in acupuncture and incorporate it into their practices. Regardless of the primary licensure, I would look for advanced and official certification to have been documented. Traditional acupuncture involves the stimulation of points by penetrating the skin with needles that are then manipulated manually or by electrical stimulation. It is one component of traditional Chinese medicine (TCM), and is among the oldest healing practices in the world. According to TCM, stimulating specific acupuncture points corrects imbalances in the flow of qi (energy) through channels known as meridians. TCM addresses the importance of balanced flow of energy through meridians the way US physicians see the importance of balanced neurology and hormones in sustaining health and healing. One of the problems you'll find is that the designation and credentials of acupuncturists are wide and varied. Listed are some of the credentials/licensure you may find:

- American Academy of Medical Acupuncture (AAMA)
- Master's in Acupuncture (MAc),
- Masters of Science in Acupuncture (MSAc, MSOM)
- Masters of Science in Oriental Medicine (MSOM)
- Masters of Acupuncture & Oriental Medicine (MSOM)
- Master of Acupuncture & Oriental Medicine (MAOM)
- National Certification Commission for Acupuncture and Oriental Medicine (NCCAOM)
- Doctor of Acupuncture & Oriental Medicine (DAOM)

As you can see, with so many designations, how would you choose whom to go to? My recommendation is to depend on the health team you have put together and look for someone who has successfully graduated from an accredited facility, and who specializes in acupuncture and/or TCM. Try to stay clear of physicians, medical or chiropractic, who have taken a certification course and wish to incorporate acupuncture as an adjunct into their practice. You wouldn't want your MD, massage therapist, or physical therapist who has taken a course in manipulation to be manipulating your spine. You would want someone who specializes in and dedicates their life and practice to neurobiology concerns via spinal health: namely, a chiropractor. In the same way, you want someone who is dedicated to the art and science of acupuncture to work with you using traditional Chinese medicine.

Physical Therapy

Physical therapy (PT) is a profession primarily concerned with the remediation of impairments and disabilities and the promotion of mobility, functional ability, quality of life, and movement potential. Physical therapists participate in examination, evaluation, and diagnosis of symptoms and symptom complexes. There are different levels of physical therapy credentials. There are physical therapist assistants (PTA), masters in physical therapy (MPT) and doctors of physical therapist (PhD). Physical therapists are not presently considered physicians; however, I want to include them in this category. First, they are direct access, meaning a person does not need a doctor's referral to see a PT. (This is true in all but two states in the US.) Second, I'm particularly impressed with postgraduate PT certification in what's called Integrated Manual Therapy (IMT). It was developed by Sharon Giamatteo, PhD. She explains: "IMT is a unique compilation of diagnostic and treatment methodology that assesses and treats pain, dysfunction, disease, and disability." It is primarily a hands-on therapy and integrates a wide range of efforts including diet, nutrition, and herbs. As chiropractic, naturopathic and traditional osteopathic would also express, IMT's philosophy is: "The body's tissue has the ability to heal on its own if given a chance and not interfered with." IMT looks to integrate how emotions and stress as well as physical and chemical influences on the body affect muscles and joints, bones, fascia, nerves, circulation, and lymphatic structures. IMT gently integrates the wisdom of the practitioner with the patient's body. These specialized techniques are offered as postgraduate work for physical therapists, medical doctors, and chiropractic physicians. However, presently they are primarily a physical therapy advanced study. All physicians treating fibromyalgia would be prudent to become familiar enough with Dr. Giamatteo's work to consider a referral when appropriate.

Failed System

Why has our system become unbalanced and failed the fibromyalgia sufferer? The failure must be shared between medical as well as non-medical specialties.

The flaws in the Western medical doctors' arena through the years are:

1. It's too easy.
   The practice of medicine calls upon people to do next to nothing and to take little or no action until diagnosis. Even

then, when it comes to treatment, it is the easiest approach to continue calling upon patients to do not much more than take their pills, promising quick-fix results. Pills usually work just to cover up symptoms.

2. The culture of medicine's commitment to an exclusive-paradigm, along with political and pharma funding throughout history, have routinely deterred if not fought against and/or blocked patients from seeking other possibilities outside of medicine. Medicine will defend its position as being "in the interest of the patient," alleging that practices not of a medical paradigm are unscientific. In actuality, the science is the science, but there is a lack of understanding of the difference in treatment, fostering poor communication—hence supporting their belief that medicine can be all things to all people. Harriet Beinfield, LAc And Efrem KorngoldL. Ac, OMD in their book *Between Heaven and Earth* pose the following question:

> "Longevity has changed little, and major illnesses such as malignancy and cardiovascular disease remain unimpeded.... Illnesses disproportionately affect the poor, major environmental and occupational causes of illnesses receive little attention and less action... Clearly, there is a crisis in health care, both in its effect upon health and in its cost... Some medical outcomes are inadequate not because appropriate technological interventions are lacking, but because our conceptual thinking is inadequate. Modern medicine directs its gaze through a microscope so that detail is gained within a restricted visual field. Specialists look at smaller and smaller fragments, gaining more and more positive information in the form of descriptive data but losing a sense of the integrity of the system as a whole. How did this medical model gain exclusive ascendance in America?"

3. The medical community, I believe with good intention, assures themselves of and believes in everything that they

say, with an arrogance they very well may deserve. Yet it doesn't serve medicine or society as assuredly. They are focused on the science and art within a relatively narrow culture. Their minds are only beginning to be open to Eastern and non-medical disciplines. However, there is a bright light on the horizon: the influx of doctors from India, China, Pakistan, and Latin America. They are trained medically but understand the value and the integration of East and West, medical and non-medical. They have helped to inspire integrative facilities within formerly exclusive MD hospitals. Dr. Kiran Dintyala, MD from Hartford Hospital in Hartford, Connecticut, noted that "Western medicine is beginning to think out of the box."

Where Are We Now?

Over the past ten years or so, financial pressures have inspired integrative facilities that combine medical and non-medical alliances. These alliances contradict the AMA's historic attitudes of autonomy and superiority. They include combining medical services with chiropractic, acupuncture, physical therapy, nutrition, and homeopathy. Sadly, it's capitalism that has driven integration rather than an innate calling to serve. It has become harder and harder for doctors of all disciplines to balance finances in light of the playing field that insurance companies have put in front of them. It's become nearly impossible for a sole practitioner to be successful and meet school loan and equipment payments, as well as overhead and malpractice insurance.

Insurance companies have serendipitously fostered more balanced and comprehensive health care. They have done this by increasing deductibles and co-pays, restricting benefits, and generally burdening the physician as well as the patient in their effort to receive and deliver comprehensive health care. This in turn has forced adaptions/creative capitalism that in retrospect I believe will prove to be a step forward to the camaraderie, inter-professional understanding, and respect that we should have been able to accomplish by physician-driven service, dedication, understanding and communication.

Non-medical

The largest group of non-medical doctors in the United States and Canada is chiropractic physicians. They also bring their share of flaws to health care.

1. It's too hard sometimes.
   Chiropractic, in many cases, is seen as too difficult. Instead of sitting home and taking a pill three times a day, the "medicine" is likely to be in-office treatment three times per week (at least initially). Additionally, patients are most often asked to participate and take further responsibility, with home care as an adjunct to treatment, addressing nutrition, exercise, and/or behavioral and environmental issues. Most people either don't want or are too busy to take that much responsibility. So they look to use chiropractic as a quick fix (aspirin chiropractic).
2. Chiropractic has a commitment to its paradigm as well. While the science is the same, the language is different, making for poor communication and misunderstandings. This is a perfect environment for each profession to remain arrogant, convinced that they can be all things to all people. Unfortunately, chiropractic is as guilty as MDs having under-referred to the other.

Shared Flaw

The flaws shared equally between chiropractic and medicine are:

- Each is doggedly committed, believing that somehow the science behind their special paradigm is unique, when in fact there is no difference. As stated above, the science is the science. However, there is a difference in philosophy and application. This is an advantage to patients as long as they can avail themselves of the best of each.
- Neither refers to the other as frequently as they should.
- Neither has the will or the financial luxury to take the time to educate people with enough substance to effectively participate in their care and advocate for themselves; consequently, there is a mystery to health care and a dependency that has not served the fibromyalgia community well. People are relegated to bits and pieces of disarticulated information through the media.

Confident Self-Advocacy in the Making

As your vocabulary and understanding of interdisciplinary possibilities improve, you will find yourself better able to communicate, asking better questions in order to negotiate your path. This will help to round out your health team, your lifestyle, family, and finances.

Plus you will have less pain, more energy, and have less need for drugs; maybe no need at all.

Diagnosis

A clear medical diagnosis must come first, ruling out all the other possibilities that could account for your aches, pains, stiffness, fatigue, digestive problems, poor sleep, mood swings, brain fog, twitching legs, tingling, numbness, burning, fatigue, etc. This should be handled by an MD. This doesn't mean that your MD should captain your ship, however. Let's put into perspective who is best suited to be the captain of your health team; that is, who would have the most comprehensive perspective of health care and be a diversified thought leader in managing your team, and at the same time be a good coach for you and help you manage the ever-changing course of fibro.

You'll generally find that a naturopathic physician will be the best candidate for the job, but you must find one who can bridge the communication gap with your MDs and of course be an "enthusiastic believer." This doesn't change the fact that with few exceptions he/she will still not be the doc to make the primary diagnosis; you'll still need your MD for that, and to manage medical issues.

If you happen to be a person who is strongly non-medically oriented, and well familiar with chiropractic, naturopathy, and/or Eastern medicine, don't turn off and close your mind to appropriate medical diagnosis and treatment; they will be necessity in the course of things. By the same token, if you are emotionally and socially committed to medical treatment to the exclusion of non-medical balance, don't close your mind to greater possibilities unless you feel great and you're back to your old self.

Allow the rest of the book to round out your understanding and bring clarity to the science, anatomy, and physiology of medicine and chiropractic. Don't be so convinced that you already know what naturopathy or chiropractic is or isn't, simply because you've been under care or someone else has tried to convince you that either one is the Holy Grail—all things to all people; they're not. By the same token, if medicine were all things to you, you wouldn't be reading this book. Be patient, and subsequently you can make up your own mind as to how chiropractic or naturopathy may change your course (or not).

The same can be said for all other disciplines and approaches that you'll read about in later chapters. We will touch on approaches that include meditation, nutrition, tai chi, yoga, and biofeedback, to name a few. Whether or not you simply stay on the same path you are on now, reading the book is guaranteed to change the conversation in your head as well as with your doctors, friends, and family.

Eastern Medical Doctors

When I speak of Eastern medicine, I'm speaking more in terms of the philosophy and the acknowledgement of its comfort speaking about "energy" as a component of health to be dealt with. The fact that there are things that take place in and around our bodies that have not been explained yet, and cannot be qualified or quantified, doesn't mean they don't exist and are not important. The West has taken them out of the equation by choice in an effort to understand and control the pieces more objectively. Objectively means "in terms of Western perspective." Therefore, the West sees the East's holistic approach as nothing more than hypotheses, experimental or unscientific.

Most people reading this book believe in God (however you personally would acknowledge God). Yet by Western scientific standards, a God cannot be.

Western medicine has a strong pull and influence when we see its amazing feats in saving lives. The emotions and finances of these accomplishments distract us from more fundamental questions of why so many people's lives are threatened prematurely in terms of quality, if not longevity. One of the reasons may be that Western medicine is amazingly accomplished as a disease-care system versus the fundamental non-medical and Eastern medical "health" system. I'm not suggesting you can tai chi your way out of fibromyalgia; nevertheless, these considerations must be balanced within a self-advocacy effort.

The Fibromyalgia Solution

Let's agree that you can't tai chi your way out of fibromyalgia, chiropractic is not the Holy Grail, and the pharmaceutical industry can create all the specialized drugs they want (and they do) and then deliver them via amazing medical doctors, yet still not resolve fibromyalgia. The fibro solution lies in a multidisciplinary approach that brings an integrative balance to you, your health, and our collective future. By now I'm sure you're recognizing the redundancy in this chapter as well as throughout the book. So humor me and let's backtrack to who has the responsibility, and how you are going to pick the right doctor.

A Question of Responsibility:

1. Who ultimately is responsible to understand and manage your fibro care? You are!
2. Which professional—medical or non-medical—ultimately should have the responsibility to diagnose fibromyalgia? A medical doctor!
3. What profession has the best vantage point to organize your personalized multi-disciplinary health team for you? A naturopathic doctor (possibly a chiropractor)!
4. Who has to do the work to find the "right doctors"? You do!

How to Find the Right Doctor

You already know the type of doctors you're looking for. Medical or non-medical, you're looking for a "believer" who is an "enthusiast." How will you find each? Many of you who are working with doctors now already know whether you have someone who can meet the challenges. You must be courageous enough not to stand on ceremony or be loyal to the doctor with whom you're working if he's not meeting your needs. And your doctor, whether medical or non-medical, is not meeting your needs if the thinking and the approach are not integrative. My suspicion is that many sufferers don't really know what their doctor thinks or knows about disciplines other than his own. So it may be time for you to re-evaluate your doctor, probing for his attitudes and understanding of other disciplines that might help you.

A word to the wise--just because fibromyalgia is predominantly considered to be under the auspices of an MD/rheumatologist does not mean that just any rheumatologist is the right one. He must still be capable of referring to, interested in, and respectful of other disciplines that offer you multidimensional and integrative options. Doctors who do a great job in the diagnosis department aren't necessarily capable of coaching your every effort to function better and live life more on your terms.

You're still going to need an "enthusiastic believer" in the chiropractic or naturopathic world who can then be your coach. When you re-interview your MD, you're looking for words that support your interest in reaching out to other disciplines and a willingness to assist you in doing so. Remember, fibromyalgia is a marathon, not a sprint. Take time to build your team and get the right doctors. You won't find them in the phone book under *"Physicians; Diversified Fibromyalgia Specialists."* You will have to depend on other Fibros or other care providers you're seeing. Don't hesitate to ask your dentist, gynecologist, or ophthalmologist. If the doctor you are working with doesn't already have this type of experience, he is probably a doctor who doesn't have as much interest in or doesn't do as much work with fibromyalgia as he says he does or as you thought he did. So you may have to start all over. It will be worth it.

The Interview

Make the Call

If you do have to start all over, take a look at the internet; you can research on LinkedIn, and the doctor's website. Check credentials, the words they use, their affiliations, bio, and practice focus. Don't be fooled by their affiliations, however. The affiliations don't necessarily make a statement about the competency or proficiency of the doctor, but they do give you some indication of what he or she has an interest in. If the doctor is a member of any fibromyalgia association or network, you can bet that she at least has more of an interest in fibromyalgia than a doctor who is not a member.

Next, you can make a phone call and chat with the person who does the scheduling. Ask questions that will give you a perspective as to how much interest the doctor has in and how much work the doctor does with fibromyalgia patients. I would then ask the office if it is possible to meet with the doctor and chat about the practice and experience with fibromyalgia before you make an official paying appointment. It seems to me that if a doctor really understands fibromyalgia patients, and the kind of attention and unique time required to help manage fibro, he or she will be willing to first meet with you informally (free). This would not be a consultation or a diagnostic visit. It would be a handshake to meet the doctor and get a hit on the doctor's attitude and bedside manner. It would be a relatively short meeting and you'd want to prepare two or three questions that you think would help target whether or not you'd want to make an official appointment. You may go through several of these interviews before you find someone in whom you believe you'd have confidence. Here are a few recommendations for questions:

1. How many fibromyalgia patients do you see in an average week?
2. Other than medication and exercise, are there any other types of doctor or therapy that might help?

Question number one: You're looking to get a feel for how many contact hours the doctor has with fibromyalgia patients. I would consider at least three to be encouraging.

Question number two: You're looking for attitude. You don't really care if your doctor personally recommends or refers you to other disciplines, but you're looking for an attitude that won't disparage other doctors or discourage/deter you from working with other disciplines. Now it certainly would be nice if your doctor already has a relationship with other disciplines, but at the very least he needs to have an attitude of acceptance and inclusion and be open-minded. You don't want someone who sees no clinical value in anything other than his own discipline.

Listen Closely

Your initial visit with the doctor will most likely be brief. The actual length of time is not as important as the doctor's demeanor. Does the doctor seem patient? Does he seem interested in you? Do you believe he has heard you? Does he seem distracted or in a hurry? Did he answer your questions clearly? Does he seem to be a good communicator? When you have the right medical doctor, everything will fall into place and you won't have to work as hard. With his experience with fibromyalgia and his understanding of fibromyalgia patients, he will customize examination and questioning procedures that will bring out the details of your case in a way that will help him decide on and direct the tests that need to take place.

In my practice, ideally I like to have the PCP onboard for general health concerns and regular physicals. And, of course, I want him to have that same open-mindedness regarding multidisciplinary value in helping the patient. Additionally, there must be open communication and understanding that there will be a rheumatologist involved for more of the specific medical and disease components involved with fibromyalgia and fibromyalgia-like or coexisting conditions. Knowing that those two components are being managed, I can then have the confidence to organize the neuromuscular/skeletal issues as well as help manage and direct other efforts, from detoxification to acupuncture, counseling, cranial work, cranial sacral work, laser therapy and nutrition, etc.

The Last Right Doctor

You'll have one more doctor to get clear about on your team. That will be the chiropractic physician or naturopath that you're either working with or whom you need to re-evaluate or re-interview with all the same criteria you used to judge your choice for medical doctor. The question that will change when interviewing the chiropractor is number two. When interviewing the chiropractor, the question will be: "Do you believe that you can thoroughly and definitively diagnose fibromyalgia, and if I really do have it, can you successfully treat it?" Fibromyalgia is not a problem that can be addressed strictly through chiropractic. If the chiropractor isn't clear as to the evolving sciences in neurobiology and the need for medical intervention, you probably have the wrong chiropractor and you'll need to continue to interview.

As I mentioned before, chiropractic addresses the finer points of neurobiology--and, of course, is a crucial component for your recovery. However, it must not be at the exclusion of a medical and naturopathic doctor's role. You should hold the chiropractor to the same open-minded need for diversity as you did your medical doctor. It's unfortunate that while chiropractic and/or naturopathy have the best vantage point for helping you steer day-to-day health options, you'll find just as many who are as closed-minded and arrogant as MDs.

The Science

The science and the need for medication and a PCP, as well as specialized rheumatologic involvement, will become clearer as we go on and discuss medications and the need for them based on what appears to be happening in your muscles, your joints, and your nervous system. Additionally, the science and the need to address your brain and central nervous system through structure (joints, muscles, ligaments, tendons, body mechanics, and posture) will become clear as well when we discuss physical medicine.

Health Costs

Just a few words about health costs in the real world: You may be disappointed to find that your insurance policy will not include/participate in any and all treatment your doctor feels you need or that you would like to avail yourself of. The reason is that somewhere along the line you will be deemed to be receiving maintenance or supportive care, wellness care, or what might fall under the term "risk and behavior." This becomes a sticky area of reimbursement and depends on how the policy you bought is written. You'll most likely have to re-sign yourself to self-funding many efforts out-of-pocket. Then there is Obama Care, assuming it is here to stay, which may come with higher deductibles and co-pays. Keep in mind that for your doctor to give you the kind of attention and time that you'll need/want to help negotiate and develop creative solutions, he will have to take time from other patients, and this will increase costs. Don't accept your insurance company playing *doctor* with your life.

From time to time, patients or even insurance company call centers will suggest that the doctor creatively code bills and procedures, suggesting that if the doctor simply changes the diagnosis or procedure codes to fit into the patient's policy reimbursement, everything will work out dandy. Creative coding is non-compliant and may be considered a federal offense/illegal if the doctor participates in any federal programs such as Medicare. These tactics jeopardize the doctor's participation with insurance companies, his or her state license, and possibly future patients' insurance coverage. I bring these matters up because it is simply naïve these days to think that insurance is there to cover everything and anything you or your doctor believe you need. Insurance is a business that sells a service contract to make a profit; a business can't make a profit if it gives more than was bought. For them it's about business/profit; for patients, regardless of what they bought, it's about health and need. Emotionally and financially they are diametrically opposed, especially when it comes to invisible disabilities, which include fibromyalgia, reflex sympathetic dystrophy, chronic fatigue, and chronic subluxation complex.

> Be prepared to put in the work and enough of your own money toward putting together a health team with diverse perspectives and opportunities to take advantage of all wisdom—not just conventional medical wisdom. Conventional wisdom has generally failed invisible disability sufferers. This brings us back to the patient having to be his or her own advocate. Doctors don't know what they don't know; the problem is that they often *think* they do know what they don't know. The patient must know.

CHAPTER 17

Diagnosis: The Story That Is Never Told!

**How is it that you believe you have the right
doctor and you've been diagnosed properly
(maybe) but you still need so much help?**

Chapter Topics:

Diagnostic Tests   *Primary Care Physician*
Fibro Impact Questionnaire *Functional Medicine*
Medical Doctor, MD   *Non-medical Doctors*
Rheumatologist, MD   *Chiropractic Doctor, DC*
Physical Therapist, PT   *Naturopathic Doctor, ND*

This section gets to the crux of the lies and the stumbling blocks inherent in traditional Western medicine. Using the word "lie" and "inherent" in the same sentence feels a bit contradictory. To me "lie" suggests intent; the word "inherent "suggests more of a natural characteristic, a right or privilege. What I really mean to say is that the characteristics, rights, privileges and paradigms of Western medicine must be rethought and retaught. They have outlived their effectiveness in health care; consequently, the inherent characteristics, rights, privileges and paradigms border on a blatant "lie." Women with fibromyalgia and chronic fatigue for the most part have already had to live with this "lie" far too long. Coming to terms with the reality of the science and times we live in and expanding our health-care perspective of possibilities is the only hope that sufferers have to effectively self-advocate. It's hard to win at self-advocacy without a complete diagnosis.

Diagnosis

Diagnosis is a process: an insightful calculated path, including and excluding possible causes, termed "differential diagnosis." This process is, in fact, an art, with one huge glitch. It is predicated on questions that develop within the confines of the doctor's clinical mind. The dilemma in diagnosing fibromyalgia, I believe, would be far from anything that you've read or heard in the past. This discussion will be politically incorrect; your doctor is likely to take exception to it. However, I'll bet it helps you to understand why you feel like you've been going around in circles to get answers.

The questions that evolve in a doctor's clinical mind can be only as resourceful as the physician's ability to diversify his thinking—to apply his art in the context of his education and experience. No one doctor or paradigm can cover the gamut of possibilities and unravel the many components and layers of symptoms that fibromyalgia sufferers live with. It's this very human and inherent inability to develop diagnostic questions outside of a doctor's education that is the glitch. Consequently many patients are swept along a diagnostic path helplessly assuming that their doctor's education, art, and paradigm cover all possibilities. The average patient is unable to pose questions herself as to whether other doctors or tests would be appropriate and needed to covers all the bases—or not.

Besides, it would be mutiny if the patient did pose questions that her doctor hasn't asked. So we have an inherent momentum and influence that has come up short clinically. The solution to this dilemma lies in the patient's ability to expand her own education and knowledge, striving to self-advocate and help steer the process. Let me give you a couple of examples of what I mean:

Example 1: Let's say you have low back pain with muscle spasms as well as pain down your legs, and it's particularly noticeable when going upstairs. You decide to seek help by contacting a chiropractic physician. After examination, a diagnosis is matched with what chiropractors do (their art and education)—namely, "physical medicine" treatment, which may include non-force manipulative therapy as well as laser therapy, ice and rest, followed by a program of home exercise and possibly referral for a massage.

The goal: to improve/correct abnormal neurobiology via the spine, helping the body to naturally reduce inflammation and re-establish painless movement. This is an artful and calculated path that has led to a diagnosis and subsequent treatment. In and of itself, this doesn't seem to pose a problem.

The chiropractor's clinical mind would rarely discuss with the patient that a medical doctor could prescribe anti-inflammatories or painkillers that may bring relief faster, nor would a patient ask. One reason is that the patient probably tried medication first (most do) but that's beside the point. Another reason is that most people go to a chiropractor because they don't want to take any more drugs than they absolutely have to, but that's not the point either. The point is that this scenario is an example of a proprietary path obligated to a specific education and professional paradigm that sets the course for diagnosis and treatment.

Example 2: Now let's take the same patient with the same low-back pain, muscle spasms, and leg pain, most noticeable when going upstairs. This time the patient consults a medical doctor first. Medical education, art, and paradigm will dictate the diagnostic process, and subsequently render a diagnosis and treatment plan as in Example#1. Medical doctors do what medical doctors do: namely, try to help a person as much as possible to reduce the pain and get on with their lives, most likely in this case through prescribing anti-inflammatories or painkillers, and possibly muscle relaxers. Subsequently, the doctor may judge that physical therapy is necessary. The goal is to reduce the pain that is the consequence of a medically diagnostic conclusion, namely inflammation and muscle spasm.

Here we have the same symptoms but a different perspective on what the cause is, and different treatment recommendations. In both cases, the patient is swept along the diagnostic path to a therapeutic regime without the advantage of adequate information to rationalize and draw any basic conclusions or generate questions in their own mind—if not in the doctor's mind—opening the door to options.

So here again we have an example of a proprietary path obligated to a specific education and professional paradigm that sets the course for diagnosis and treatment. This is simply not good enough for fibro sufferers; it's too shallow and limiting.

However, this is not the end of the story, but rather, the beginning of the problem. Let's now say the symptoms subsequent to treatment return, as they tend to do with fibromyalgia.

Now the patient must enter into another path with inherent momentum that is too shallow and limiting and had already come up short the last time around. The process is repeated and completely controlled by the doctor each time, due to two main factors.

Doctors, all doctors, have the responsibility to explain the diagnostic process and treatment options, and most of them do. However, doctors most likely will have the discussion within the paradigm of their discipline, and that's the point: "within their discipline." That is the box from which all reasoning/thought springs. This is just not good enough. The patient is doomed to repeat a clinical path—and often the same outcome—over and over, until they are frustrated enough to take their own initiative and find an alternative, another type of doctor with a different paradigm.

Fibromyalgia patients run around in frustrated circles trying to get answers and help until they break out of the "one doctor" management model. One doctor means only one paradigm. Ninety percent of medical doctors have medical-culture blinders on. They are locked into a Western medical paradigm, as we discussed; hence they limit possibilities, which is detrimental to the fibromyalgia sufferer's future. Non-medical doctors are no less blinded by their paradigm. However they refer to MDs more frequently, which is encouraging.

You will read time and time again that I believe a medical doctor, in particular a rheumatologist, should take the primary role in fibromyalgia diagnosis. The roles may reverse when we discuss long-term management of symptoms and the layers of physiological dysfunction accounting for chronic fatigue, myofascial pain syndrome, irritable bowel syndrome, etc., when a *health* plan must be put in place rather than the medical diagnosis and management of symptoms only.

But let's stay on point. We're talking about getting to a proper diagnosis first. In the grand scheme of things, we have to consider that there are some doctors who are best suited to order the tests to diagnose fibromyalgia. But different doctors may be best suited to order the tests that help direct and manage the health concerns of a fibromyalgia case. This means muscle, spine, and painful-movement issues, and functional issues such as diet, digestive/gut, and energy. (One caveat here: we will assume the diagnostic process did not uncover another medical condition that must be dealt with medically.) This whole section is to clarify that some conditions are medical and some are other than medical. The reality is that a medical doctor is incapable of diagnosing a chiropractic problem. The impediment to health care and the success of a fibro case specifically, is when MDs and DCs think they can autonomously diagnose and treat all aspects of a Fibro's case.

Definitions
Diagnose: To identify the nature and cause of something, in our case distinguishing one disease from another. To distinguish fibromyalgia from chronic-fatigue syndrome or rheumatoid arthritis, depression, etc.

Disease: Disturbance or loss of proper function, with measurable signs and symptoms.

Pathology: The understanding of the cause of the disease, especially as it applies to the structure and function of cells, nerves, tissue, organs, as well as musculoskeletal movement, as in kinesio- pathology.

Syndrome: Several clinical signs and symptoms coexisting that may or may not be related.

Symptoms: Observations reported by the patient.

Signs: Observations by someone other than the patient

Fibromyalgia Diagnosis

The diagnosis of fibromyalgia (identifying the cause) leading to a label of "fibromyalgia" has not yet completely crystallized. Contemporary neurology, as aforementioned, is very close to a unifying theory, however. Between advances in specialized scanning and laboratory studies, a clear objective diagnosis may be in our hands before you finish reading this book. But for now, the evaluation of structure and function of cells, nerves, tissues, and musculoskeletal movement takes us a long way toward devising physical and behavioral treatments, as well as drugs and emotional therapies, to help fibromyalgia sufferers.

What's more exciting is to use the same science to help prevent fibro—in effect, inoculating younger people who might be environmentally or genetically predisposed, thereby avoiding having to go down the same path as a parent or grandparent.

The Tests

There are many tests to be considered in the diagnostic process. A patient is unlikely to find any one doctor who would or could consider all the possible tests covering the range of physical, emotional, and chemical considerations. This, as we have discussed, is unfortunate because it puts an extra burden on the sufferer to learn and continue to self-advocate. However, once one self-advocates for a team of doctors who will communicate with each other, the job will become much easier. There are three layers of diagnostic and testing considerations.

1. The first layer of the testing process will be to order common medical diagnostic lab tests and likely will

progress to more specific tests to include or exclude fibro as a possible diagnosis. These tests will hopefully be ordered by a medical rheumatologist. The referral to a medical rheumatologist will most commonly be made by a PCP or chiropractor. Don't assume that a referral from one doctor to another means you have the right doctor; you'll still want to keep in mind what we've discussed in "Finding the Right Doctor."

2. The next layer of tests for consideration will generally be best handled by a doctor who specializes in functional medicine. This could be (in order of consideration) a functional medical specialist, a naturopath, and possibly a chiropractor.

3. The third layer—and arguably the most empowering components of the testing and diagnostic process—will necessitate a chiropractic physician who specializes in fibromyalgia and chronic-pain conditions or a physical therapist with special training in integrative manual therapies.

Conclusions

While lab tests are necessary they are unlikely to be definitive of the cause of chronic pain and the plethora of symptoms. Tests conducted on the first and main layer will help to eliminate conditions other than fibromyalgia that could account for symptoms. Therefore, we understand that fibromyalgia is a diagnosis by default/judgment simply because nothing else could explain the symptoms. Therefore, the primary medical goal in testing is to eliminate possibilities of such things as cancer, rheumatoid arthritis, lupus, and connective-tissue disease, to name a few.

Your second layer of tests will help to decipher complications and coexisting conditions or fibromyalgia look-alikes. These conditions include chronic fatigue syndrome or myofascial pain syndrome, as well as metabolic problems—e.g. irritable bowel syndrome, dysbiosis, toxicity issues, etc.

The third layer of tests necessitates an additional physician and focuses on the physical and functional components of painful movement, nerve irritation, and muscle and joint problems as they relate/affect the central nervous system. This understanding will shed light on perpetuating factors and complicating or exacerbating factors, as well as how congenital, developmental, or past injuries such as whiplash or abuse could have triggered fibromyalgia in the first place. These issues fall under the auspices of osteopathic and chiropractic diagnosis. There tends to be some confusion as to how chiropractic diagnosis relates to the chronic pain of fibromyalgia, so let's elaborate.

Using back pain as an example, lab tests can confirm that there is excessive inflammation and that various other diseases do not exist. An MRI may show a bulging disc, degeneration, or mal-positioning, any one of which may be judged as the cause of low back pain. A chiropractor will be able to determine if that's true, or if the pain is in fact coming from some other tissue, such as spinal joints, nerves, or ligamentous structures--either at the site of the pain, or possibly far removed; for instance, low back pain may be coming from the neck, and vice versa. This could be crucial to diagnosis and greatly change the treatment protocol, reducing the need for drugs, hence improving the clinical outcome with more conservative care. If this diagnostic step is missed, it can lead to permanent idiopathic pain that is unaffected by medication in any permanent way. Also, you'll remember that we discussed subluxation complex and its direct causal relationship via the spine to issues of central neurology, driving fibromyalgia within the brain circuitry. Chiropractors are the only physicians qualified to diagnose and treat subluxations.

Physical
Before lab tests or imaging has been ordered, a thorough history and physical examination, including assessing tender points, will commonly be conducted. The typical eleven out of eighteen possible tender points will be considered indicative of fibromyalgia, by most general practitioners. However, these tender points as originally defined by the American College of Rheumatology are nearly useless and given little to no diagnostic value. This has been confirmed by the most recent definition of fibromyalgia, in 2010, which basically states that fibromyalgia is depicted by pain that exists above and below your waist, as well as to the right and to the left of your midline. The rest is up to the doctor's judgment.

We won't discuss the rationale and the implication of every possible test; rather, I will cover the most important and common tests likely to be ordered. Additional tests will be decided by the individual doctor's judgment in respect to their particular paradigm. That means the most appropriate doctor noted when we described the three different layers of testing. I have listed the tests, as well as an indication of the doctors who are best qualified to order and interpret the tests.

Keep in mind that what I'm trying to put in perspective is that different doctors have different thought processes. For instance, it's not that a chiropractor couldn't order liver tests or a test for lupus; it's simply that your medical doctor is best-educated/suited to order, interpret, and subsequently manage a positive finding. By the same token, a medical doctor's education and daily paradigm makes him unsuited to diagnose subluxation in consideration of the spinal relation to issues of central neurology driving fibromyalgia.

The following chart is meant to help put in perspective the best doctor for the job. However, the possible tests and or physician specialties are not limited to this chart; rather, it depicts the most common that a patient will encounter.

Best Doctors for the Job:
Medical=MD, Chiropractic= DC, Physical Therapist=PT, Naturopathic =ND

TESTS

	Medical	Functional MD	DC	PT	ND
Complete Blood Count	✓	✓			
Fasting Blood Sugar	✓	✓			
Liver Tests	✓	✓			
Arthritic Panel	✓	✓			
Epstein-Bar	✓	✓			
Lupus	✓	✓			
Lyme Test	✓	✓			
C Reactive Protein	✓	✓			✓
Homocysteine	✓	✓			
Nutritional Panel		✓	✓		✓
Adrenal/Cortisol		✓	✓		✓
Thyroid		✓	✓		✓
Food Sensitivities		✓	✓		✓
Heavy Metals		✓	✓		✓
Digestive Stool Analysis		✓	✓		✓
Orthopedic Test	✓		✓	✓	
Neurological Evaluation	✓		✓		
Kinesiology			✓	✓	✓
Posture			✓	✓	
Joint/Movement			✓	✓	
Subluxation Complex			✓		
Gait/Posture			✓	✓	
Old Injuries			✓	✓	
Muscle Test			✓	✓	
Life Style & Diet		✓	✓	✓	✓
Radiology					
X-Rays/CT Scan	✓	✓	✓		
MRI	✓	✓	✓		
\					
EMG	✓	✓	✓		
Qualitative Sensory	✓	✓	✓		

Your Body

Because the first visit can be a bit nerve-racking, at least for most patients, some valuable information might be left out. You'll have a lot to talk about with the doctor, and he will also have a lot of questions for you. Being prepared with these forms helps you to clarify your thoughts and feelings as well as reduce possible misunderstandings of exactly what you're going through. Prepare these forms ahead of time and keep the master copy for yourself. Every doctor or therapist you go to is going to want basically the same information. You'll find that many times your copies suffice—but if not, you'll be able to fill out their paperwork quickly when you can refer back to what you prepared, and not have to rethink everything. The diagram below does a great job. It is a variation of a form originally designed by Dr. Paul St. Amand MD.[66]

Use the Letters Below to Indicate the Type and Location of Your Sensations Right Now

A= ache　　　B=burning　　　N=numb
S=stabbing　P=pins and needles　O=other

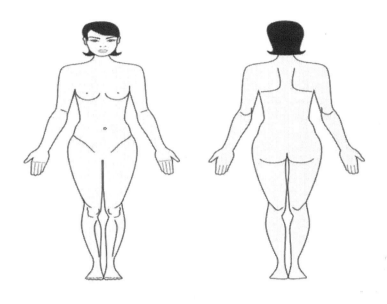

Fatigue	Hunger Tremors	Eye Irritations	Bloating	Chemical sensitivity
Irritability	Palpations	congestion	Constipation	Poor balance
Nervousness	Panic Attacks	Abnormal tastes	Diarrhea	Light irratation
Depression	Frontal Headaches	Gas	Salt craving	Odor Irratation
Insomnia	Occipital Headaches	Depression	Pungent Urine	Sound Sensitivity
Poor concentration	Sweating	Ringing ears	Bladder infections	Rashes
Poor Memory	Dizziness	Numbness	Vulvodynia	Sounds
Anxiety	Vertigo	Restless Legs	Weight Changes	Allergies
Sugar Cravings	Blurred Vision	Nausea	Bruising	Pain

Check off anything you experience

Fibromyalgia Impact Questionnaire (FIQ)

The fibromyalgia impact questionnaire is something you may want to download and provide to you doctor. It was developed by Robert Bennett, MD. If you go to my website; fibro-doc.com you will find a link to the questionnaire under Resources.

Your doctor may already use it or be happy to consider it in your case. It was developed with the intent of understanding the scope of fibromyalgia as well as the patient's response to therapy. It has been shown to have validity and reliability in understanding therapeutic outcomes. Dr. Bennett has been one of the driving forces in research and understanding of fibromyalgia. He's a professor of medicine at the department of medicine of the Oregon Health and Science University of Portland, Oregon. If your doctor is unfamiliar with this question-naire he may retrieve/read about it at; *Robert Bennett, MD, FRCP, FACP, Professor of Medicine, Department of Medicine (OP09), Oregon Health and Science University, Portland, OR 97329, USA. E-mail: bennetrob1@com-cast.net Clin Exp Rheumatol 2005; 23 (Suppl. 39): S154-S162.© Copyright CLINICAL AND EXPERIMENTAL RHEUMATOLOGY 2005.*

Diagnosis and Tests

I hope that this section will help to mitigate misconceptions, in-cluding the secret shortcomings of doctors and doctoring. So many patients fall victim to being swept along a diagnostic path that has inherent momentum and misguided influence, reducing a patient's ability to step back and find the right doctoring team, subsequently improving the chances of winning what could be a lifetime battle. More importantly, I believe it's clear that there is no one doctor who is likely to unravel all the components and layers of symptoms that fibromyalgia and chronic fatigue sufferers live with. This awareness alone will help patients ask better questions of doctors and open the sufferer's mind to seeking a multidisciplinary approach even if and when a doctor is unaware or unwilling to co-manage the recovery.

During quiet time, over a cup of tea at home, prepare to communicate your feelings and symptoms. Don't assume that the doctor will ask all the right questions or that you won't leave something out when you hear the words, "How can I help you?" Bring your completed form as provided above to each appointment, ready to explain and ask the important stuff unemotionally. You will feel less stress and be able to self-advocate the encounter while helping to steer the next step.

CHAPTER 18

Functional Somatic Syndromes

Reality Check

I've included this abstract "Functional Somatic Syndromes," from Pub-Med. I take exception to it; it's too strong an assertion and it is generally irresponsible. Further, it disregards, if not belies, accepted neuro-bio-physiology. The abstract speaks of the perpetuation and amplification of symptoms due to psychosocial factors as if they were contrived, with no basis in reality. Regardless of the author's credentials, it feels that they've made a mockery of sufferers and evolving sciences. However, the abstract offers insight for those striving for self-advocacy. The author's attitude is something that fibromyalgia sufferers are better off to be aware of than not, as they are likely to be faced with it from time to time. I realize that this abstract will be insulting to many; it is to me. However, we should take into consideration that it was written through a division of psychiatry. It is another example of paradigms in the world of doctoring that support my somewhat obnoxious insistence that reaching your best level of health requires multidimensional/multidisciplinary (medical as well as non-medical) involvement.

Empowerment comes with knowledge; sometimes we must set aside the established authority of someone's degree, white coat, or stethoscope and weigh their words.

Ann Intern Med. 1999 Jun 1;130(11):910-21.

Functional Somatic Syndromes.

Barsky A.J, Borus J.F.

Source

Division of Psychiatry, Brigham and Women's Hospital, Boston, Massachusetts, 02115, USA.

Abstract

The term functional somatic syndrome has been applied to several related syndromes characterized more by symptoms, suffering, and disability than by consistently demonstrable tissue abnormality. These syndromes include multiple chemical sensitivity, sick building syndrome, and repetition stress injury; the side effects of silicone breast implants; Gulf War syndrome, chronic whiplash, chronic fatigue syndrome, irritable bowel syndrome, and fibromyalgia. Patients with functional somatic syndromes have explicit and highly elaborated self-diagnoses, and their symptoms are often refractory to reassurance, explanation, and standard treatment of symptoms. They share similar phenomenologies, high rates of co-occurrence, similar epidemiologic characteristics, and higher-than-expected prevalences of psychiatric comorbidity. Although discrete pathophysiologic causes may ultimately be found in some patients with functional somatic syndromes, the suffering of these patients is exacerbated by a self-perpetuating, self-validating cycle in which common, endemic, somatic symptoms are incorrectly attributed to serious abnormality, reinforcing the patient's belief that he or she has a serious disease. Four psychosocial factors propel this cycle of symptom amplification: the belief that one has a serious disease; the expectation that one's condition is likely to worsen; the "sick role," including the effects of litigation and compensation; and the alarming portrayal of the condition as catastrophic and disabling. The climate surrounding functional somatic syndromes includes sensationalized media coverage, profound suspicion of medical expertise and physicians, the mobilization of parties with a vested self-interest in the status of functional somatic syndromes, litigation, and a clinical approach that overemphasizes the biomedical and ignores psychosocial factors. All of these influences exacerbate and perpetuate the somatic distress of patients with functional somatic syndromes, heighten their fears and pessimistic expectations, prolong their disability, and reinforce their sick role.

Nice, eh ?

I would love to hear your comments about this abstract.

E-mail me if you like, via www.fibro-doc.com

INSIGHT # 5

VISION, CHOICE AND ACTION

LIVING BY CHOICE,
NOT REACTION

WHAT YOU CAN DO FOR
YOURSELF RIGHT NOW

Vision without action is merely a dream.
Action without vision just passes time.
Vision with action can change the world. — Joe L. Barker

CHAPTER 19
Understanding Brain Power

Chapter Topics:

    Optimism   *Secrets*
    The Future   *Memory/Pain*
    Avoid Overwhelm   *Cognitive Neuroscience*
    Values and Beliefs   *30-Day Challenge*
    Negative Emotion   *Yoga, Tai Chi, Qigong*

Optimistic?

We've already discussed some of the emotional components of dealing with fibromyalgia—as well as any other health or life issue, for that matter. With fibromyalgia, there's never a shortage of symptoms that we might try to address. Today it's your left knee, tomorrow your shoulders, and for the rest of the week it's fatigue that you're fighting from the first thing in the morning to the last thing at night, to say nothing of everyday life issues such as challenges with the children, marriage/communication, and balancing the checkbook this month.

Some of us learn optimism, most likely due to the influence of parents. Optimists believe that there are opportunities everywhere they look. They have a sense of confidence and a lack of fear. And, although you may be tired of the quote "Optimists see the glass as "half-full," it's like they have a special filter that doesn't allow emotional toxins to get to them. Those who haven't learned optimism might see the glass as "half-empty." There is no filter; stuff gets through to them. To pessimists, everything seems to be confusing and overwhelming; they generally feel like most efforts will end in failure. Even when something good is accomplished, they see the next problem coming right at them (Let's face it; we can always find another problem, especially if we are wired that way). Pessimists feel as if they have few if any choices and no "wins."

Natural-Born

I suppose some of us are natural-born optimists or natural-born pessimists. Natural-born optimists have natural filters and can manipulate massive amounts of information. We are constantly being bombarded with information that's meant to control our thoughts, direct our attention, and persuade or dissuade our judgments, leading us to fulfill agendas that are not our own. As you search for your personal answers to fibromyalgia, you will, hopefully, find a way to ask one of the most important questions that can be asked in an effort to have a sense of control/empowerment and peace of mind (optimism).

Natural-born pessimists would be people who have legitimate hormonal or brain chemistry imbalances, such as a serotonin or dopamine deficiency, that shape perceptions and judgments negatively. I believe there are far more pessimists who technically would be considered hormonally imbalanced than have learned pessimism. Also, they are likely not to have been exposed to tools that empower and develop peripheral vision, healthy filters, and an ability to ask empowering questions that shape their point of view in a healthier, happier direction. The question is: "What can I do to control my own thoughts today?" Another way to put this would be: "How can I train/control my attentions to better serve me and my needs, wants, and desires today?"

The next question you'll ask yourself will be, "How can I control my thoughts and not be led blindly, when fathers, mothers, teachers, preachers, television, friends, newspapers and magazines, my computer, or even doctors attempt to persuade or dissuade my thoughts and feelings?" You'll pose this question only when you come to the realization that there is a choice—and telling you that there is a choice is my most important message. Further, you don't have to live a reactionary life at the mercy of powerful influences around you that push and pull you in different directions. Those other influences and the people who deliver them have their own fears, opinions, agendas, paradigms, etc. They want you to join them; you don't have to.

The Future

Tony Robbins says, "The height of insanity is doing the same things the same old way and expecting different results." With fibromyalgia, much of the research that you're likely to read (other books, websites, newsletters, etc.) is redundant. You'll hear different words, different stories, and different anecdotes, but they tend to all revolve around the same basic data: fears, opinions, agendas, exercise, medication, and paradigms. On this path your future is destined to repeat itself; your future is almost prewritten. Sit in on a support group sometime. Ninety-five percent of what you know, everyone else knows. The conversation from one support group to another is the same.

290

It's not just the substance of the information you've been exposed to, but who has delivered it and by what medium is what makes a difference. These different factors will determine what messages have the most influence on your thoughts. For instance, "Vitamin B6 will cure fibromyalgia." If this quote was in black and white print, it would have a certain degree of influence on your subconscious mind. However, if it was in bold, **"Vitamin B6 Will Cure Fibromyalgia,"** it would have a different impact on your brain. Let's take it a step further and add, **"Dr. Norman Nutflamer, from the University of Breganhammer, found that Vitamin B6 will Cure Fibromyalgia."** You can see how it starts to take on more validity and has a different influence. Better yet, how about the real-world example we used in an earlier chapter: We were told by people whom we "believed" to know the truth, "Stay away from fats." We heard this for two decades. We believed it, but why? Because the degree of influence came from the big, bold money voices from the pharmaceutical/medical world and when combined they are hard not to believe. (As you know, they were wrong.) And then we've all heard that if you repeat a lie often enough, it becomes the truth. It's scary to think how committed we are to our beliefs and hang onto them, in many cases for a lifetime. Yet we aren't even aware of where they came from.

We can rewrite an almost certain future (as Landmark Education would put it) by posing the aforementioned question: "What can I do to control my own thoughts and beliefs?" So let's get back to the question at hand: "How can we train/control our own attention to better serve us, and our needs, wants, and desires? How do we direct what we're going to pay attention to, believe and act on?" And as fathers, mothers, teachers, preachers, friends, television, newspapers, magazines, computers, and doctors attempt to persuade or dissuade us, what if we were aware and in control, enough so that we could formulate new beliefs and more resourceful values to change the personal struggle with fibro?

Do you see how the answer to these questions could then change your life and your future? Might you be more optimistic and successful in anything and everything you do? Might you be a better communicator, personal-relationship builder and, more importantly a health-team builder? Would reducing the stress that fibromyalgia and confusing input from others cause you to feel as if you're a more natural-born optimist, and more in control of your life and destiny? Might you forge on with confident self-advocacy?

I think so.

Avoid Overwhelm

This section is meant to be a window into the brain and help to explain why we are the way we are. We will take a look at some fundamental neurology and how it's possible for us to make conscious efforts in shaping the way the brain works and ultimately controlling stress, avoiding overwhelm, and reducing pain.

Values and Beliefs

Have you ever noticed how easy it is to become overwhelmed by everyday life? Life happens on a backdrop of accumulated beliefs, values and experiences that color our judgments and everything that we do, think and feel. Unfortunately, most of us have some beliefs, values, and experiences in the past that weigh on us and negatively affect us in the present. They negatively color how we see things now, how we evaluate things, how we process and deal with problems and ultimately how we experience life.

This all takes place within the brain automatically.

Negative Emotions

Dr.Van Mittendorf and Dr. Lumley's research at the University of Utrecht in the Netherlands looked at how negative emotions, specifically anger and sadness, affect us. What they found was that "The experience of both anger and sadness amplified pain in women with and without fibromyalgia. The occurrence of anger and sadness appears to be a general risk factor for pain amplification." Their findings built on prior research that has shown that anger, sadness, resentment, disappointment, and fear can lower pain thresholds.

Secrets

This chapter will seem at times mind-bending, at others times encouraging. Many of the ideas are taken from *Incognito: The Secret Lives of the Brain,* by Dr. David Eagleman, neuroscientist.

It should be clear by now that the perception and experience of pain takes place within the circuitry of the brain. Eagleman brings to light that secrets are unhealthy for brain circuitry. That's right: "secrets," like something you don't tell, feelings and thoughts that are unrevealed, kept unknown, and unacknowledged. Neurobiological research has documented that when someone suffers some type of emotional trauma--let's just use an extreme example such as rape or incest—the victim will commonly feel shame or guilt and subsequently lock the event and all the feelings away as "secrets."

The longer these thoughts and feelings are allowed to be harbored in a victim's head and heart, the more chance there is for permanent corruption of brain circuits. It's hard to believe, but this may in fact be more damaging in the long run than the original incident that's being kept secret.

Conversely, when victims confess to what happened, share their feelings, or put them in writing—effectively releasing the secret—it affects the nervous system in such a way that health improves. They are happier, more productive, and have less need to visit doctors. Their stress levels, measured by blood tests, are consistently improved.

This makes a case for the value of friends, relatives, and counseling—people that you can confide in and who will be supportive. It makes a case for journaling as well. Journaling is a habit we strongly recommend on a daily basis, at least in the beginning when you are putting together your health team and working your way through this book. You can say anything to your journal. It will never criticize you. It will never challenge your thoughts, discourage you or push you to share more than you are ready to. Journaling is a tool to get all of the secrets out of your head. Another interesting process is to write a letter—it could be to yourself, someone dead or alive, to God or to the universe. Journals are a great place to release secret sadness and feelings you've never had a chance to come to terms with or express. It could be that you have suffered emotional hurt, physical pain or have been abused in some way; you may have suffered broken promises, disappointments and fear. Possibly you have feelings of being a victim, or you feel guilt or shame, jealousy or anger, and believed that you needed to bury it all.

A great example of the power of letter writing is Stacy, a 47-year-old woman from Connecticut who happens to be a patient of mine. As a child, she was abused on a repeated basis by a close friend of her father, but she never shared the abuse with anyone. She kept that dark secret hidden. It wasn't until thirty-eight years later, when I encouraged her to write a letter to her deceased father, that it came out. The cathartic effect truly changed her life for the better. She experienced such relief that I asked her to write a second letter to me—to share the positive effects of the first letter in which she finally unloaded the secret she had kept bottled up for so long. Here is the letter that she wrote me:

Dr. Langone,

After I considered writing my story, it made me very nervous. Several times I thought about starting my story, but I would get nervous and sit down and cry. I can't believe I did it, but I'm glad I did. I was kind of scared and I was afraid of other people reading it and what they would think. The first person I shared it with was my husband and it served as a great forum for us to come together and talk more about the situation, and since then he has been much more understanding. I have not been covering things up or denying things as much, and I can be much more real and much more myself now that he understands, so it's brought us closer together.

I also let my mother read it and she was surprised and had no idea of most of the things that I shared with her. We had a good cry together and that's brought us closer as well. I then shared my story with other people in the family, a cousin and a niece, and they were amazed as well.

It's not only helped my relationship with them, but it's helped my life in general, because now that they understand better it makes it easier to be myself and they have gone out of their way to help me more.

The last thing that has made things better for me is having gotten it out of me it has helped me to have more of a forward perspective of life and stop looking backwards and rehashing things. It's as if through telling the story I have dumped it or got it out of me or got over it. I know I'll never get over everything in the past completely, but in a way I feel like it has, or I have. I'm lighter, emotionally lighter.

If you would like to read Stacy's original "Letter to my father," it is posted with her permission on our website: www.Fibro-doc.com

How Does This Work?

Eagleman posed the question, "How do these findings really work in the brain, and what is a 'secret,' neuro-biologically speaking?" In his book he discusses the term "rival networks" in the brain. This means that within the brain, systems exist that are hard-wired and compete with each other. Hard-wired, meaning innate, preprogramed, the way our affinity to sweet-tasting things are hard-wired. You may notice this with simple decisions like will you choose chocolate or strawberry ice cream today; or it may be a more complex battle like, do you ask a question that has been gnawing at you or do you keep it to yourself for fear of embarrassment or rejection? It may also be seen in a heart-mind tug-of-war that you're engaged in where you know by sharing your feelings someone else may be hurt while at the same time understanding that if you don't get it off of your chest, it'll eat you alive. There have been many instances in the past when fibromyalgia sufferers have kept their pain, emotions, feelings, and thoughts buried inside rather than risk the pain they anticipated if they were to share their feelings. If this is something you have done, I should warn you that it greatly increases brain and emotional stress, which may lead to your nerves becoming more sensitive, leading to amplification of your perception of pain. When we talk about these emotional components, such as what's happening in the brain or the neurology of emotions and health, it's not voodoo. It's not esoteric. It's not religious. It's neurology. It is biology. With this knowledge, we have two choices. Either we take steps to reduce neurological negativity and actually help to heal the brain (or more precisely, change the brain), or we allow it to continue to wreak havoc in brain circuits and our lives, creating more pain, fatigue, and a plethora of other symptoms that fibromyalgia sufferers live with.

Can You Keep a Secret?

"A man who can keep a secret is wise,
but not as wise as a man who has no secrets to keep."
—*Edgar Watson Howe*

"Some people are constitutionally incapable of keeping a secret and this bias may tell us something about the battles going on inside them and which way they tip. Good spies and secret agents are those people whose battle between rivals (should I tell or should I not tell) always tips toward long-term reward/value hence choosing to not tell."[28] When the average person chooses not to tell a secret, it is because he or she fears that the consequences of sharing will create more emotional pain than holding it in. This perception may be rooted in a fear of hurting someone else, embarrassing themselves, or exacerbating a problem. Eagleman notes that it is far easier to tell a secret to a stranger, because their reaction doesn't matter. It's simply a cathartic exercise, which may be one reason that so many religions believe in confessing sins, thereby causing a shift in the conscious and subconscious brain as well as a positive shift in hormones. There's an interesting website, www.PostSecret.com, where people can go to post/journal secrets and feelings, saying anything they want and basically putting secrets out there to the world with no fear. The simple expression of a secret is healing; it reduces stress, and it's a nice cheap way of performing your own hormone therapy.

Eagleman's book has a section entitled "Why Do We Have Consciousness At All?" He discusses that there are blueprints and mapped-out circuits in the brain that respond appropriately and automatically, such as "I push, you pull." They are called "zombie systems." An example of this is that when you put salt in your mouth, saliva starts to secrete. But if we were nothing but zombielike hardwired circuits, what would be the reason for consciousness? [28]

Neuroscientists Frances Crick and Cristoff Koch report that "consciousness exists to control and to distribute control over automated alien systems." The "alien systems" they speak of are the zombie systems that Eagleman discusses. These are the circuits in the brain that seem to function on their own, in the exact same manner that fibromyalgia circuitry seems to be functioning completely on its own with no conscious control of suffering. So why is it that a conscious mind can't do a better job of controlling this automatic system that seems to generate pain on its own? Or is it possible that it can? Well, we will discuss in later chapters how researchers are beginning to develop ways of controlling the conscious mind to do just that by studying the brain via MRI imaging. The hope is that with some training a person can consciously re-pattern a zombie system, which in turn will reduce or control their pain.

When these zombie systems are running smoothly and in an appropriate manner, we love them because they make life easy. When we have to develop a new pattern (learning) there is a lot more work, brain activity, and energy that must be expended if things are going to change for the better. For instance, let's say you're trying to become a better golfer or tennis player and you want to develop a better swing, to strike the ball and control shots.

How do you do that? Well, it takes a lot of energy, a lot of consciousness and a lot of repetition. I've read that Tiger Woods, before a golf tournament, will go to the driving range and hit 1000 balls to help reinforce the circuitry of a successful swing pattern. It seems to have worked pretty well for him. Some learning takes less conscious effort and, automatically through innate zombie systems, learn/reinforce all on their own. In the same way there are unperceived programs running in the background of your computer that result in a more efficient and faster computer?

You may remember my example of remodeling our kitchen and moving our knives on the counter from the right side to the left side of the cutting board. After six years, the knives have been on the left three times longer than on the right. Yet my brain still hasn't completely re-patterned. Some bio-neurological influence caused the imprint to not fade. It may have to do with the emotional state or the context in which I first learned or decided to put the knives on the right. Or it may have to do with more primitive zombie circuits dictating that logically they really should be on the right, which won over my new logic and decision to place them on the left. One way or the other, the point is that circuits must be retrained. Notice I said circuits plural.

Another example was going to a movie and feeling fear when a roaring saber-toothed tiger jumped out of the screen or to be brought to tears by a sad story. There are zombie circuits wired to feel emotion even when we know they are completely contrived on the screen.

Question?

Q#1: In spite of the fact that the threat of being attacked by a saber-toothed tiger every time you leave your cave has diminished (at least for some of us), is it possible that competing and rival circuits matched up against each other for protection and survival in a hostile world just can't let go? And can preprogrammed protection circuits simply not be reprogrammed in spite of evolution having given us confidence to use consciousness and deductive reasoning in an organized, lawful, and relatively safe environment?

Fibro Question?

Q#2: In spite of the fact that intellectually we know that a light touch on a leg won't generate pain (at least for most of us), is it possible that Fibros are stuck in an automatic zombielike state in which primitive circuitry wins over evolution and intellect, insisting on a response to being touched that is locked into prehistoric alarm called PAIN? Or is fibromyalgia the result of a brain gone wild, a sick brain that science would identify as being in a neuro-pathological state, most recently termed "central sensitivity syndrome"?

It seems that the answer to the questions posed are all "Yes." It is possible that the chronic pain and dilemma of fibromyalgia comes from one or both possibilities:

1. Some Fibros, in fact, may have an amazingly efficient brain stuck in a primitive commitment to protect and survive in a hostile environment: "*It's not safe to be touched.*"

2. Some Fibros may have a brain that has made the transition to a more safe sane society (evolutionary success) but the brain circuits have been corrupted and the person is now considered to have a sick brain or "central sensitivity syndrome."

Now What?

For now, let's accept that harboring secrets will negatively influence circuits of the brain, fibromyalgia and your life. Secrets will create stories, confusion, fears and other negative emotions that color everyday relationships—your relationship with yourself and with others.

Memories and Pain

The hippocampus is a structure within the brain that is very important for remembering, from where you were, to what you were doing when something important happened—in other words, providing memory and context. For example, remembering where you were and what you were doing on September 11th, 2001 is a function of the hippocampus. One of the reasons that we remember that day so clearly has to do with the amygdala, another brain structure very close to the hippocampus. The amygdala does its job by adding emotional components of memories. It's like the hippocampus records memories in black and white and the amygdala adds emotions, drama, and colors, cementing in the memories.

This means that the remembering machinery in your brain works better, lasts longer, and has a more profound effect when a strong emotional component accompanies it. Together they can imprint memories and, subsequently, those memories are easily retrieved, last longer, and fade less over time. Memories, when retrieved, can bring back or even exaggerate reactions, perceptions, and experiences with emotion. Like 9/11--it's hard to forget feelings, images of where you were, what you were doing and whom you were with when you first found out. To erase or lighten the load of a memory like this, a person would have to put in a lot of work, assuming it's even possible. A lifetime of emotional traumas like physical or emotional abuse, rape, incest, humiliation and rejection during our school years, inferiority complexes, and insecurities cause our emotionally charged memories to vividly contribute to this sick-brain concept that won't let go. Or, at the very least, the brain encourages and reinforces the necessity for our primitive circuits to prevail. One way or the other, change is necessary.

So now that we're all depressed and confused, thinking that there's no hope for the brain, let's begin to understand what we can do on our own to influence the brain and its recovery.

Contemplative Neuroscience

Contemplative neuroscience is an evolving understanding and study of the brain. It seeks to understand how self-directed thought and activity can influence the brain. It offers us the potential to control and change everything that we have spoken of so far in this section, in the same way that experience, the media, and unintentional thoughts and activities (life) influence the brain. For better or worse, the brain is always being influenced, constantly changing and adapting. So why not decide that we're going to consciously participate in shaping, controlling, and redirecting how we think and feel? The brain's ability to change is called "neuroplasticity." And when we say change, we mean literally change our brain matter, circuits, and communication between circuits. With some effort, the amygdala and hippocampus will talk to and influence each other differently, helping to reduce physical and emotional pain. Through neuroplasticity, the physical form and size of the brain can change—adaptation at its best. Self-directed neuroplasticity is exactly what we want to participate in to help manage and resolve fibromyalgia.

Sounds like a pretty good trick, doesn't it? It amuses me to think that there are those who believe that contemplative practices are religious simply because someone participates in them intentionally. There is a contemplative component to almost everything that we do. Some would argue that if it's not conscious and intentional, it's not "contemplative." I would argue that there is a subconscious, prewired, and zombielike contemplative mechanism in place. Further, there are physical efforts of a contemplative nature, as well as purely thoughtful efforts.

Physical Efforts

I would like fibro sufferers to take away from this chapter the reality that stress and overwhelming pain can be influenced by choice, and to have confidence that the brain and nervous system can be controlled. We should not give up. Further, drugs may not be as necessary as we have been told.

The activities that are the least problematic for Fibros to participate in to self-manage pain, energy, mood, and even painful emotions are meditation, prayer, yoga, tai chi, and Qigong. These don't have the drawbacks and side effects that more intense physical exercise has; nor do they come at a high cost compared to counseling in cognitive therapies.

Some of these practices date back 5000 years. We need to choose our words carefully, because Western scientists have the need to understand in Western terms, as we discussed above. Interestingly enough, The National Institute for Health, in 2011, allocated $541 million to similar studies having to do with alternative medicine and complementary sciences, searching to understand in Western terms.

Many people close their minds to the term meditation because they feel that it could somehow compromise their religious beliefs. However, most of these practices have evolved as a spiritually-centered physical activity; they are not religious. Western societies are built on a mentality of active "doing," "creating," "building," "physically demonstrating results," etc., and judge their reality accordingly. Depending on our senses to confirm reality, of course, seems to make perfect sense—however, there's some debate. Traditionally we recognize our senses as sight, hearing, taste, smell, and touch; additionally, we are reasonably comfortable with including temperature, movement, pain, and balance as senses. This mindset helps to explain why the West has been so detached, and why it rejects practices and activities that don't fall into Western definitions and modes of proof or confirmation.

Many people with fibromyalgia are initially unable to participate in the kinds of exercises that are common in Western medicine; however, they are very capable of practicing meditation, prayer, yoga, tai chi, or Qigong and, surprisingly, can accomplish almost all that physical exercise can offer and, in some instances achieve better results in managing their pain. Some of the activities I mentioned involve sitting postures, breathing exercises, sounds, words, singing, chanting, or guided imagery; they are sensory and mindful exercises. These different exercises calm the nervous system, stimulate endorphins, and manage the experience and perception of pain, while stimulating the immune system. This all happens by calming and helping to modulate areas of the brain such as the hippocampus and amygdala.

All of these practices can be done in a community setting with classes, or at home by following instructions or through the use of DVDs. They have a physical, psychological, social, and spiritual component.

300

Through them you can expect nothing less than improved health with very little inconvenience or cost.

Yoga

Studies have shown that yoga in as few as ten sessions can reduce the pain of fibromyalgia.[3] Women with fibromyalgia will typically have adrenal exhaustion, demonstrated by lower than average cortisol levels. This can contribute to pain, fatigue, stress, sensitivity, and thyroid stress. Yoga relaxes the sympathetic nervous system, lowers heart rate, and increases oxygenation of the blood, while raising cortisol levels and helping to balance the hypothalamic-pituitary-adrenal axis.[8]

Tai Chi

Tai chi is another mind-body practice that originated as a martial art in China, and like yoga, incorporates slow gentle and controlled movements combined with focusing/clearing the mind, breathing, and relaxation techniques. Fibromyalgia impact questionnaires have documented improvement in sleep and depression, as well as mental and physical components of pain and stress in as little as 10-12 weeks.[72] Dr. Ron Glassy has studied similar practices and reports an enhancement of the flow of cerebral spinal fluid due to the improvement in posture and spinal mechanics also enhancing serotonin and endorphin production, both of which improve mood and the feeling of well-being.

Qigong

Qigong is a practice that is similar to yoga and tai chi. Qigong has many forms of relaxation and mind/body coordination. Slow, gentle movements are well-tolerated by people with chronic pain and offer relaxation, mood enhancement, and reduction of pain as well as improved sleep patterns. In a study completed at the Department of Clinical Psychology at the University of Uppsala, Sweden, it was found that Qigong has a positive and reliable effect on fibromyalgia syndrome, and that 93 percent of participants can tolerate and complete the activity. All participants reported a feeling of contentment. Qigong simply means "energy work" and is an ancient energy healing system used for centuries in China. It is a form of daily exercise routines integrating physical postures and breath awareness. When practiced daily, it helps to build an individual's energy, called "chi." It also helps to build stamina, increases vitality, helps support the immune system, improves awareness and overall well-being, and reduces stress.

Along with my daily Western-style exercise regime, I incorporate one day of yoga per week and have found it to have amazing rejuvenating effects. It has helped to improve my balance and my coordination, posture and flexibility. I would encourage everyone, particularly fibromyalgia sufferers, to choose one of the practices that we've discussed and give it a try.

Thoughtful Efforts

During preparation for Thanksgiving meal, a teenage girl observed her mother in the kitchen cutting off the last four inches of a leg of lamb. Then she began to season it, and grease the pan. As her mom slipped the lamb into the oven the teenager asked, "Mom, why do you cut the end of the lamb off?"

Her mother replied, "That's just way you do it, honey; it's a family recipe."

The girl replied, "But why?"

Her mother said, "I'm not sure exactly why, but that's the way my mother taught me. But now that you are asking me, I will ask Grandma."

They went into the living room to ask Grandma. "Grandma, in your recipe for lamb, why do you cut the end of the leg of lamb off before you season and cook it?"

"It's just the way you do it; that's the recipe that my mother taught me," she said.

Great-grandma was due to come shortly, so they decided they would wait and ask her. After she arrived, they posed the question, "Great-grandma, why do you cut the end of the leg of lamb off before you season it and cook it?"

Great-grandma answered, "You have to cut it off or it won't fit in the pan."

And so it goes. Generation to generation beliefs, habits, and perspectives are handed down as truths; recipes for lamb, recipes for life. But not all of them are positive, resourceful, necessary, or even understood.

I'm a big believer in not letting the past take an unhealthy toll on how we experience the present and not letting the past paint a picture of fear that overwhelms us when we look to the future. In order to be more successful, with life in general, but more specifically in our concerns with fibromyalgia, an effort must be made to let go of negative influences in the past that sabotage our health and our happiness in the present. Unfortunately, negative beliefs are likely to be carried forward in the head and heart as "stories" that surface from time to time, sometimes helpful in supporting present reality, but sometimes sabotaging health and happiness. Nevertheless, they are part of our foundational beliefs and values; they tweak our zombie system.

We bring these stories forward into everyday life and believe them as if they were true since the beginning of time and always will be true—something that cannot even be considered changeable. Let me give you an example. Let's say you are 11 years old and you bake a pie. Your father makes a comment that you'd better marry someone who can cook because you can't. So, for the rest of your life, your "story" about yourself is that you can't cook. Your identity is now your "story" and you stay away from cooking and entertaining. Why? Because you know you can't cook. So now you are 35 years old and you ask yourself, "I wonder why I cannot cook?" It's simple; your father told you 24 years ago that you can't cook. Additionally, you spent the past 24 years trying to win your father's approval and you generally have low confidence and self-esteem in everything you do and the decisions you make. You do this in spite of the fact that we would agree that the past is the past. Can you relate to this?

So the question is: Why? Why do we let the past have so much power in our lives? Why do we carry forward these negative beliefs, values, thoughts, and perspectives? Maybe the more empowering question is: What if we just started fresh every day? Dale Carnegie, a master in managing relationships, wrote about living in day-tight compartments. What if we were able to give up/let go of the past stuff? How would that change our lives? Would it change the quality of life today and tomorrow? What possibilities would it open? Might you have a better relationship with your father? Could you bake a pie? What would a little more self-confidence mean to you? Take a second and consider how all this stuff could relate to stress, to your health, and to fibromyalgia.

Quite a few years ago I went through an educational process called the Landmark Forum. This educational process opened my mind in areas that I didn't think needed opening. I had an opportunity to step away from myself and take a look at the past rather than just owning it forever. I realized what a joke I had played on myself by taking the past and dragging it forward into now and thinking that all my learned values and beliefs from the past had to be part of today. It is as if once you learn that the world is flat, the world will always be flat, and every day that you set sail in your world is based on that belief.

After going through this process, I customized some self-talk points for myself, the basis of which are teachings of the Forum. We will go over them in a minute.

Mind Control
How much do you think the way we experience life is of our own creation? Are we just kind of going along, being pushed and pulled, reacting and putting out fires? Think about getting up in the morning and how many influences are trying to get your attention and trying to get you to think, believe, accept, and value that which they think is important for you to think, believe, accept and value. We're talking about a type of brainwashing. We get up in the morning and listen to the radio, television a mobile devise and we're inundated with negativity and fear. They tell us how we should expect to feel today—"The pollen count is high; prepare for eyes to water; we will sneeze all day." Announcers plant insecurities about finances, about our weight, how we look. And then every person we meet throughout our day has an agenda. They try to sell us something or to talk us into something. Did you ever have relatives try to control you, pull you down, and suck you into their space and their stuff? Then we read or hear the news, and there's more negativity. Every store window is begging for our attention: "Buy me!" And how is it that there is an urgency every day to buy before the sale ends? How do retailers stay in business when they constantly sell at 50 percent off? When do we decide to play a role in controlling our own minds and our own thoughts? Do we even have any say?

Self-Talk
Below I have a list of affirmations or self-talk points, a form of contemplative neuroscience. Most of the points that I'm going to review are taught by Landmark Education. Landmark's goal is to supply "innovative programs to live an extraordinary life." Part of me hesitates to share these points, because we humans have a tendency to prejudge. Our judgments, of course, are based on our past, our beliefs, and our values. Tony Robbins, and many other authors, have written

about these concepts extensively. Most people, when first exposed to the thoughts I've listed below, will either accept or dismiss them immediately, one by one. Their decisions reinforce/confirm and help them to hang onto their own "stuff" (beliefs and values) no matter how invalid their own stuff might have been in the past. We self-validate as a default. It's easier to hang on to our beliefs than it is to open up and take the chance of experiencing the vulnerability that comes with change. So my fear is that some readers will turn off and hit the default icon to self-validate, hence invalidating not only this section, but possibly other parts of the book that don't immediately match what they already think, believe, comfortably accept, and value.

Over the last 20 years, I've found that the least successful patients—the patients who are stalled, stuck, and getting nowhere—are the ones who are steadfastly committed to their beliefs and values, cutting off the end of the leg of lamb and not knowing why.

One of the default beliefs that most people hang on to is that they believe they have an open mind. This is comforting and gives permission to remain closed. I'll ask you to step past your comfort zone and give yourself the opportunity to at least consider my recommendations to hopefully help open the door to critical thinking and questioning of yourself first, and then rethink and begin to question the healthcare community that you must deal with along your fibro path. I realize this is a tall order. I fight the battle every day—most of us do. This section's purpose, as it applies to fibromyalgia, will reveal itself as you read on and implement your personal health plan and negotiate the medical community.

Before I get to my recommendations, I have to admit that I'm guilty of having prejudged many of the points that I will make below before I gave myself or them a chance.

My recommendation is to take each of the next 30 days and, first thing in the morning, privately read out loud each point as listed below. Do nothing more than that. You don't have to accept, reject, judge, or believe them. They don't have to become part of you any more than anything else you hear, see, or are exposed to during any other of your day's activities. Think of them more as browsing through a department store of possibilities; you don't even have to linger on any one of them (unless you wish to). And rest assured that at the end of your 30 days of browsing you will have not lost yourself; you can pick up from where you left off when you bought this book and continue on the same path you've been on if you believe your defaults are working for you. My goal is not to win you over or change who you are. My goal is simply to create possibilities of brain power.

The 30-Day Challenge.

Jack Canfield, one of the authors of the *Chicken Soup for the Soul* books, shared a study done by NASA many years ago. The study was to determine the effect that weightlessness might have on the brain when everything seems to be upside down. Astronauts were given concave -lens glasses and told to wear them all their waking hours. The glasses made everything appear to be upside down, simulating a weightless environment. As you can imagine, this posed quite a challenge in negotiating everyday life. But, as time went on, the brain had the ability to make changes that allowed perceptions, eye-hand coordination, and spatial relationships to adapt and ultimately have the same efficiency that you and I have: the brain "righted" things. They found that the tipping point, the shift, came at 30 days. By the 30-day mark, an astronaut's brain and central nervous system had changed; brain circuits effectively reoriented themselves.

The study was very clear that it takes 30 days for the brain to allow the astronaut the choice to accept or reject the information as useful and adapt it, or not. Not 20 days, not 24 days, not 29 days; exactly 30 days: 30 consecutive days, to be more precise. Napoleon Hill was a personal success coach and great motivator. One of his famous sayings was: "What the mind can conceive and believe; it can achieve." In the world of neuroscience and as it applies to our subject, if Napoleon Hill were to rewrite his quote it might be: *"What a man can conceive or experience, the brain will believe and rewire itself to achieve."*

How Does This Apply to Fibromyalgia?

There are many ways that the brain can be reprogrammed to re-map and remake itself. But first let me give you two other examples of the power and the validity of the brain's ability to adapt and reprogram. Fibromyalgia and neuropathic pain are believed to be examples of the same neurological glitch/adaptation that we've been speaking of. With some aspects of fibromyalgia, the brain doesn't really get it wrong as much as it simply reads what the experience is, and that experience is "pain." The brain then believes this is the way it's going to be and should be. In response, the brain sensitizes itself and basically reprograms itself to be more efficient, helping to self-actualize pain. This will be covered in more detail in various parts of the book; in particular, look to Chapter 24, "New Science, Real Hope." Another example might be a two-year-old child who is scared out of his diapers by a dog barking and running at him. A child's brain experiences the alarm and fear and imprints it into the nervous system. The brain then believes that any and every dog poses a danger. The child now grows to be a 6'3" 230-pound football-playing adult. When the neighbor's six-pound Chihuahua barks at him, he cowers and feels the same alarm/ fear he did as a child. Of course he passes it off as "I just don't like dogs."

We're simply going to take advantage of the brain's ability to adapt and use it to our advantage. But remember our discussion about how emotions cement in memories. One of the reasons a 230-pound guy could fear a six-pound Chihuahua for a lifetime is that there was a strong emotional component to the original experience. This means it will take longer to un-program and reprogram because, at least for now, we don't have the emotional glue component.

I'm going to do some paraphrasing and take information as well as words from Landmark Education principles and incorporate them into the challenge of giving your brain the opportunity to live a less re-active life. Take five minutes quietly and privately every morning and recite out loud the ten points provided as an opportunity to choose what you will expose your brain to, in lieu of outside influences that are competing for your attention. If a point does not strike an emotional chord of value/importance to your brain, it is less likely to do anything but pass through. In the meantime, you'll give yourself a gift of a simple technique that will help you work toward regaining power, control, and focus. I'm not asking you to necessarily agree with any points listed, but simply to take a leap of faith and give your brain the opportunity to clarify your vision and take things that you might now see as upside down and right them.

The content of your thoughts and personal beliefs can be proven by a single indicator – your current result.
—James A. Ray, *The Science of Success*

Ten Points

Recite the following phrases. Don't judge or rationalize any of them. Do this one time per day in a quiet, controlled environment. No interruptions, no cell phone. Each time you sit down to do this, you'll work your way through the list three times. I recommend simply reciting it on the first run-through. On the second run-through, take a moment to think about what you are saying--and if there's any area of your life that it applies to, it will immediately resonate with you. In the third and final run-through, just recite as you did on the first run-through. We get feedback from people who have practiced this; they tell us they can't understand why, but they love it and life improves. If you find this to be true, after 30 days it may be a practice that, once a day or once a week, you'll look forward to doing.

1. My goal, life vision, what I choose for myself in the future, and what I am committed to achieving can be mine simply by choosing and then sharing my thoughts with others.
2. The past does not have to equal the future. The future is a clean slate, a blank canvas.
3. I give up having to be right all the time and making others wrong. I do not find fault or criticize.
4. I speak honestly, clearly, straightforwardly, and powerfully; then I take what comes.
5. I give up trying to fix, change, or improve things; instead I look to what is possible in the future.
6. I see present reality distinct from the fears, preferences, disappointments, opinions, and agendas of others.
7. I see the simplicity of present reality distinct from my own fears, preferences, disappointments, opinions, and old baggage.
8. I give up the interpretation that "there's something wrong here"—some things just are what they are. They have no meaning unless I give them meaning.
9. I have no attachment to outcomes; I flow through the process with simplicity.
10. I honor my word and my calendar.
11. I am grateful for _____.

When you feel grateful, you become great;
it eventually attracts all things.
—Plato

> Having a sense of how we tick encourages self-help practices. Focusing on the things we can do daily to control overwhelm and to work toward a better life is self-advocacy at its best; it brings power and confidence, energy, less pain, and more fun. All other things will seem to fall into place more easily.

CHAPTER 20

Adrenal and Thyroid Stress

Chapter Topics:

Stress: HPA
Adrenals
Carbs, Fats, and Protein
Lifestyle

Stress: Thyroid, HPT
Substance P
Serotonin

Stress: HPA—Hypothalamus-Pituitary-Adrenal Axis

The endocrine system is a system of glands that secrete hormones to help control metabolism. It functionally integrates itself with the nervous system, which, as the master-control system, plays a direct role in the synthesis and release of hormones. Like the nervous system, the endocrine system is involved with every aspect of function: disease, illness, and recovery. In particular, we're going to talk about the relationship between the hypothalamus, the pituitary gland, and the adrenal glands (HPA). These three glands communicate with each other to orchestrate, balance, initiate, and modulate all systems of the body. There is a crucial and delicate balance among the three relating to fibromyalgia.

We'll discuss each one separately so you can get a good sense of where they are and what they do, and then we'll talk about how they integrate with each other and can directly relate to what a fibromyalgia patient experiences.

If you refer to the figures below, you can see the positioning of the glands that we're talking about. The hypothalamus is part of the brain. The pituitary and the adrenal glands are not part of the brain. The pituitary gland dangles down just beneath the hypothalamus and is considered the master-control gland. The adrenal glands are located one on each kidney.

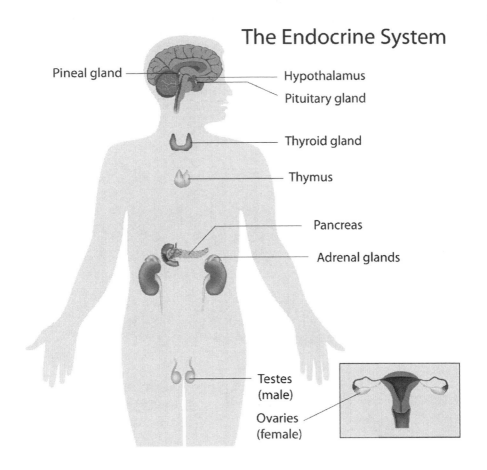

The Endocrine System

Pineal gland

Hypothalamus

Pituitary gland

Thyroid gland

Thymus

Pancreas

Adrenal glands

Testes
(male)

Ovaries
(female)

The coordination among these three glands, along with the nervous system, will in large part dictate how the body, physically and emotionally, will respond to and handle short-term as well as long-term stress. By the way, as a reminder, anytime we say stress we're talking about physical, chemical and/or emotional stress. It wouldn't be hard to suspect that the balance among these three glands could be upset by a disaster (like an earthquake, the death of a loved one or an auto injury). What's less obvious, and most commonly relates to fibromyalgia, is insidious and chronic stress that overloads the system and causes one or more of these glands to become fatigued, upsetting a subtle balance between them.

Symptoms that are indicative of an upset in this balance are fatigue, irritability, difficulty concentrating and difficulty sleeping, all of which fibromyalgia patients experience regularly, lack of sleep being one of the most concerning. Additionally, we find that the general function and reparative capacity of muscles, tendons, joints and ligaments suffer.

HPA, Axis Diagnosis

Before we get into understanding how we might decipher the culprits that upset this triad, let's get a little bit more clarity about what each component is and does.

Hypothalamus

The hypothalamus is part of the brain. Its responsibility is to help coordinate the nervous system with the endocrine system (hormones). It creates and secretes neurological hormones that either turn on or turn off the pituitary, as well as adrenal hormones. The hypothalamus controls things such as body temperature, hunger, thirst, energy, sleep, biorhythms, and circadian rhythms. In general, it communicates with all other glands, directly or indirectly. As we discussed earlier, shift workers challenge biorhythms, so you can see how that will affect the hypothalamus, which will, in turn, affect the pituitary gland and the wake-sleep cycle.

Pituitary Gland

The pituitary gland secrets hormones and is located conveniently just below the hypothalamus. It generally is not considered to be a part of the brain, however. There are small tubes that allow hormonal and neurological communication (neurotransmitters) to move back and forth between the pituitary gland and the hypothalamus. The hormones that it secretes are meant to help balance all functions of the body. In spite of being under the control of the hypothalamus, it is considered to be the master hormonal gland because it secretes up to nine different hormones. Its secretions help to control growth hormones and blood pressure; they participate in pregnancy and childbirth and the production of breast milk. They modulate the sexual organs and thyroid gland, pituitary hormones and kidneys and help to make endorphins. Endorphins relieve pain and alter mood; they affect all cells in the body and all areas that generate or transmit pain—this is crucial to our study of fibromyalgia.

Adrenal Glands

Located one on each kidney, the adrenal glands are responsible for releasing three broad categories of hormones. They are the body's own anti-inflammatory pharmacy. These are steroids derived from

cholesterol. We're most concerned with the stress hormone cortisol, which is involved in the metabolism of fats, proteins and carbohydrates, helping to generate energy for muscles and mental acuity
when a protective and active response is called for, such as a "fight-or-
flight" response. The second stress hormone we are concerned with is
dehydro-epiandrosterone or DHEA. DHEA helps to modulate normal
daily hormone cycles.

I find that the culprit in upsetting the balance of the HPA axis in
reference to fibro is most likely the adrenals rather than the pituitary
or hypothalamus. Luckily it seems to be the easiest to treat as well. For
this reason we're going to spend some extra time talking about the
adrenals so we can understand how easily they can be improved to
directly affect fibro.

During a normal/healthy response to stress, the adrenals will secrete stress hormones, cortisol and DHEA. As the stress subsides, the
adrenal glands recover and reset, readying themselves for any future
stress that may come along. This is similar to the way you would be
out of breath after running a mile. Then, huffing and puffing, you
walk around a little bit and catch your breath; you recover and you are
ready to carry on. However, if stress levels stay high for long periods
of time, the adrenals will be unable to catch their breath and may
become locked in a state of hormone overproduction. This is called
adrenal exhaustion.

Common Causes of Adrenal Stress

Stress comes from emotional, physical and chemical pressures.
Let's call them toxins. Individually and collectively, toxins raise the
allostatic load (the cumulative load which stressors exert on human
physiology).

Emotional toxins are things like anxiety, fear, anger, worry and
guilt.

Chemical toxins are literally that: chemicals, air pollution, preservatives, food additives, sugar substitutes, MSG, high carbohydrate and
high glycemic index diets, alcohol and drug consumption (prescription, nonprescription, social drugs—even vitamins).

Physical toxins refer to physical exercise, overuse, physical trauma like a whiplash, strain/sprain or athletic injury. We will include

chronic pain from subluxations, postural and structural problems, in this category.

Stages of Adrenal Exhaustion
Stage I

In this first stage approaching exhaustion, the adrenals are forced to overproduce hormones to deal with chronic, unrelenting stress. Eventually as they get fatigue they'll enter Stage II.

Stage II

In Stage II, the adrenals are unable to keep up with the demand and cannot produce adequate amounts of required hormones. So they sacrifice the production of DHEA and focus on cortisol production, setting the stage for Stage III.

Stage III

Adrenal exhaustion has progressed to where there is an inability to produce cortisol or DHEA in sufficient amounts. As a result, the body cannot recover from stress and the symptoms of adrenal exhaustion become more obvious. Some of the symptoms will include:

- Blood sugar imbalance
- Depression
- Digestive disorders
- Fatigue
- Excessive sweet cravings
- Headaches
- Pain on movement
- Thyroid disorders
- Neck, shoulder and back pain
- Poor memory
- Sleep disorders

It's clear how the adrenals directly participate in the symptoms of fibromyalgia. Some people who have been diagnosed with fibromyalgia do not really have classic fibromyalgia; rather, they have adrenal fatigue, if not exhaustion. It's pretty hard not to be under stress on a regular basis, considering the state of the world and having to live under the stress of finances, job, world, and weather calamities as well as family matters, relationships, and general physical as well as dietary stressors. To backtrack just a little bit, cortisol plays a very important role in keeping the body's immune system intact. When the adrenals aren't functioning correctly they challenge the immune system, which further deteriorates and complicates the picture of fibromyalgia, encouraging autoimmune and inflammatory diseases as well as chronic fatigue.

Terms

There are two terms I want to bring up that relate to adrenal exhaustion; you may find that they apply to other topics that we'll discuss: anabolism and catabolism.

Anabolism, or an anabolic state, is when a person's body is healthy enough and balanced enough to be repairing and rebuilding its tissues. The body is continually regenerating itself and repairing as necessary—everything from blood vessels to heart tissues, bones to nerves. In an anabolic state, the body balances mental function, enhances memory, and manages inflammation: muscles, tendons, ligaments, and joints can repair and give the opportunity to have pain-free movement without medication.

Catabolism, or the catabolic state, is when the body is breaking down; it literally begins to consume its own resources. The word catabolic comes from the Greek for cataclysm, which means disaster. If we spend too much time in a stressful state (adrenal exhaustion), catabolism is encouraged and has disastrous effects on the body. The aging process in itself is a catabolic process. So in adrenal exhaustion we see people who are unable to recover from stress; they have more illness, degenerative diseases, age faster, and have more pain. In most cases, this leads to taking more drugs, if not addressed by natural means early enough.

Tests

There is an adrenal test that would most likely be ordered by a chiropractor, functional medicine MD, or naturopath. We use ZRT Laboratory out of Beaverton, Oregon. The graphic below depicts the results of such a test, which helps to evaluate a catabolic state requiring intervention. The middle line is the average/reference line. We look for readings above/below to understand the patient's condition.

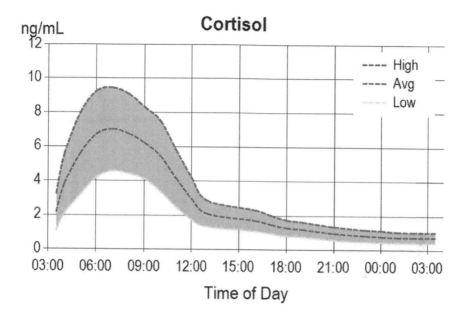

The test is done over a 24-hour period, providing accurate and comprehensive measurements of cortisol levels throughout the day. It detects the amount of cortisol present in the body during different times of the day. The normal trend of cortisol is to start at its highest level in the morning and gradually decrease till midnight. However, some conditions can lead to improper secretion of cortisol. More often than not we are looking for stress-induced cortisol imbalances that may account for fibro symptoms, reported as an excessive (high reading) or insufficient (low reading) of cortisol levels.

Protecting Your Adrenals
Reducing Physiological Stress

For now, let's discuss the one area that we can all take charge of to improve and work toward healthier adrenals, living in an anabolic state. Keep in mind that managing the adrenals and the hypothalamic-pituitary-adrenal axis (HPA) is crucial to general health and improving fibromyalgia.

The first thing we can do is to manage our diet. Details of managing diet and body chemistry are in several areas of this book. A great complement to this chapter would be Chapters 8 and 22.

Controlling blood sugar plays a vital role in managing the adrenals. We manage blood sugar primarily by eating the right foods at the right times of the day. When blood sugar isn't managed, energy systems aren't managed and adrenals will be overtaxed even if emotional and physical stress levels are normal. Low blood sugar in and of itself can cause everything from headaches to brain fog, sweet cravings, nervousness, possibly depression--and, more importantly, can lead to adrenal exhaustion and a catabolic state, as we discussed.

Our diets really do need to be balanced. All three food groups should be consumed to reach a blood sugar balance. This means carbohydrates, fats, and proteins. We'll cover these here in just a general way. Keep in mind that there are very few thoughts or recommendations in this text that apply to every person in every situation. Person-by-person customization is necessary. This is why and where the health team that you have worked to put together will pay off.

Carbohydrates
The understanding of carbohydrate and blood sugar importance and management is crucial to managing health/fibro. They are arguably the two most important yet neglected and abused components of health and healing. Diabetes is diagnosed as the 7th leading cause of death in the USA and 8th in the world. Blood sugar and carbohydrate consumption are directly associated with the other leading causes of death, as well as every other defined disease or condition the body fights. These issues deserve a minute for a quick review.

Becoming familiar with the term glycemic index is important. Glycemic index refers to how fast a food turns to sugar in the body after it is consumed. The higher the glycemic index, the faster it turns into a sugar. The faster it turns into a sugar, the more insulin the body has to produce, and as a result stores more fat (refer back to Chapter 8 for more clarity). This scenario causes blood sugar to drop, triggering a counter-regulatory effort by the adrenal glands to stimulate the production of more cortisol. This doesn't upset the balance, because it is the way it's supposed to work in short spurts of necessity. However, when high-glycemic carbohydrates are consistently overconsumed, the system becomes exhausted. Adrenal glands become fatigued. Cells resist the overexposure to insulin, and the hypothalamus becomes almost indifferent to cortisol's signals. Subsequently Stage III adrenal exhaustion ensues.

So it would seem that carbohydrates in and of themselves do not cause inflammation the way a strain/sprain or infection would; rather, they upset the innate mechanism that controls physiological inflammation. This can show up as puffiness or increased arthritic types of aches and pains. The message is: Stay away from high-glycemic carbohydrates. As a side note, don't be fooled by foods that boast of using whole grains or multigrain (they just sound like they should be healthier; remember there have been millions of dollars spent to convince us we are doing a good thing). If they have been processed in any way, the glycemic index will rise to an unhealthy level.

Admittedly, this is an oversimplification of managing blood sugar and the toll that stress can take on the HPA axis. Nevertheless, doing better is an effort that we can all make with the confidence that it can only help. Vegetables are relatively complex carbohydrates (lower glycemic); they are chock full of fiber and vitamins. Most would agree that they are considered good for us. They help to maintain pH balance in the body as well as add valuable minerals and enzymes (if not overcooked). As a general rule, the lowest glycemic index vegetables are grown above ground, such as broccoli, lettuce, cucumbers, and cabbage. The vegetables that are grown below ground (root vegetables such as potatoes and carrots) tend to have a higher glycemic index. When we contrast vegetables with grains we find that corn, rice, bread, pasta, bagels, and all grains are considered to have a very high-glycemic index. The healthiest diets are those that include mid-and low-range glycemic index foods and restrict high-glycemic foods. You'll be way ahead of the game simply by committing yourself to removing grains from your diet, at least for now.

Remember "glycemic load." This refers to the net results of slowing down digestion and the speed at which the food turns to sugar, by adding fats, proteins, and fiber to a meal. The transformation from food to sugar slows down, and puts less of a load on the pancreas as well as the adrenals. Paying attention to meals fiber content, fats, and protein will help reduce glycemic load.

Proteins

Lean protein should be eaten more frequently than high-fat proteins; range-fed or wild animal proteins are far more desirable than farm-raised. The same holds true for fish: wild-caught cold-water fish is a better choice than farm-raised. Other sources of great protein are eggs, nuts and seeds. Some grains, such as amaranth and quinoa, have relatively high protein, offer a good percentage of fiber, and are more alkalizing.

Fats

I have found fats to be the most misunderstood type of food. We've been misled for years, having been told that fats are something we should stay away from. If you'd like to clear up the controversy and the general medical information that we've gotten over the last 25 years in reference to heart disease and cholesterol and fats, read *The Great Cholesterol Myth*, by Jonny Bowden PhD and Stephen Sinatra MD. In the meantime, know that we cannot be healthy without consuming fats, properly termed "essential fatty acids." Good fats are essential for hormone balance, cellular activity, cellular metabolism, and neurological function. There are two, possibly three disasters that have taken place in the last 20 years due to what allopathic medicine has claimed about fats. One is that cholesterol is necessary to maintain proper hormone production. The reduction in good fats has sabotaged many women's hormones, affecting mood and energy and creating miserable menopausal years. This is likely to take two generations to reverse. I further suspect that this is one of the contributors to women being the highest population of fibromyalgia sufferers.

The second issue has to do with vitamin D. As of this writing, nearly everyone in the medical community now realizes that most of the population is deficient in vitamin D. Vitamin D deficiency affects sex hormones as well as reducing the body's ability to manage pain. We've been told one of the reasons for low vitamin D is that we don't get enough sun, but it's not that simple. For the body to produce vitamin D, there must be adequate amounts of oils/fatty acids in and on our skin in order to synthesize healthy levels of vitamin D. We have discussed previously that vitamin D is more a hormone than a vitamin. There is debate as to whether or not surface skin oil is necessary to generate D. While the jury is still out, it doesn't make sense that the body cooks up the D with the skin's surface oil and then goes through an absorption process. I do think many are obsessed with washing with soap and can dry out skin, but I don't think we have to let oils build on the skin's surface to be safe. Photo receptors in the cells of epidermis will generate D as long as there is antiquate cholesterol.

The third issue is that the same people who for decades have been telling us not to eat fat are now realizing that enough of the proper fats are essential to controlling healthy levels of cholesterol. Cholesterol is a necessary part of the body's natural anti-inflammatory and blood-sugar management system. By restricting and\or lowering cholesterol with medication, we leave ourselves open to many other illnesses and inflammatory conditions. Cholesterol, for the most part, is at best guilty by association in reference to how it clogs arteries and causes heart disease.

As it applies more directly to fibromyalgia, fats help to lower the glycemic load of foods. Essential fatty acids (good fats) are found in seeds, nuts, and plants, as well as respected oils such as olive oil, avocados, and fish (salmon and sardines, etc.). Bad fats, which we discussed in Chapter 15, are found in poorly stored or handled foods that may cause rancidity. Hydrogenated/high trans-fat products as well as saturated fats are harmful (vegetable oils in particular) and cause inflammation and system breakdown. These are found in adulterated fats as in chips, crackers, and fried foods. Animal fats and dairy are generally bad when not raised wild.

These are the major dietary considerations to improve adrenal function and help the body deal with stress and repair, creating an anabolic state. If your health-care provider suspects adrenal insufficiency, he or she can order a test as discussed above. Many cases can be handled with nutritional and dietary changes, as well as some lifestyle modification.

Lifestyle Modification

The areas of lifestyle and behavior that we could change to support the adrenals include getting enough sleep and maintaining a regular wake/sleep cycle. This means trying to go to bed at approximately the same time every night and getting up at approximately the same time every morning.

The next would be regular exercise. The exercise should be something that you enjoy and that you can do consistently and safely. We find the people who have the best result with exercise carve out a specific time of the day that they can dedicate to exercise on a regular basis. Exercise should include aerobic as well as anaerobic activities. Aerobic exercises increase oxygen consumption and raise our metabolic rate, like walking and swimming. Anaerobic means "without oxygen" such as resistance exercises like lifting weights, resistance bands, etc. Remember that consistency is more important than anything, and overexercising can work backward and create a catabolic state, meaning tearing the body down and in turn stressing the HPA axis. Consult your health-care provider for more specifics for your situation. But read Chapter 21 first.

Emotional Stress

Emotional stress can be helped by exercise. Real exercise has an emotional and spiritual component to it that enhances brain function and relaxes the nervous system. Additionally, I'm a big believer in counseling, journaling, praying, and meditating as options for releasing thoughts, confusions, emotional baggage, fears, jealousies, and guilt. These provide a way of venting and reorganizing thoughts and feelings. They are active, productive, and have been clinically shown time and time again to reduce stress. Let's keep in mind that any time we talk about stress we're not just talking about some emotional component that has no cellular, neurological, or physical relationship. Stress means increasing allostatic load, as in physically and energetically wearing down the nervous system, the hormonal system, and all the other systems required for a balanced healthy body and life.

Supplements

There are some creative supplementation theories to affect the hypothalamus and pituitary. However, more commonly it's accepted that nutritionally we have the opportunity to influence the adrenals. Discuss with your health care provider preferred supplementation for you in light of any tests that have been done, and other nutritional efforts that have already been undertaken. Without getting into the biochemistry, I'm going to name just a few things that we've seen to be supportive of the adrenal glands. B complex vitamins are very important, as well as minerals. Many researchers and doctors in the field are finding that taking extra biotin is effective along with choline, inositol, Siberian ginseng, rosemary leaf, rutin, DHEA, and pregnenolone. These suggestions are only to help you further research, formulate better questions, and improve your vocabulary when speaking to your health care provider. I would also suggest that you look into formulas that are considered to be "adaptogenic." Adaptogenic herbs can help strengthen the patient's ability to respond to both daily and chronic stressors. I use a product by Moss Nutrition called HPA Select and, for patients wanting to deal with stress plus lose weight, I suggest trying ACTS (Adrenal, Cortisol, Thyroid, stress Support) by TLS (see appendix). Research of the herbal extracts in these formulations has suggested the ability to support and enhance healthy cortisol regulation, mental alertness, restful sleep, immune resistance, and healthy mood, all of which help to modulate the HPA axis, having direct influence on fibro.

Thyroid

All stressors prompt the brain to release chemical messengers that tell the pituitary to instruct the adrenals to "make cortisol." In turn, these messengers reduce thyroid stimulating hormone (TSH). The thyroid is responsible for how quickly the body utilizes energy, makes proteins, and how it handles other hormones that come from the adrenals and the hypothalamus. It's the largest hormone gland in our body. It's located in the throat behind what you might call your Adam's apple. It has two lobes and it looks like a butterfly.

Hyperthyroidism

Hyperthyroidism occurs when your thyroid is overactive, possibly creating a condition like goiter. In goiter, a person's eyes protrude a little bit; there are heart palpitations and excessive sweating, diarrhea, weight loss, muscle weakness, sensitivity to heat, and possibly increased appetite. It's most commonly seen in an autoimmune disorder called Graves' disease.

Hypothyroidism

Hypothyroidism is the underproduction of thyroid hormones due to stress, but it may also be due to congenital factors or autoimmune diseases such as Hashimoto's or iodine deficiency. It is also seen, as you might expect, in the removal of the thyroid or cancerous thyroids.

Frequently iodine deficiency is noted as being related to poorer countries where nutritional deprivation is obvious. However, it has been my experience, and the experience of many colleagues, that iodine deficiency is extremely common in relatively affluent countries as well. Lower than optimal iodine consumption can cause subclinical hypothyroidism that undermines metabolism. It's most often not recognized as hypothyroidism—at least not in early stages. There is a subtle and insidious progression, noting that a person is unable to control weight as they would like to, or is tired, maybe balding, or has intolerance to cold. Often symptoms are chalked up to age or everyday stress, as if the symptoms don't matter. Iodine tests are very simple and supplementation is very effective.

Deficiency in iodine opens suspicion that other elements are lacking as well that further handicap the thyroid. One study by Dr. Lowe, 1998–1999, suggests that thyroid insufficiency all by itself could be enough to induce fibromyalgia. Additional supplementation has been found to be very helpful, with a protocol similar to adrenal supplementation. Consider B complex vitamins, as well as adequate minerals and antioxidants.

Both the adrenals and thyroid will benefit from regular meals. A breakfast that includes protein, fats, and minimal complex carbohydrate within the first hour to hour and a half after rising is helpful to reduce systemic stress after fasting overnight. Go easy on the caffeine, and no simple carbohydrates.

Substance P and Serotonin

It's interesting to note that we don't have confirmation as to whether adrenal fatigue/exhaustion causes fibromyalgia or fibromyalgia causes the adrenals to malfunction. Nevertheless, their relationship remains necessary to support. The adrenals do play the more obvious role in affecting the thyroid. Hypothyroidism may be the explanation as to why low serotonin and high Substance P levels are common to fibromyalgia patients.[16] The hypothalamus and pituitary are intimate with the thyroid, and that relationship in itself is intimate with the HPA axis. Sounds confusing, but the bottom line is that the thyroid is accepted as having a more direct causative relationship to fibromyalgia.

The neurological and hormonal changes in Fibros are different from the general population in respect to how they respond to chronic pain and stress. In fibromyalgia, the thyroid becomes hypo-functioning when under chronic pain and stress, serotonin is likely depressed, and Substance P will tend to rise. This relates to symptoms of fatigue and sluggishness, constipation, achy muscles, tenderness and stiffness, muscle weakness and depression, as well as pain, stiffness, and swelling of joints.

In the non-Fibro population the thyroid becomes excited/hyper-functioning, as you expect to see, when exposed to chronic pain and stress. [71]

The Rest of the Story

Adrenal Fatigue vs. Hypothyroidism

There is an extremely important correlation and understanding about the interaction and interdependency between the adrenal glands and the thyroid. The medical community is generally geared to recognize low body temperature, fatigue, poor weight management, increased sluggishness, and various aches and pains as being a signal that there is a thyroid problem. Yet 70 percent of people taking thyroid replacement medication continue to complain of symptoms.[1] Let's take a look at the correlation between adrenal fatigue and hypothyroidism.

Adrenal Fatigue vs Hypothyroidism
The following table contrasts Adrenal Fatigue to Hypothyroidism

Characteristics	Adrenal Fatigue	Hypothyroidism
Body		
Weight	Difficulty Controlling	Generalized Weight Gain
Temp regulation	On the High side	On the Low side
Mental Function		
Mental Function	Brain Fog	Sluggish
Depression	Sometimes	Frequently
Appearance		
Eyebrows	Normal	sparse outer 1/3
Hair	Thin at hair lines, possible loss	Coarse but Thin
Nails	Thin, brittle	Normal to thick
Around Eyes	Sunken	Puffy
Skin	Thin and Dry	Normal
Mental Function		
Mental Function	Brain Fog	Sluggish
Depression	Sometimes	Frequently
Body Awareness		
Fluid Retention	No	Yes
Pain	Headaches, muscular aches	Joints, muscles
Reactivity	Heightened and hyper-reactive	Hypo-reactive
Ligament Weakness	Unable to hold chiropractic adjustments	Unable to hold chiropractic adjustments
History		
Infections	YES, candida, yeast, bacterial	Occasionally
Chronic Fatigue	Yes	Yes
Hypotension	Often	No
Blood Sugar	Frequently Hypoglycemic	Normal - Hyperglycemia
Gut	Irritable Bowels	Constipation/sluggish
Mal-Absorption	Yes	No
Sleep	Wake up 2-4 am	Loves to Sleep
Temperature	Intolerance to Cold	Intolerance to Heat
Food Craving	Craves salt, loves sweet	Loves Fats

In a clinical setting, many symptoms are first recognized/considered to be a thyroid issue. Laboratory tests are conducted on the thyroid, and thyroid medication is prescribed. So why doesn't this solve the problem? Hypothyroidism can be primary or secondary. Primary hypothyroidism may be due to congenital or developmental abnormality of the gland or in response to environmental damage, such as from taking medication. Secondary hypothyroidism is due to a problem with the pituitary gland.

This helps to explain why 70 percent of people will still have symptoms even if medication is prescribed and lab tests show that the thyroid hormones have increased to close to normal. Dr. Lam, board certified in anti-aging medicine by the American Board of Anti-Aging Medicine, reports that when the adrenals reach the secondary stage of exhaustion, the adrenals will try to rest.

When the adrenals rest, thyroid hormone production slows body metabolism. Thyroid symptoms appear and thyroid medication will be prescribed. This approach works directly against the adrenals and frequently sets the stage for an adrenal crisis. This is due to the fact that thyroid medication is meant to soup up the thyroid and increase metabolism, the exact opposite of what already weakened and fatigued adrenals need. This common clinical approach fails to control the thyroid or the symptoms, and further weakens the adrenals. Frequently, more medication or different medication will be prescribed, insisting on treating thyroid alone to resolve symptoms. This is a common scenario, causing frustration and aggravation of fibro symptoms.

Some patients describe feeling wired, tired, or living in constant fatigue; they report being unable to fall asleep and feeling anxious throughout the day. All at the same time, their adrenals continue to weaken. It's my recommendation that if you believe you fall into this category, discuss with your PCP a second opinion by a board-certified anti-aging medical physician/endocrinologist.

Eliminate Toxins

Eliminating toxins, as discussed in Chapter 12, will go a long way to support your hormonal systems. This includes dietary toxins/preservatives, which includes processed and prepared food, drink, and alcoholic beverages. Refrain from using artificial sweeteners and, at least temporarily, get as many grains out of the diet as possible, especially wheat. Don't forget environmental toxins such as smoke, electromagnetic exposure, noise, and anything else that stresses your senses.

> Seek a second opinion from a functional MD or naturopath if you can't seem to get your stress/adrenal or thyroid under control. In the meantime, work toward controlling overwhelm, restrict carbohydrates, and support your system with supplements.

CHAPTER 21

Exercise/Fibro-cise

Chapter Topics:

Made to Move	*Aerobic vs Anaerobic*
When and Where	*Out-of-Control Wins*
Is It Worth It?	*Act and React*
Fibro-cise	

Made to Move

We're going to spend what may seem to be a disproportionate amount of time discussing exercise. I hope that the perspective I share and the words I use will ultimately bring commitment and consistency of exercise into your life, for the simple reason that we humans are made to move. We are made to lift, push/pull, reach, and climb. Movement inspires proper physiology; it fine-tunes and helps to coordinate all systems and functions of our body, including hormones and attitude. Many of the diseases that we suffer from in the modern world are due to living a life that contradicts what we've been made for: "movement." Don't take this section lightly or assume that you've read it all before and know everything there is to know about exercise. Words to the wise, however; don't think exercise is the Holy Grail. Valerie Martin, a Transitions Lifestyle Systems health coach, would say: "You can't exercise your way out of a poor diet." I believe the principles in this section, along with nutrition/lifestyle changes, can change your life and the course of fibromyalgia for you. I know that's a tall order to fill. Hang in there and read it all, then consider going to our website www.fibro-doc.com and giving us some feedback that we can post to inspire other readers.

Exercise and muscle physiology provide fundamental insights regarding why fibromyalgia sufferers have such a difficult time with muscle strength, endurance, and pain. Your grasp of this will help bring perspective and understanding of recommendations and science that will be shared in other chapters, in particular when we discuss nutrition. Our experience is that the more that patients become familiar with anatomy and physiology of the body, the better chance they have of following through with self-management issues.

Definition

You'll find that everyone has an idea of what exercise is, with formal definitions offered by authors, dictionaries, and doctors. Dorland's medical dictionary defines exercise as: *The performance of physical exertion for the improvement of health or the correction of physical deformity.* I'm not sure that this is the definition we want to work with. Let's try this one:

Motion by voluntary contraction and relaxation of muscles. Is this too vague? How about this:

Exercise is an activity that is voluntary, with the intention of improving and/or maintaining one's ability to adapt and survive and to reproduce.

While all of the above are true, I'm not sure that any one of them is resourceful enough to meet the challenge that fibromyalgia sufferers live with. I think we need a definition that's specific to fibromyalgia and chronic fatigue. I'm going to offer my definition, but before you read any further, take a moment and write your own personal definition of exercise in the space below.

Exercise is:

_____

_____

_____

_____

_____

For our purposes, I would like you to consider adopting this definition: *Exercise is a voluntary active exertion that is above, beyond, and in addition to activities of daily living, with conscious intent to improve physical, mental, and social well-being.*

Let's break it down a little so we really get a practical sense of what physical, mental, and social well-being mean to us.

PHYSICAL: To move and negotiate the activities of daily living without injury. (Activities of daily living are things like putting on socks, climbing stairs, bending down to put a pan away, taking groceries out of the trunk of your car, caring for your home, and performing your job.)

MENTAL: The facility of thought, emotions, and activities. This is the integration of your life, feelings, desires, reason, memories, and motivations to attend to your life with contentment.

SOCIAL: The integration of self into relationships with other living things that have the capacity to learn, reason, and feel.

I often hear people say, "I get plenty of exercise. I tend my garden, I work around the house. I am moving every minute of every day." However, domestic activities and work responsibility do not necessarily constitute exercise; they rarely completely fulfill our definition. Gardening, for instance, will be considered exercise only if it meets our definition and not simply because a person was active, moving, and working. That's not to say that gardening can't be exercise, but if it doesn't meet our definition, one could work in the garden all day and it may all add up to feeling worse. We're going to discuss the subtle and practical aspects of exercise success.

Why, What, When, and Where of Exercise

There is no shortage of books and opinions giving us exercise suggestions and explaining how important it is to all of us. Frequently a patient will sit across from me and explain that he has either read about exercises, or his doctor gave him exercises and he does them faithfully and in fact loves them, explaining that "they really work." My question to him is, "If they are working, why are you here?" And he says, "Well, I am no better; I think I am getting worse." So how can exercise be so beneficial when it does not really seem to get you anywhere?

One reason is that fibro physiology does not tolerate the waste products and toxins that the body generates when exercising. So, at best, most patients only temporarily feel better from the results of exercise: relaxing the nervous system, increasing circulation, stimulating endorphins, and escaping from life. However, in the long run, waste products and toxicity win, due to their lingering and cumulative negative effects. I am guessing that you're all too familiar with pain, soreness, and fatigue that return after your efforts.

Sorting It Out

As with any project, we need to sort out the *why, when, what,* and *where* to be able to formulate a plan, follow through, and succeed. In this case, to succeed means success based on our definition above. Without these crucial components being thought out, you are likely to fail, as about 80 percent of those who embark on such a program do. This is more than understandable when you consider that the average fibro sufferer is beaten down by pain, brain fog, and lack of energy. On top of that, there is the subtle yet piercing attitude of those around you who wonder why you refuse to exercise: "She doesn't look like there's anything wrong with her. Why isn't she exercising? Is she lazy?" They simply don't understand the pain and suffering that you are going through.

Personal

The first step in the process is to find your personal *Why* to help motivate you. As Tony Robbins has said, "If you have a big enough *Why*, you can do anything." We covered this back in our chapter on Fibro men. It will be your personal *Why* that serves as the driving force for you to exercise, even on the days when simply getting out of bed seems like a monumental challenge.

Your personal *When* is the target time to exercise that will give you the best chance to make it happen regularly to gain the maximum result for a resistant body and mind.

Your personal *What* refers to what exercise you should do or what equipment you should utilize in your specific case.

Your personal *Where* determines that if you're going to exercise, where you will do it and why it matters.

Why

The power to succeed in any human endeavor or to meet any challenge lies in the reasons/motivation behind our efforts. The *Why* of exercise has one personal factor and five scientific factors.

In the book *Man's Search for Meaning* by Viktor Frankl, he wrote about how he survived a Nazi concentration camp by creating a *Why* every day: a reason to live, to try—a reason not to give up. It would have been much easier to give up, Frankl noted, and most did. According to the Book-of-the-Month Club and the Library of Congress, Victor Frankl's *Man's Search for Meaning* is one of the top ten most influential books in the United States. If you've never taken the time to read it, now would be a great time to do so. Your personal *Why* will apply in every area of your life and every area of your fibro challenge.

So what's the reason to get philosophical over exercise? It is just exercise, after all. The reason is that exercise is the single most manageable personal effort to help ourselves and enhances the success of all other efforts. In my opinion it even comes before nutrition.

PERSONAL WHY. We could speak of *Whys* in terms of beliefs, reasons, or responsibilities. However you choose to look at them, they must be compelling and strike an emotional chord. While I will offer *scientific Whys*, make no mistake about it—your *Personal Why* is the *Why of Whys*. Stop for a minute and make a list of the five most important people in your life, the ones who make your life worth living.

_____

_____

_____

_____

Now circle the one who is most important to you, and imagine the sky's opening up and a voice thundering down to announce that your special person will be taken from you forever. And that the only way for you to get that person back would be for you to commit to exercise 30 minutes every day for the rest of your life. I'd say that is an overwhelmingly emotional reason to exercise. My question is: Could you and would you exercise 30 minutes a day for the rest of your life?

That's your big *Why* if you believe that it is the only way to keep that person in your life who matters the most to you. It's up to you to think it out and find other reasons why improving your health is more important than just improving your health. I hope this makes sense. I'm just trying to prove the point that you could and would exercise regularly if you found a big enough *Why*. Right now you're limited more by your mind than you are by your body. Did you ever notice how motivated and committed to success people are when looking forward to going to a class reunion, because they want to lose 10 or 20 pounds and look good?

Your big *Why* does not have to stay constant. You could play leap-frog with your *Whys* and create a new one every six months, every year, or every week if you want; whatever works for you. You have to be clear on your big *Why* if you ever hope to have success over the long haul. So

I challenge you to look at your priorities and values in life to find your motivational *Whys.*

You have already compiled a list of the most important people in your life. Now go through that list, and for each person write out three to five reasons why that person needs you to be healthier. What would it mean to that person if you got worse and couldn't be part of his or her life? Maybe one of the people on that list is your daughter. She needs you to be there. She needs you to be emotionally and energetically available and healthy to help her negotiate the challenges and heartaches of life. Perhaps you have a parent on your list who is getting on in age and you want to be able to help her take care of herself and live as independently as possible. Your partner in life may be on your list. Many couples find that they are drifting apart due to lack of active participation like they had in the old days. Any of these can and should be a motivating factor for you. There are social reasons, domestic reasons, and sexual reasons. List three to five reasons for each of the five people. Go for it and see where it takes you.

Next step: Make a list of five other priorities in your life that are not people. Follow the same steps as above. Prioritize these. Job/career—you may find that you need more energy and mental sharpness for your job than you currently are able to put out. Maybe you fear losing a promotion or, worse still, you might lose your job if you're unable to improve your energy and your effectiveness. Another heading may be that you love to travel and you envision seeing more of the world as you age. If you are serious about accomplishing everything on your little bucket list, you need to find the *Whys* in your life. If you find your *Whys*, then you will find yourself and the motivation you need to succeed. Don't confuse responsibilities with *Whys*. Responsibilities can feel like *Whys*, but may hold resentment or other emotions that will work against your success.

Is It Worth It?
There are four factors why exercise should be a #1 priority for fibromyalgia suffers, most of which your doctor may not know or explain to you.

1. Pain Management. The movement of joints stimulates special nerve endings called mechanoreceptors. These mechanoreceptors, when called into service by movement, inhibit pain, improve coordination, and decrease muscle tightness; they also stimulate neurotransmitters and endorphins. Because this directly affects the brain, it's especially important for fibromyalgia sufferers as they attempt to control pain levels. This assumes that they don't have any joint restriction. However, endorphins are short-lived and they need to be stimulated on a regular basis to enjoy the effects. This cannot be accomplished on a regular basis until abnormal joint movement is corrected.

Joint restrictions may first need to be addressed by a chiropractor, osteopath, or a physical therapist before beginning.

Controlling pain and inflammation requires controlling blood sugar too, and exercise is particularly effective in doing so. When blood sugar is high, moderate exercise can help to reduce it. The physiology of reducing blood sugar by exercise is an issue of how well our cells utilize insulin. Research is striving to come to a conclusion as to whether high-intensity interval training or moderate-intensity interval training would best serve the diabetic and non-diabetic population to control blood sugar. Exercise increases cellular sensitivity to insulin for approximately 12 to 24 hours after exercising. Those with Type II diabetes are helped by the increased sensitivity of cells' ability to utilize insulin. Note that people with diabetes should avoid exercise during extreme hyperglycemic episodes. This is due to the potential complications associated with ketoacidosis. Always discuss exercise with your doctor before beginning.

2. Emotional Leverage. Endorphins and other chemicals secreted during exercise may make you happy, help you think more positively, and stimulate areas of your brain that will allow you to think more clearly. There was a study done that showed that ten minutes of walking improved a person's mood and outlook for up to two hours; not a bad payback for ten minutes of effort.

Another emotional advantage is that exercise is a way to nurture "self." Giving yourself special time puts the universe and everyone around you on notice that it's about "you" for a change. This is why it has to be voluntary (an option) driven by your personal *Why*, so you don't feel that it's your responsibility. I'm sure you already have enough "responsibility" in your life. Exercise offers a chance to further focus the mind and keep the mind centered on health as a priority, plus it activates higher centers within the brain, which helps dissuade pain circuit imprints. In the early stages of your recovery, exercise is one of the few action steps that you can have complete control of; you don't need to depend on anyone else.

Go back to the definitions we gave earlier. Exercise must be above and beyond your normal activities/responsibilities, to fulfill the emotional component. Also, to fulfill a physiological need, exercise should take you above and beyond your normal everyday exertion. By doing so, you increase strength and endurance so that everyday exertions/activities in the future become easier, with less chance of injury. Exercise will make life easier to live emotionally, and easier to live physically.

3. Cellular Energy. Exercise stimulates every cell in the body to do a better job. When the demand is created, cells will look for ways to be more efficient at using nutrients and creating more energy. This assumes that you are providing adequate vitamins, minerals, enzymes, proteins, fats, etc., in your diet.

When cellular energy goes up, your energy goes up. Healthy cells make for healthy tissues. Healthy tissues build healthy organs. We need healthy organs to build healthy systems and overall health.

There are 15 systems in the body that exercise will help to build. You may have been diagnosed with a coexisting condition that makes you particularly interested in enhancing one or several of the systems listed:

Circulatory System: Exercise strengthens and helps circulate more oxygenated blood to the brain and all parts of the body, while carrying away carbon dioxide and other toxins.

Digestive System: Exercise helps the efficiency of digestion and the successful absorption of nutrients into the tissues, while helping to eliminate waste.

Endocrine System: The endocrine system includes the glands of growth, metabolism, emotions, biorhythm, and reproduction. Exercise triggers chemical and neurological messengers in the brain to stimulate, balance, and coordinate all the hormones needed to successfully adapt to our internal and external environment.

Immune System: The immune system is a defense system against infection and disease. Exercise stimulates and helps to regulate automatic responses to inflammation, chemical stressors, and bacterial, viral, and fungal invaders.

Lymphatic System: The lymphatic system is another defense system that deals with toxins; it produces disease-fighting antibodies. It also assists in the distribution of fluids and nutrients to tissues. This is an amazing system that deserves proper credit for all that it does. The lymphatic system deals with waste products and fluids of the system. It has two times more volume than there is blood in the body. Lymph bathes every single cell in the body. Unlike blood in the circulatory system, the lymphatic system does not have a pump. This system uses muscular contractions and gravity to move and effectively pump its fluids around the body. By exercising consistently, you help the lymphatic system to be more efficient and not stagnate.

Muscular System: Muscles give the body shape and help us not to fall over. This system is responsible for voluntary and involuntary movement. An arm or a leg muscle is an example of a voluntary muscle. Heart muscles and blood vessels, as well as the intestinal tract, are examples of involuntary muscles. Exercise strengthens and stimulates muscular systems. Keep in mind that each of these systems in our list is crucially important to each of the others. All of them have reciprocal, complementary responsibilities. As an example, you might not think of muscles being important in the regulation of chemicals, hormones, and brain function, yet they are.

Nervous System: The brain, spinal cord, and peripheral nerves are included in the nervous system. Exercise stimulates nerves and fine-tunes the nervous system, which helps regulate all brain-to-body and body-to-brain functions and communication, including coordination and perceptions of the body in time and space as it integrates us with our environment and emotions.

Reproductive System: Exercise stimulates a healthy, happy, and driving force to perpetuate the species.

Skeletal System: The skeletal system is the framework providing levers, triangulation, and mechanisms to tolerate vectors of force and gravity; it is rich in calcium and mechanical wizardry. It helps achieve effective movement and stability. It also provides compartments for our organ systems to reside in. Exercise helps bones to be strong yet elastic, with the ability to absorb shock, similar to the frame of a good racing bike. Unlike a bike, of course, bones are living communication networks, and along with the joints of the skeletal system, they help to manage brain function and health.

Respiratory System: Exercise strengthens the respiratory system's responsibilities of oxygenating blood, while expelling waste products (mostly carbon dioxide).

Excretory System: Exercise helps to massage the large and small intestines for better absorption of nutrients, while selectively eliminating toxins.

Integumentary System: This system includes skin, hair, and sweat glands. Exercise helps to increase the system's efficiency with the excretion of waste and the management of body temperature. It also helps to evaluate our environment, assessing danger while improving coordination and balance.

Fascial System: The fascial system was once seen as being included in the integumentary system. However, fascia is a specialized system of the body that has an appearance similar to a fabric/sheet woven of one continuous strand. Fascia is very densely woven, covering and interpenetrating without interruption every muscle, bone, nerve, artery, and vein, as well as all of our internal organs including the heart, lungs, brain, and spinal cord. It has intelligence and communication throughout. It helps to protect, organize, and modulate all it comes in contact with.

Urinary System: Exercise helps to improve the movement of fluids so that the kidneys, urethra, and bladder can more efficiently eliminate waste products, while balancing crucial elements such as calcium and phosphorus.

Sensory System: This system includes sight, smell, taste, hearing, feeling, and balance. Exercise sharpens each while improving the neurological coordination and integration of all.

5. Consciousness. Exercise helps direct the mind and helps focus on self. One of the most common characteristics of fibromyalgia sufferers is that they tend to put themselves last. They look to take care of everyone else and deny or turn a blind eye to themselves, as my grandmother used to say. Fibros feel guilty when they take time or financial resources from the family to take care of themselves, even though they would do anything to help anyone else in their family. When you exercise regularly, you are able to focus more on yourself—but not as a victim. It's important to understand that's not being selfish; it's part of the healing process. You will become more aware of other things that are necessary to drive your recovery, such as meal preparation, nutrition, food choices, getting proper rest, and even personal time. Exercise will help to steer you and multiply every effort in reaching your health goals.

What

Patients ask me what exercises will be most beneficial. My answer always is, "Whatever you will do and can do consistently." We are going to talk about different types of exercise and equipment. In that discussion, we will look at aerobic, anaerobic, and reactive exercises. For now, think about something that you enjoy doing and that you will do on a consistent basis. It could be walking, swimming, biking, yoga, exercise bands—the choices are endless. You don't have to worry about doing any harm; just listen to your body and choose what hurts the least. As time goes by, you will progress to a more complete program and understand that hurting does not always mean you are doing any harm. For now, keep it simple and make it easy.

When

The *When* of exercise success is simple. You can do it at any time, as long as it's the same time every day. I have noticed that the most successful patients or athletes pick a specific time each day that they are able to fit exercise into their lifestyle. This will be a time that they can control and call their own every day. You must put everyone in your family on notice that exercise time is "your time."

Your first step is to make a decision about a sustainable *When* based on your goals and your values: your big *Why*. Regularity counts. Regularity means your brain gets it; in time, your brain will automatically tell you to exercise—and obviously when. The *When* is now easy; it's the same time every day. It will be as automatic as getting up in the morning and going to the bathroom, washing your hands and face, or having a drink of water. You may want to piggyback the time you choose with watching TV or listening to music, maybe sipping a cup of tea at the same time. Whether it is the first thing you do in the morning or if you have to squeeze time in at lunchtime or in the middle of the afternoon, pick a time and stick with it. For some of you, that time might be when you get home from work, or just before you go to bed. Exercising just before you go to bed is not generally recommended. However, considering the oddities in body chemistry with fibromyalgia, I've seen patients who do best by exercising before they go to bed. No harm will come from it, so it may be worth a try if that is the time that is most convenient for you. Now write this time down and put it on your refrigerator, your mirror or another place so that both you and your family know that it is your time. This will help to keep you committed, and it will also reinforce for your family how important this is to you.

Remember that for now, your exercise is going to be simple and easy. You want to get to the point where your exercise and exercise time are on autopilot so that day to day there is no decision to be made. Reaching exercise autopilot is likely to take 6 to 12 months, but when you hit it you will love it.

Where

The *Where* of exercise is just as crucial as the *When*. Many people will make the mistake of picking their *Where* based on what they believe is the right place to exercise. Having watched many of my patients experiment with this, it seems that most often the first choice is not the correct one. I suggest a little honest introspection; a lot of compromise may be necessary for you and your family to carve out a *Where* that is sustainable over the long haul. It may end up being a space in your home. Perhaps you'll have to paint your treadmill blue to go with the drapes in your living room. There are always health clubs, but I've found that, at least in early stages, joining a club is not a sustainable commitment for Fibros.

It may be that you are the type of person who needs a companion or an exercise teammate. If so, find one! Facilities like Curves or Workout Express may be a great option also. There are no sweaty guys, no waiting in line for equipment and no confusion as to what you need to do. Most gyms, even the "sweaty" ones, will have some type of circuit training that can be completed in a very efficient manner—often 30 minutes and you're done. Keep in mind that consistency and sustainability should be your primary focus. For those readers who elect to go to a gym, you will need an alternate plan if there is inclement weather. For those times, it will be important to have an at-home option so as not to break your pattern.

As far as in your home goes, you will want it to be comfortable and convenient enough but yet in-your-face enough that you cannot ignore it—and, of course, it needs to fit into your lifestyle. As mentioned earlier, consider piggybacking. In neuro-linguistic programming, this is called neuro-association. This means to link one activity with another activity that is already programmed to happen automatically in your life. This goes back to when I made a suggestion earlier about exercising when you first get out of bed in the morning, when you first get home from work, or just before you go to bed; in this way the exercise will be linked to that event. When you utilize one of these suggestions (or another link that you may create), you will increase the chance of success!

I'd like to reiterate something mentioned at the beginning of this section. Exercise and muscle physiology are fundamental to the understanding of why fibromyalgia sufferers have such a difficult time with muscle strength, endurance, and pain. Your understanding of how cells generate energy—all cells, not just muscle cells—will help bring perspective and understanding when we discuss nutrition and will help you make distinctions when you read the section on Real Science/Real Hope, as well as our coverage about relentless pain, co-existing conditions, and the nervous system gone awry.

Fibro-cise

Fibro-cising considers that proper and comprehensive exercise stimulates the master control system of the body aka central nervous system. This fine-tunes and modulates all brain-to-body and body-to-brain communication necessary for proper function of all systems of the body. Necessary also to manage pain, improve mood, and increase energy, and to help us get a better night's sleep. Accordingly the nervous system must receive stimulation from muscles, joints and connective tissue, as well as from our senses. The more diverse the movements we choose in our exercise program, the more valuable the stimulation. The more diverse the movements, the younger and better shape the brain will stay in, helping to slow down the aging process. As we age or face health challenges choosing the most effective exercises becomes more crucial to satisfy the nervous system's dependency on movement. In turn, this will help to improve the nervous system's management of strength, balance, and coordination that we so often see fail prematurely. So what is the answer?

It is important to exercise both sides of the body, as well as the upper body and lower body. Okay, so practically speaking, what does this all mean? It means that walking is better than stretching. Walking with your arms moving, with a light weight in your hands, would be better than just walking. Swimming is better than walking because you are getting more coordination, upper and lower body activity, and you are using more muscles. Through this you are stimulating more neurological function simultaneously, and this is a good thing. Cross-country skiing would be better than biking because you are using more muscles above the waist and below the waist, as well as more core muscles. Remember, at least initially, controlled activities are safer and more doable. They should be simple and easy, and done at the same time every day.

Flexibility

I am a fan of being flexible, but I have found that most patients do better with minimal stretching. Flexibility seems to come automatically with increased activity. There is an emotional danger with flexibility that allows people to think that they are actually getting the exercise they need because they stretched. In the initial stages, this may not be a bad thing when you are shooting for behavior modification and carving out a time and a place to exercise. Being told that stretching is a great way to reduce injury and to warm up for an activity has brought much controversy. I have found that the best way to warm up for any activity is to begin to go through the motions of the activity slowly, without strain. This will warm up the exact muscles and the areas of the body that you will be using when you get into the activity you are prepping for. Additionally, it will recruit and warm up auxiliary muscles. The better time to stretch is after you have completed your activity and are cooling down. During this cool-down period, stretching will help to reduce some of the soreness that you might develop within 48–72 hours. Here again, I must caution you. I would rather see you cool down by minimizing the intensity and the speed of your chosen activity as a way to cool down, just as you did in the beginning when you warmed up. Flexibility will come as you increase your activity.

Yoga

Yoga is not the same as stretching, although it will require you to stretch. Yoga should be approached slowly and methodically; it's likely you'll need some coaching. Live instruction or DVD training will work. Yoga satisfies the need for flexibility, balance, and strength, as well as spiritual and mental relaxation when practiced properly. Activities like yoga, Qigong, and tai chi can be great adjuncts to any exercise program, but cannot satisfy all the neurological and physiological needs that need to be met to improve your health and meet all the criteria and definitions that we mentioned earlier.

Aerobic vs. Anaerobic Exercise

The average person has about 50 percent of what are called fast-twitch muscle fibers, and about 50 percent of slow-twitch muscle fibers. There are some people who have a genetic predisposition to have more of one than the other and these folks are liable to excel in particular types of athletics. However, for the rest of us, the split is about 50–50. Slow-twitch fibers help with your endurance level. Their source of energy requires oxygen. Fast-twitch fibers, as you may have deduced, are for quick response. They don't have time to utilize oxygen; they need to fire powerfully and quickly as in "right now." They do this without oxygen (anaerobically). However, they tend to fatigue quickly because they use up the energy inside the muscle itself. Both types of muscle fibers can improve by training them regularly.

When most texts discuss exercise, they break it down into these two categories: aerobic and anaerobic. However, of equal importance to aerobic and anaerobic exercises are something that I would call reactive exercises. These are especially important as you age with a fibro body, and we will get to them shortly.

Aerobic

Aerobic activities include things like walking, swimming, biking, dancing, elliptical machines, etc., and should account for about 30 percent of our exercise efforts. Aerobic activities involve slow-firing muscles that with practice can improve efficiency in creating energy, leading to better endurance levels. To do this, a constant supply of oxygen is required. Flexibility of the spine and the ability of your chest to expand and then recoil/retract under muscular contraction and tissue elasticity are crucial to oxygenation. This type of exercise is usually moderate in exertion, but done over a relatively long period of time. It increases heart rate and circulation, tones vessels, and stimulates all kinds of good chemicals in our bodies. Some, such as endorphins, reduce pain and improve mood; others will stimulate the immune system. You probably have read that for maximum benefit you need to raise your heartbeat to a certain level for a particular amount of time. I don't want you to worry about that for now. It's more important, as we said, to accomplish behavior modification with regularity and consistency. It is best to simply participate in some aerobic activities and worry about heart rate at a later time.

Anaerobic

Anaerobic literally means without oxygen. It is high-intensity, short-burst exercise that utilizes muscles and the energy stored in those muscles. The most common form of anaerobic activity is resistance exercise, like lifting weights or using some type of controlled machine resistance or resistance bands. Building strong muscles will increase metabolism, which helps to burn more calories between workouts even when you are not moving much. This is a great way to help control weight, give your body shape, and feel more confident. Anaerobic exercise also stimulates the hormones necessary for all physiological goals in fibro cases, and should account for another 30 percent of your exercise efforts. Research shows that even people who regularly exercise are likely to miss the boat, spending too much time doing aerobics and not enough time building muscle mass (anaerobics). Muscle mass is a better indicator of future health than BMI and helps to manage blood sugar and metabolic set-points, which are important if energy and controlling weight are of concern. So you may need to cut the walking short, get off the treadmill, and pump some iron to condition/recondition those weak muscles, increasing energy and supporting a healthier metabolism.

Out of Control

As you become more active, don't be afraid to lose control (sounds like fun!). When we say to "be out of control," we mean try activities that will challenge the nervous system in a way that causes your body to react, and react quickly. Some of these reactions may deal with judgment; other times it may be something automatic, like a reflex, but that always requires movement. These activities may include playing ping pong, dancing, badminton, or having a game of catch.

Reactive Exercises

It is not often that we read about reactive exercises and certainly not in respect to their benefits for fibromyalgia or chronic fatigue. Reactive exercises, aka responsive exercises, are primarily aerobic in nature. They hold a unique neurological complexity that helps not only in conditioning for strength and endurance, but that also helps to condition and protect the spine, preserve posture, improve balance, and reduce injury. Reactive exercises literally ward off some of the conditions we see as part of the aging process—neurologically, physically, and cognitively.

This type of exercise has to do with the training—or we could say programming—of the nervous system, called neuroplasticity. Neuroplasticity is the nervous system's ability to learn and adapt. We have discussed this in several previous chapters. With these exercises, we want the nervous system to learn (relearn or preserve might be more accurate) how to respond more quickly/automatically and efficiently to a condition, a circumstance, or a stimulus. In contrast, when we spoke of aerobic and anaerobic exercise, we were talking about controlled activities—that for the most part mean controlling body movements by conscious choice. This assumes that your aerobic activity has not progressed to playing tennis or basketball, which would then combine aerobic and reactive activities. Automatic muscle reactions and body mechanics are important when balance is required in order to react and avoid injury. Fibros already have difficulty with movement, strength, and endurance. Imagine how important these considerations become in later life.

As children or young adults, reactive activities are part of everyday life. We play soccer, baseball, basketball, and field hockey. These activities are all about action and reaction, using fast-twitch and slow-twitch fibers aerobically and anaerobically, all accomplished by youthful neurological circuits. As our lives change and we get into our 20s, 40s, and later, we participate in fewer and fewer of these types of activities. Probably the most important point about reactive exercises as they relate to fibromyalgia is that they encompass all of the senses, which in itself helps to condition the nervous system and slow down the aging process. Simultaneously we are conditioning the nervous system and all the chemicals and neurotransmitters that are involved in managing pain. Consider all of the calculations and senses that have to be in place to catch a ball. There is eye-hand coordination--you must judge the speed. Your muscles have to flex and they have to move quickly. The complexity of muscle firing and neurological response and sense coordination far surpasses walking on a treadmill for 20 minutes, or lifting a weight over your head. Plus this diminishes conscious pain and builds confidence in your body, more like your younger days.

So you could join a football team, participate in combat karate, or play soccer—but as a fibro sufferer, you may have to tone it down. Simply playing catch, learning how to juggle, playing ping pong or badminton—even dancing will do the job. Keep in mind that these activities should be done regularly. You'll notice that these activities usually require social interaction, assuming the interaction is not with a robot or computer game.

What About Pain?
Most fibromyalgia patients will complain of low back pain from time to time, so we are going to use low back pain and low back injury as an example. For our purposes, it does not matter whether it is an acute injury, an old injury, fibro-back, or some combination thereof. Patients will typically refer to themselves as having a bad back and they will say, "Well, this is something I have to live with," or they may say, "It's my fibromyalgia." This leads to activity avoidance, more deconditioning, loss of energy, and a negative self-image. We've all experienced pain causing fear, avoidance,

and anxiety. The good news is that the exercise strategies we have discussed so far are a great way to get the ball rolling and get back to being more active, however slowly that may be. Fear and avoidance of activity would be looked at clinically as yellow flags. Yellow flags are management and motivational issues, and unless they are dealt with, they will lead to further physical and emotional deconditioning and pain. Fibromyalgia and many coexisting conditions may then worsen as an adaptive/compensatory problem rather than a true source of the problem.

One of the main points in this section is that if your exercise program is taken slowly and methodically, and done in a timely manner, you will incorporate all of the components we have discussed and your confidence and willpower will improve. In *Rehabilitation of the Spine*, Dr. Craig Liebenson speaks of the advantages of participating in rehabilitation in spite of the pain. He states, "The biopsychological approach teaches us that the old adage, 'Let pain be your guide,' can actually reinforce illness behavior such as fear avoidance." So we find that a contemporary approach to fibromyalgia management through exercise would strive to reassure patients that they do not have a disease such as a tumor, infection, or fracture that exercise may make worse. Rather, staying active will actually help recovery. Learning that pain does not always warn of impending harm or damage can empower patients to remain active, avoid disability, and prevent fibro pain from becoming progressive or physically and emotionally disabling.

The importance of exercise cannot be denied; however, attending to toxicity issues and blood sugar management will be the only way to fully benefit from you exercise efforts.

Would it be too corny to borrow a saying from NIKE?
Just Do It!
Exercise pays! Carve out some time for yourself and fill it with exercise.
Be committed: *Just Do It!*

CHAPTER 22

Nutrition: the Rest of the Story

Chapter Topics:

    Acid-Alkaline Balance   *Coffee and Pain*
    pH Affects Everything   *Osteoporosis*
    Fats/Oils   *Arthritis / RA*

Books about nutrition number in the millions. They don't all agree, but many have common themes and fashionable concepts depending on what's hot in the media, health news, discoveries or people's needs, concerns, and fears. We have touched on some of these topics in previous chapters, hopefully in an interesting way that added perspective and depth to concepts you are already familiar with or concepts/science that you were unaware of, but will now help you to turn a new page in confident self-advocacy.

Acid-Alkaline Balance

For this discussion, let's stick mostly to subclinical imbalances, meaning those that undermine physiology and subtly cause changes that show up as other conditions that need to be addressed, such as fibromyalgia and chronic fatigue, as opposed to a formal diagnosis of acidosis, alkalosis, or malnourished syndrome. As an example, respiratory acidosis may have symptoms of shortness of breath, chronic cough, fatigue, abnormal muscle control, decreased stamina, sleeping problems, sneezing, and increased carbon dioxide levels, etc. Respiratory alkalosis is hyperventilation, where we might see tachycardia, tremors, dizziness, mental confusion, convulsions, numbness and tingling, and decreased carbon dioxide levels. The signs and symptoms of these conditions become relatively obvious. But we are concerned with the subclinical challenges of balancing pH and the way it relates to fibromyalgia.

Our bodies work very hard to stay chemically in balance. When this balance is upset, it sets the stage to challenge the immune system and opens the door to a myriad of diseases and illnesses, often in very subtle ways.

The human body does an amazing job of regulating blood pH between 7.35 and 7.45, regardless of what we eat. However, it does this at a high cost; the body's protective mechanisms will encourage storing fat as protection to absorb toxins when body chemistry becomes too acidic. It does this to help protect vital structures and functions. Improving diet and enhancing body chemistry (balancing acid/alkaline food intake) will help the body to be willing to reduce fat storage. Additionally, when the body becomes too acidic, oxygen levels drop, which reduces the cell's ability to produce ATP, causing poor muscle recovery and loss of stamina, and leading to fatigue. This condition also encourages fungus, mold, parasites, and bad bacteria as well as viruses to flourish. Fibro and chronic fatigue sufferers can help their bodies by eating a diet high in fresh fruit and vegetables and by drinking plenty of water, with a reasonable consumption of protein and enough saturated and unsaturated fats, as well as avoiding processed foods, coffee, alcohol, and tobacco. The recommended ratio of acidic to alkaline foods in the diet is 20 percent acidic and 80 percent alkaline foods.

The focus on fresh fruits and vegetables is because they have a high concentration of minerals. It's minerals that help to alkalize. Most people's lifestyle will not allow for adequate quantities or quality of fruits and vegetables. Growing conditions, depleted soil, imported foods, and cooking practices make it difficult for most people to get high-quality and absorbable vitamins and minerals in their food. For the same reasons, it's difficult to put together a precise acid/alkaline food chart to guide choices. Supplementation of minerals, in particular calcium, is recommended. Calcium and other minerals buffer an acidic pH, meaning that they help move body chemistry toward alkaline. When we don't consume enough minerals—again, in particular, calcium—the body starts to liberate calcium from bones, tissues, and teeth to neutralize acid and toxins. This is a safety mechanism because pH balance is so crucial to life. However, it takes its toll not only on teeth and bones (osteoporosis) but on cellular energy, and muscle function and strength, as well as the body's ability to manage pain.

While an imbalanced diet may be the greatest stress on a Fibro's body chemistry, there are many other sources that generate acid. A genetic predisposition is one, along with cellular malfunction. Exercise, emotional stress, poor (generally shallow) breathing, hypoglycemia, and diabetes are also contributors to acid production. Counterbalancing these acid-producing factors is the reason to strive for 80 percent of the diet to be alkaline and/or to supplement. Keep in mind that not all supplements are created equal. You can depend on a chiropractor, naturopath, or nutritionist to be aware of which nutrition companies have high-quality and highly absorbable products.

Diet

In this section, we are going to look primarily at the way diet affects pH. Inferior diet plans will neglect pH control and contribute to the overweight and diabetes crises that are currently facing many modern societies.

All foods, after being consumed, will contribute to the acid side or the alkaline side of body chemistry. You would think that something like a lemon, being so acidic, would cause the body to be more acidic. However, this isn't the case. The digestive process leaves in its wake what's called an "ash," similar to a combustion engine of a car leaving hydrocarbons as a byproduct of the combustion of fuel.

With foods, the more mineral content, the more the byproduct is an alkaline (higher pH) ash. The more processed a food is, and devoid of minerals--as is the case with processed food and drink, and most canned, bagged, jarred, boxed foods or fast food--the more acidic (lower pH) the ash will be. A typical American diet, for instance, is an acid-generating machine, with overconsumption of sugars, processed foods, salts, coffee, and an abundance of carbohydrates. Diets dominated by protein are often highly acidic as well, due to not being balanced with mineral-rich foods. For the sake of this conversation, we have to include the huge volumes of alcohol, medication (prescription as well as over-the-counter), synthetic vitamins, and tobacco, along with more genetically modified foods and manipulated oils and chemical additives than we are aware of—all of which generate acid.

The charts below are offered as a tool to put foods by pH in perspective. My research has shown arguable variations in pH charts. This is due to many variables in the way foods are grown, the regions, shipping and processing issues, etc. I've adopted the following table from Dr. Russell Jaffe. I believe it does a great job. As with most health care issues, it's not an exact science. However, the relativity is accurate and useful. For further information you could either e-mail me or go to Dr. Jaffee's site: http://www.drrusselljaffe.com/#/publishedscience

Food Category	Most Alkaline	More Alkaline	Low Alkaline	Lowest Alkaline
Spice/Herb	Baking Soda	Spices/Cinnamon Valerian Licorice •Black Cohash Agave	•Herbs (most): Arnica, Bergamot, Echinacea Chrysanthemum, Ephedra, Feverfew, Goldenseal, Lemongrass Aloe Vera Nettle Angelica	White Willow Bark Slippery Elm Artemesia Annua
Preservative	Sea Salt			Sulfite
Beverage	Mineral Water	•Kambucha	•Green or Mu Tea	Ginger Tea
Sweetner		Molasses	Rice Syrup	•Sucanat
Vinegar		Soy Sauce	Apple Cider Vinegar	•Umeboshi Vinegar
Therapeutic	•Umeboshi Plum		•Sake	•Algae, Blue Green
Processed Dairy				•Ghee (Clarified Butter)
Cow/Human Soy Goat/Sheep				Human Breast Milk
Egg			•Quail Egg	•Duck Egg
Meat Game Fish/Shell Fish				
Fowl				
Grain Cereal Grass				Oat 'Grain Coffee' •Quinoa Wild Rice •Amaranth Japonica Rice
Nut Seed/Sprout Oil	Pumpkin Seed	Poppy Seed Cashew Chestnut Pepper	Primrose Oil Sesame Seed Cod Liver Oil Almond •Sprout	Avocado Oil Seeds (most) Coconut Oil Olive/Macadamia Oil Linseed/Flax Oil
Bean Vegetable Legume Pulse Root	Lentil Brocoflower •Seaweed Nori/Kombu/Wakame/Hijiki Onion/Miso •Daikon/Taro Root •Sea Vegetables (other) Dandelion Greens •Burdock/•Lotus Root Sweet Potato/Yam	Kohlrabi Parsnip/Taro Garlic Asparagus Kale/Parsley Endive/Arugula Mustard Greens Jerusalem Artichoke Ginger Root Broccoli	Potato/Bell Pepper Mushroom/Fungi Cauliflower Cabbage Rutabaga •Salsify/Ginseng Eggplant Pumpkin Collard Greens	Brussel Sprout Beet Chive/Cilantro Celery/Scallion Okra/Cucumber Turnip Greens Squash Artichoke Lettuce Jicama
Citrus Fruit Fruit	Lime Nectarine Persimmon Raspberry Watermelon Tangerine Pineapple	Grapefruit Canteloupe Honeydew Citrus Olive •Dewberry Loganberry Mango	Lemon Pear Avocado Apple Blackberry Cherry Peach Papaya	Orange Apricot Banana Blueberry Pineapple Juice Raisin, Currant Grape Strawberry

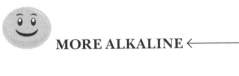

MORE ALKALINE ←————————————

Food Category	Lowest Acid	Low Acid	More Acid	Most Acid
Spice/Herb	Curry	Vanilla Stevia	Nutmeg	Pudding/Jam/Jelly
Preservative	MSG	Benzoate	Aspartame	Table Salt (NaCL)
Beverage	Kona Coffee	Alcohol Black Tea	Coffee	Beer, 'Soda' Yeast/Hops/Malt
Sweetner	Honey/Maple Syrup		Saccharin	Sugar/Cocoa
Vinegar	Rice Vinegar	Balsamic Vinegar	Red Wine Vinegar	White/Acetic Vinegar
Therapeutic		Antihistamines	Psychotropics	Antibiotics
Processed Dairy	Cream/Butter	Cow Milk	•Casein, Milk Protein, Cottage Cheese	Processed Cheese
Cow/Human	Yogurt	Aged Cheese	New Cheese	Ice Cream
Soy		Soy Cheese	Soy Milk	
Goat/Sheep	Goat/Sheep Cheese	Goat Milk		
Egg	Chicken Egg			
Meat	Gelatin/Organs	Lamb/Mutton	Pork/Veal	Beef
Game	•Venison	Boar/Elk/•Game Meat	Bear	
Fish/Shell Fish	Fish	Mollusks Shell Fish (Whole)	•Mussel/Squid	Shell Fish (Processed) •Lobster
Fowl	Wild Duck	Goose/Turkey	Chicken	Pheasant
Grain	•Triticale Millet	Buckwheat Wheat	Maize Barley Groat	Barley Processed Flour
Cereal	Kasha	•Spelt/Teff/Kamut	Corn	
Grass	Brown Rice	Farina/Semolina White Rice	Rye Oat Bran	
Nut	Pumpkin Seed Oil	Almond Oil	Pistachio Seed	Cottonseed Oil/Meal
Seed/Sprout	Grape Seed Oil	Sesame Oil	Chestnut Oil	Hazelnut
Oil	Sunflower Oil	Safflower Oil	Lard	Walnut
	Pine Nut	Tapioca	Pecan	Brazil Nut
	Canola Oil	•Seitan or Tofu	Palm Kernel Oil	Fried Food
	Spinach	Split Pea	Green Pea	Soybean
Bean	Fava Bean	Pinto Bean	Peanut	Carob
Vegetable	Kidney Bean	White Bean	Snow Pea	
	Black-eyed Pea	Navy/Red Bean		
Legume	String/Wax Bean	Aduki Bean	Legumes (other)	
Pulse	Zucchini	Lima or Mung Bean	Carrot	
Root	Chutney	Chard	ChickPea/Garbanzo	
	Rhubarb			
Citrus Fruit	Coconut			
	Guava	Plum	Cranberry	
	•Pickled Fruit	Prune	Pomegranate	
	Dry Fruit	Tomato		
Fruit	Fig			
	Persimmon Juice			
	•Cherimoya			
	Date			

MORE ACIDIC ⟶

pH Affects Everything

Anytime our pH is challenged, it will cause all cells in our body to overwork, which subsequently opens the door for cells to mutate, as well as encouraging pathogenic organisms to thrive. This forces enzymes and oxygen delivery systems as well as the kidneys to overwork. Reduced oxygen delivery can encourage degeneration. Dr. Otto Warburg was awarded the Nobel Peace Prize for the discovery of how oxygen deficiency can encourage the growth of cancer. When pH is off, the body becomes more acidic, and cancer cells thrive.

Other research has documented that low pH changes the electromagnetic characteristics of fat cells and cholesterol in the body, in turn allowing blood cells to become tacky and stick to the walls of arteries. This is one of the processes that have been implicated in heart disease.

When body chemistry becomes too acidic, it can convince our brain that we are hungry, and cause headaches, drowsiness, or neurological changes. When chronic, it will pollute tissues and compromise nerves and nerve function, potentially over time triggering fibromyalgia in those who are genetically predisposed and most susceptible. For a diabetic whose body chemistry is out of sync, there is a real danger of a diabetic stroke or death due to acid levels spiking (low pH).

High pH, aka Alkalosis

Alkalosis (high pH) is not as much of a concern for Fibros, but worth noting. The most common cause for a body ratio that is more alkaline is hyperventilation—however, for Fibros, diet is still the issue. Another possible risk for increasing the body's pH is through specialized home water processing that adds minerals to the water. If these filters are used in a complementary way, they may help the average person keep body chemistry in line by filtering out toxins and mitigating poor diet habits—the most common of which, of course, is a high-carbohydrate diet. There is a danger in overutilizing these filters, however. Symptoms may begin subtly, experienced as fuzzy thinking, mental confusion (fibro fog /brain fog), increased emotional sensitivity, and numbness and tingling. I've read reports and testimonials touting the improvement in health after beginning to utilize these special water-processing units. My suspicion is that the perception of improved vitality has to do with simply increasing water intake and decreasing negative drinks such as sodas and coffee. Additionally, being well- hydrated will help to increase energy and reduce hunger. This makes it easier to cut down on carbohydrate consumption, which is primarily wheat and sugar, both of which commonly challenge and encourage chronic pain and fatigue.

Diabetes, Kidneys and pH

The kidneys and the pancreas team up to manage pH balance. The pancreas secretes chemicals called bicarbonates to alkalize the small intestine after the acidic breakdown of food in the stomach. When the pancreas malfunctions, as it does when a person has diabetes, and/or if it is further challenged by a high-carbohydrate diet, the kidneys may become overworked in their effort to help raise pH and maintain the acid-alkaline balance.

Every cell in the body has the ability to protect itself by creating bicarbonate chemicals to raise pH when it senses low pH in fluids and blood. Our lungs have the ability to decrease acid as well. They do it by exhaling carbon dioxide, which gets rid of acid, and hence raises pH. Let's consider exercise for a minute. Fibromyalgia sufferers are frequently told to exercise, so let us begin to look at the effects that this may have on their condition. During exercise, breathing becomes faster and hopefully deeper. This increases oxygenation of the blood cells, while also increasing the amount of carbon dioxide expelled in order to reduce the acids created by the exercise (for example, lactic acid) that are produced due to increased cellular metabolism.

In spite of the increase in respiration rate, many continue to breathe rather shallowly. The struggle causes relative acidosis during exercise. For Fibros, this is particularly egregious because muscle tissue is already hypersensitive, making it difficult to tolerate the excess acid produced by exercise. This not only discourages patients from exercising, but exacerbates muscle and nerve sensitivity. This is an important concept, which helps to explain why fibromyalgia patients are not overly successful with exercising.

Fibromyalgia

So let's get back more specifically to our topic: fibromyalgia. Remember that when our physiology is challenged with a highly acidic diet (carbohydrates), inflammation and pain are encouraged. If that is not counterbalanced by increasing alkalinity (eating more fruits and vegetables), we cause our organs and our cells, our lungs, kidneys, and pancreas to overwork. This is one of the ways to encourage all the negative neurology and physiology associated with fibromyalgia. So in spite of the fact that fibromyalgia is not generally considered an inflammatory disease, chronic inflammation can mount, inspire, and conspire with coexisting conditions like chronic fatigue, arthritis, and myofascial trigger points, encouraging, perpetuating, or possibly triggering fibromyalgia.

We will recycle the visual used back in Chapter 13 of a balanced meal as it holds true for acid/alkaline concerns, as well as general nutrition and toxic concerns.

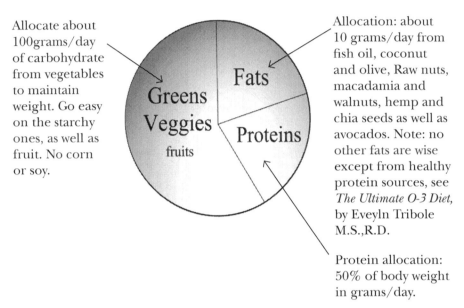

Allocate about 100grams/day of carbohydrate from vegetables to maintain weight. Go easy on the starchy ones, as well as fruit. No corn or soy.

Allocation: about 10 grams/day from fish oil, coconut and olive, Raw nuts, macadamia and walnuts, hemp and chia seeds as well as avocados. Note: no other fats are wise except from healthy protein sources, see *The Ultimate O-3 Diet,* by Eveyln Tribole M.S.,R.D.

Protein allocation: 50% of body weight in grams/day.

A Cobb salad is a good visual concept of the approximate desirable ratio of alkaline-forming foods and acidic-forming foods. At any given meal, if we remember that our diet is best to be about 60 percent alkaline and 40 percent acid, then we want to try to conceptualize that with each meal. Sources will differ on their recommendation of alkaline/acid-forming foods. There is a range that's healthy, depending on the person. However, keep in mind that good fats, while being relative acid producers, have anti-inflammatory advantages that net a systemic advantage. Therefore, there is no need for most to shy away from consuming them. Plus, they add taste and satisfy the hypothalamus, reducing the urge to eat carbohydrates.

Summary
Your best shot at managing body chemistry is to shoot for the 60/40 rule. Eliminate processed foods, alcohol, tobacco, and as much

medication as possible. Drink plenty of water and supplement your diet with a natural mineral complex. Additionally, make every effort to control stress and avoid overwhelm. Exercise modestly but regularly, and pay close attention to maintaining a deep and rhythmic breathing pattern throughout the day--not just during exercise. This will relax muscles and promote clear thinking. Adhere to the parameters as outlined in this section, and exercise will be more enjoyable and productive for you.

Fats

Much of what you're going to read in this section you've probably heard before. I hope that I can put it together in a way that will motivate sustainable dietary habits.

There are only three types of food: carbohydrate, protein, and fat. Fats are necessary if we are to be healthy. Fats do four things, the most important of which with fibromyalgia in mind is maintaining the integrity of cell membranes (Letter C below). This is due to the necessity for Fibros to increase energy, reduce inflammation and pain, as well as manage brain function. This responsibility requires unadulterated fatty acids.

A. Fats balance body chemistry

B. Fats balance blood sugar

C. Fats are necessary for cell-membrane health

D. Fats are necessary for hormone balance

E. Fats are anti-inflammatory medicine

Cells and Fibromyalgia

Every cell in the body, except blood cells, produces energy within little cellular power plants called mitochondria. The term for the energy produced in the mitochondria is adenosine triphosphate (ATP). Brain and muscle tissue house the densest population of mitochondria, in anticipation of needing the most energy. Studies have shown that in fibromyalgia sufferers' ATP levels are reduced by approximately 20 percent.[66] Think back to how many chapters/topics in this book we have talked about muscle and cell energy ATP. Just about everyone and every topic relates to energy/ATP production.

Mitochondrion

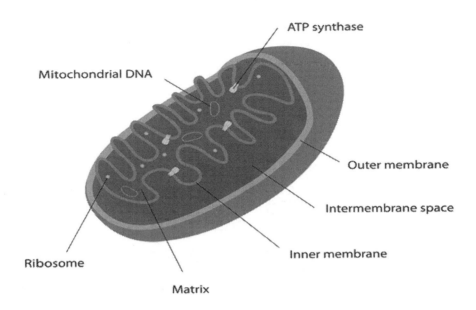

All cells use glucose and amino acids for energy, with some cells heavily relying mostly on fatty acids. This is particularly important to fibromyalgia and chronic fatigue sufferers in that between meals, cardiac muscle cells meet 90% of their ATP demands by using fatty acids rather than glucose. In some situations, the utilization may fall to about 60%, depending on the nutritional status and muscle demands. Skeletal muscle also depends primarily on fatty acids during rest, normal everyday activities, and conservative-intensity exercise. As exercise intensity increases, cells look to glucose to help out.[76] We can easily see how the intake of adequate fats in the diet or lack thereof plays a role in CFS and fibromyalgia. It's all about cellular energy.

When mitochondria don't generate enough energy, there is a lack of energy for brain and muscular functions. Considering that every cell utilizes the same energy pump, a lack of energy in all tissues, organs, and systems of the body could account for any one or all of the symptoms in fibromyalgia. This theory is the basis of Dr. St. Amand's guaifenesin protocol.

The outer membrane of a cell is alive and biologically active. The membrane, said to be the "brains" of the cell, separates the interior of all cells from the outside environment. The cell membrane is selectively permeable to ions and organic molecules; it controls the movement of substances in and out. The cell membrane, as well as the membrane of the mitochondria within the cell, is made up primarily of saturated and unsaturated fats, as well as proteins.

There are three membranes (outer, inter, and inner) which nutrients must cross to enter the inner sanctum where ATP production takes place.

If any of the membranes have been corrupted by an imbalance of Omega-3 and Omega-6 fatty acids or by trans-fats, transport and exchange across the membranes will compromise the biological brains of the cell. I share with you these details only to emphasize the importance of high-quality balanced fats and proteins in the diet, without which all cellular functions will be compromised.

Essential Fatty Acids

All dietary fats are a blend of saturated and unsaturated. Unsaturated fats include poly- and mono-unsaturated fats. Omega-3s and 6s are types of polyunsaturated fats and the two that we are most concerned with. They are the most important fats to humans, referred to as "essential fatty acids," or you might see them termed "parent essential oils," because they are essential to life hence it's essential to consume them. Omega-3 fatty acids are primarily alpha-linoleic acid. Omega-6 fatty acid is primarily linoleic acid. If the proportion, the quantity, or quality of these fats in the diet is improper or altered due to heat or processing, they will work against health. Fatty-acid abnormalities are linked to diabetes, inflammatory conditions, heart disease, cancer, and neurological disorders which would include fibromyalgia, chronic pain, and fatigue.

To understand how these fatty acids relate and why they're important to our topic, we need to discuss inflammation. Inflammation is a healthy and welcome component for our immune system's response to injury and illness. However, we want it to do its job and then turn off. If our cells themselves are ill, they create their own inflammation constantly.

Omega-6 fats are termed pro-inflammatory because they contribute to the inflammatory response in a typical diet. Omega-3 fats have an anti-inflammatory effect, helping to balance Omega-6 fats.

If diet causes cell membranes to lose balance between 6's and 3's, the inflammatory response can overreact and then possibly not turn off, creating a state of chronic inflammation/pain. Many people's diets are likely to be 75 percent or higher in pro-inflammatory Omega-6 fatty acids, with only 25 percent or less Omega-3 anti-inflammatory essential fatty acids. The target ratio would be 50/50. When the percentage of 6s in the diet goes up it surpasses/competes with 3s; then inflammation goes up--and with it, the risk of disease.

It's important to know if your body chemistry is pro-inflammatory (too much Omega-6) so diet can be adjusted. We use Lipid Labs out of Minnesota to evaluate a person's ratios. They have a home blood-spot test to determine the ratio of Omega-3 to Omega-6. (See appendix for testing information.)

Farming and agricultural techniques have destroyed the balance of many foods, including green leafy vegetables, animal meats, eggs, fish and vegetable oils that are rich in Omega-6 fats. Ratios are skewed from a 50/50 healthy ratio to 20 to 1, or 95 percent Omega-6. This is not good.

Livestock raised in a more natural environment, with minimized grain feeding, will bring the balance and ratio closer to 4:1. North Dakota State University conducted a study on the nutritional differences between grass-fed and grain-fed bison. The grass-fed bison had Omega-6 to Omega-3 ratios of 4:1, while the grain-fed bison had ratios of 21:1.

The longer cattle are fed grain, the greater the fatty acid imbalance. For instance, after 200 days in the feedlot, grain-fed cattle have Omega-6 to Omega-3 ratios that exceed 20:1. Many cattle are fed 200 days or more in the United States, which makes for nice fat beef, while at the same time beefing up the bottom line for farmers, stockholders, and—indirectly--retailers.

There are the same concerns with chicken and pork. Preferably they would be raised eating vegetables high in Omega-3 fats, along with insects and lots of fresh green grass, supplemented with fresh or dried fruit and small amounts of corn (hopefully not genetically modified). Food retailers, you'll notice, are starting to respond to consumer demand. High Omega-3 eggs and grass-fed beef are becoming more available. However, costs can be prohibitive for many families because natural agriculture is more costly to produce. Additionally, retailers may tweak the price up for the minority of people who are driven and committed to breaking away from the pack. There is also a boutique perception that helps consumers tolerate a bump in price. Your best bet would be to find farmers in your local area who are committed to natural and organic production. This will save some money and reduce the risks involved with shipping and too many people having to handle the product. Local farmers will usually be able to give you great package prices for storage in your own freezer. Wild game meat would be a great choice if you can get it.

The Fish Solution

Fish is generally seen as a healthier food choice compared to grain-fed beef, and is heavily promoted as a good source of Omega-3 fats. There are, however, concerns about mercury accumulation in the fish. Young, wild-caught cold-water fish are the best choice. Farm-raised fish may be less susceptible to mercury contamination, but are generally an inferior source due to questionable toxicity levels. Many fish farms feed the fish grain or the carcasses of their dead playmates, once again possibly raising the ratio to 20-1.

Dr. Michael Dobbin informed me of a company that cans only young, wild-caught fish to help reduce the fear of the accumulation of toxic mercury levels. The company's name is Vital Choice (www.vitalchoice.com). A great resource to learn more about fats and food sources is the Weston A. Price Foundation (www.westonaprice.org).

We have all heard the terms "saturated fats" and "unsaturated fats." There's no need to get into the chemistry of what makes them saturated or unsaturated—suffice it to say that a practical understanding is simply that unsaturated fats are considered to be flexible and liquid at room temperature; saturated fats are rigid and solid at room temperature. As we go on, you'll see that we need both. Saturated fats, up until recently, have been thought to raise cholesterol and put us at risk for heart disease; we have been told not to consume them. However, we now know this to be untrue. Most of the research done in the past was conducted with flawed/adulterated fats, netting invalid results. Consequently, study results showed that blood cells don't seem to like solid fats. Under dark-field microscopy, the blood cells of a person who over consumes adulterated saturated fats can be seen to be sticky and lethargic. They will tend to look as if they are clumped together, not moving independently. The sluggishness reduces their ability to transport oxygen throughout the body. In a typical diet, bodies tend to be overburdened with saturated fats, primarily from animal meats and dairy products that have been manipulated either during growing, processing, cooking, or they are simply too high in Omega-6 and people overindulge. However, as mentioned earlier, we must have them in our diet—and in fact, more than what we've been told in the past. New science recommendations are as follows:

1. Stop using vegetable oils (corn, safflower, and sunflower).
2. Avoid tofu, soy, corn and peanut-based products.
3. Consume no fried foods, even if fried in good-quality olive oil. High heats will break down the oil and sabotage any inherent value of the original oil. Having said that, if you must fry, follow the directions closely for oil temperature and consider using coconut oil, peanut oil, avocado oil, or animal fat from grass-fed sources. Proper temperature when frying will help reduce the fat being soaked up like a sponge; plus it will maintain fatty acid value.
4. Eat as many leafy, dark green vegetables as you can, such as kale, broccoli, and spinach. Give algae/kelp a try. Eat fruits such as mango, papaya, and kiwi (all preferably organic).
5. Do not consume trans-fats or partially hydrogenated fats. The only way to successfully avoid them is simply to decide that you're not going to eat any prepared foods: no boxed, bagged, jarred, engineered, or fast food. Otherwise you simply can't avoid bad fats, unless you plan on studying every label and you're prepared to research and understand every single ingredient on the label. Consider that anything labeled zero trans-fats or zero hydrogenated fats cannot be trusted to mean zero. Also, some additives have trans-fats within the FDA's acceptable limits. Once the additive is added to the primary food, it's hidden in the recipe. Only the FDA or the manufacturer will know the details of this, and you may never have the information. Having said that, there is hope; the Food and Drug Administration recently announced that all artificial trans-fats are to be taken entirely out of the food supply and is pushing the industry to reformulate the remaining products that still have them. While this is good news, the industry is not about to give up profit advantages from using certain fats, and will find a way to adhere to the law yet prevail. Best advice: stick to my recommendation above. This also helps to eliminate many other chemical/toxic concerns.
6. Consume olive oil, avocados, raw nuts and seeds, as well as butter, coconut oil, and fat from grass-fed animals daily. If you are a vegetarian, be careful to eat high-quality vegetables and lots of them, as well as raw seeds (flax and

chia) and nuts. Concentrate or you will overdo bad carbs and pay the price. Carbs up = inflammation up. It will take a lot of Omega-3 to balance.

7. Minimize or eliminate dairy products, with the exception of buttermilk and natural plain yogurt.
8. Consume cold-water wild fish at least two times a week (young salmon is the best).
9. Eat salmon, cod, herring, sardines, and mackerel.
10 Do your best to eat red meat that is grass-fed and range-raised. However, you're better off to eat farm-raised animals rather than over consume carbohydrates. You can't make up for the farm-raised negativity by upping your fish oil supplements.
11. After understanding fats and adjusting your diet, consider no longer taking supplements intended to boost EPA and DHA. These supplements are normally unnaturally high in potency of fish oils and, unless prescribed based on blood tests as described in Chapter 15, have a negative value, based on the most recent studies.

Eat Fats

From *The American Journal of Clinical Nutrition*, Volume 80, September 2004, we read about "Health Effects of Saturated Fatty Acids": "The approach of many mainstream investigators in studying the effect of consuming saturated fats has been narrowly focused to produce and evaluate evidence in support of the hypothesis that dietary saturated fat elevates LDL-cholesterol and thus elevates the risk of cardio arterial disease (CAD). The evidence is not strong, and, overall, dietary intervention by lowering saturated fat intake does not lower the incident of nonfatal CAD; nor does such dietary intervention lower coronary disease or total mortality.

"Unfortunately, the overwhelming emphasis on the role of saturated fats in the diet and the risk of CAD has distracted investigators from studying any other affects that individual saturated fatty acids may have on our body. If saturated fatty acids were of no value or were harmful to humans, evolution would probably not have established within the mammary glands the means to produce saturated fatty acids that provide a source of nourishment to enhance the growth, development and survival of mammalian offspring."

Many studies have found an inverse proportion between fat intake and health. The less fat people consume, the more their health is in jeopardy. As far back as 1953, the third edition of *The Vitamins in Medicine* reported a study in 1929 by Burr; it was found that animals on a fat- starvation diet developed:

- Dryness and roughness of skin, resulting in eczema
- Seborrhea
- Nails and hair that lacked luster, became brittle and split easily, or fell out
- Pituitary insufficiency
- Sterility
- Prolonged gestation
- Severe nephritis, leading to death

In *The Archives of Internal Medicine*, 1992, William Castelli, director of the Farmington Study reported: "In Farmington, Massachusetts, the more saturated fat one ate, the more cholesterol one ate, the more calories one ate, the lower people's serum cholesterol.... We found that people who ate the most cholesterol, ate the most saturated fat, and ate the most calories weighed the least and were the most physically active."

The moral of the story is "eat fat."

Trans Fats/Partially Hydrogenated Oils
Chronic inflammation plays a role in most chronic diseases such as heart disease, diabetes, Alzheimer's, and fibromyalgia. An annual physical is likely to involve blood tests for a factor called C-reactive protein, which is a warning signal that inflammation exists. We covered some of this in Chapter 15.

Trans-fats and partially hydrogenated oils come in the form of vegetable oils that include safflower, soy, sesame and sunflower. Due to these oils being almost everywhere in foods, we suggest that you eliminate them from your diet completely. Know that you're bound to get some even if you shoot for zero.

Good Fats
Butter, beef tallow, lamb tallow, and lard
Chicken, goose, and duck fat
Cold-pressed olive oil, sesame oil, and flax oil
Tropical oils, such as coconut oil
Marine oils, such as cod liver oil
Seeds and nuts

Bad Fats

All partially hydrogenated/trans-fats, including margarine and shortening

Industrially processed vegetable oils, especially soy, safflower, corn, peanut, cotton seed

and canola.

All fats heated to breakdown temperature, especially polyunsaturated oils.

Fish Oil Supplementation

When supplementing, target fish oils with 1000-2000 of EPA, DPA and DHA per day, as well as 2000mg of ALA per day. Green vegetables are also a good source of plant-based Omega-3. Veggies typically have a balanced ratio of Omega-3 and Omega-6, as well as being a good source of antioxidants, fiber, nutrients, and live enzymes. Your health care provider may recommend more or less depending on your profile, and if you have any bleeding issues or are already on an anticoagulant.

Choosing a high-quality Omega-3 fish oil can be a little tricky. You can buy oil supplements almost anywhere; however, the quality becomes a concern. The old saying "You get what you pay for" comes into play. When selecting a high-quality fish oil supplement, consider the following, directly from "Lipid Labs":

Choosing an Omega-3 Fish Oil

Omega-3 supplements vary widely in molecular form (bioavailability), purity and freshness (contaminants, taste), type of processing, and company commitment to sustainable fishing practices.

Triglyceride Form: Both short- and long-term studies suggest that triglyceride-form EPA and DHA may be incorporated into cell membranes more efficiently than when consumed as ethyl-esters.

Molecular Distillation: This process removes oxidized by-products, heavy metals, and other contaminants without damaging the structural integrity of important EPA and DHA fats. The result is fish oil that has a fresh, clean taste and is safe for people of all ages. Purity should be verified through independent third-party laboratory analysis.

Magnesium and D-Ribose

Now that we know how to support the gateway into the mitochondria in hopes of generating the energy needed to run each and every aspect of physiology, let's recognize two crucial substances that may be contributing to your pain and fatigue.

Magnesium and D-ribose have been studied in the effort to rejuvenate the heart muscle. After a heart attack, there is very little time to re-energize heart cells before severe and permanent damage will occur. New studies have found simple and cheap nutrients that support mitochondria production of ATP, helping to spare the heart muscle and repair damage.

This science has been successfully applied to understand and treat fibromyalgia and CFS. We covered magnesium in Chapter Five when discussing chronic fatigue syndrome. Let's now cover D-ribose and how we could diagnose "Failed Mitochondrial Syndrome" and possibly the underlying glitch in physiology accounting for loss of neurological integrity (pain, stiffness, fatigue, and mental fog) in fibromyalgia.

Glucose is one of the raw materials cells need to drive the production of ATP. However, the process may be too slow in some cases to meet demands when stressors, injury, or disease calls for the body to produce therapeutic levels of ATP. D-ribose is a simple sugar and offers a more efficient energy source to drive ATP production compared to glucose. Dr. Julius G. Goepp, MD reports the need for supplemental D-ribose of 5 grams/day for healthy individuals, 10-15 grams/day for athletes, and 10-30 grams/day for heart patients, CFS and Fibros. He does note a couple of problems with supplementation, however. The first is gut fermentation; the second is if a person is sensitive to corn.

1. **The fermenting gut**. If there are bad bacteria or yeast in the upper gut, D-ribose may be more efficient at causing fermentation, hence producing more alcohol and gas. In this event he suggests reducing the daily dosage and holding it in the mouth as long as possible – some will be absorbed through the oral mucosa. Space doses throughout the day.
2. **Corn sensitivity**. D-ribose is derived from corn, so if you have a sensitivity to corn, you may have an allergic reaction, restricting usage. There doesn't seem to be a corn-free source of D-ribose.

Test
The tests that we are going to discuss to understand mitochondrial function and energy production were developed by John McLean Howard, biochemist. Although we've discussed primarily magnesium

and D-Ribose to increase ATP production, Dr. Howard explains that there are three possible explanations of mitochondrial failure and loss of cellular energy, all of which his test measures. The first measures levels of ATP in the cell, which he explains as a magnesium-dependent process. The second aspect of the test measures the efficiency with which ATP is made within the mitochondrion. If this is abnormal, it may be a result of magnesium deficiency, low levels of Co-enzyme Q10, vitamin B3 (NAD), or of acetyl L-carnitine. The third possibility is that the protein that transports ATP across mitochondrial membranes is impaired, so this too is measured in the third part. The lab we use Genova Diagnostics out of Asheville, NC.

Genova offers a convenient home urine test with specificity for mitochondrial dysfunction. It measures urinary organic acids. Organic acids are metabolic products and byproducts left over from bodily functions. Organic acid testing has the ability to detect dysfunction of mitochondrial energy production, as well as the presence of functional nutrient deficiencies and toxins that are adversely affecting detoxification pathways. Genova also has tests that cover all of Dr. Howard's research. (See appendix.)

Supplementation

For general supplementation to increase muscular energy, repair, and recovery look to magnesium, D-Ribose, branch chain amino acids BCAA, and antioxidants such as CoQ10 and OPC-3. Discuss with your doctor initial dosing and timing, then guide upward as you monitor your energy and stamina. Check-in at www.fibro-doc.com for webinars and resources to further understand specific mitochondrial enhancement and supplement formulas customizable to your needs. Don't hesitate to email me with questions at fibro.epc@comcast.net.

Keep in mind that our discussion is about mitochondrial insufficiency as opposed to mitochondrial disease. Mitochondrial disease is due to inherited as well as possibly spontaneous genetic mutations.

Conventional teachings as well as our discussion has over simplified mitochondria as "energy factories", when in fact mitochondrial DNA allocates less than 5% of its responsibility for energy production. The other 95% holds responsibility in embryonic development and throughout life in all functions of the body. Because mitochondria perform so many different functions in different tissues, there are literally hundreds of different mitochondrial diseases. I felt that a distinction was in order, however further discussion is beyond this writing.

Coffee

Coffee is considered a stimulant drug. Although it is not as addictive as a drug like cocaine, it nevertheless has an effect on neurotransmitters that bring pleasure and behavior modification. Dopamine, for instance, is a neurotransmitter and is best known for its role in pleasure, motivation, and motor control. Recent evidence suggests that it is also involved in pain modulation. Fibromyalgia patients are found to demonstrate abnormal dopamine response to pain, hence in a roundabout way bringing coffee into the conversation.[73]

It has been reported that in addition to a stimulating effect on the adrenal glands, coffee activates an enzyme that enhances ATP production, further accounting for the apparent energy uplift most drinkers experience. I say most, because some people whose adrenals and mitochondria are in failure seem to get no kick out of coffee. They can drink a cup of coffee at bed time and still sleep. For everyone else, Dr. Sarah Myhill suggests trying a cup of black organic coffee with a teaspoon of D-ribose for a CFS/fibromyalgia pick-me-up. However, this is a Band-Aid approach for the most part. I would shy away from the coffee, for the following reasons.

Coffee is considered a psychoactive drug; it crosses the blood-brain barrier, acting primarily upon the central nervous system, where it affects brain function (possibly resulting in alterations in perception, mood, consciousness, cognition, and behavior). The higher the level of caffeine, the more psychoactive it appears to be, having a more profound effect on the central nervous system. Some people are more sensitive to caffeine than others. Coffee drinkers who switch to decaf for perceived health benefits will not necessarily be free from many of the effects of coffee, although their pleasure centers will certainly not be stimulated as strongly.

In and of itself, coffee is acidic; additionally, it will trigger the stomach to release gastric acid. How does coffee do this?

Coffees oils are acid-based and are an irritant to the lining (mucosa) of the stomach. Some evidence shows that decaf coffee is even more acidic than regular coffee due to the type of coffee beans that are usually used. It makes sense that the consumption of coffee could aggravate conditions such as acid reflux or gastro-esophageal reflux disease (GERD). The increased acidity could irritate not only the stomach lining, but the lining of the small intestine just outside of the stomach as well. This irritation can set the stage for bacteria to flourish and lead to an ulcer, further upsetting digestion and confounding the symptomatic picture

Coffee stimulates another neurotransmitter: adrenaline, which in turn stimulates the release of insulin, causing a relative hypoglycemic state (low blood sugar). Between these two reactions, initially there will be an increase in energy and tension with a mild rise in blood pressure, followed by a drop in blood sugar, sometimes termed "rush and crash effect." This can tax the adrenals. The brain may interpret this as being tired, hungry, having a sugar craving, or needing another cup of coffee. Tampering with blood sugar and challenging the adrenals are sure ways of adding challenge, confusion, and/or complication to a Fibro's life. While the main symptoms are pain and fatigue, the "rush and crash effect" of stimulants may create a downward spiral of fatigue, brain fog, and loss of motivation.

Coffee and Pain

You may be tired of reading this, but let's backtrack for a quick review. The experience of pain takes place over special pathways (nerves) that transmit signals to the brain. Nerves use chemicals, termed neurotransmitters, to push the signal of pain along the nerve. Neurotransmitters work at intersections/gaps along the same pathway, or intersecting with another nerve. It is at these intersections/gaps, aka synapses, that nerves have a chance to adjust the signals as needed, increasing or decreasing the intensity, possibly even determining if there's any need for the signal to continue to the brain or not. In order for this to take place, the receiving side closest to the brain (see post-synaptic nerve, B, in the figure below) must have an available friendly site, called a "receptor site," to accept the neurotransmitter and support the continuity of the communication's intent to reach the brain.

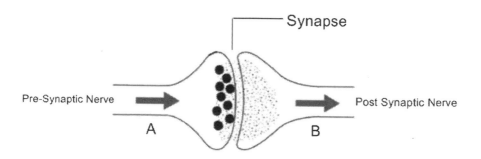

Synapse

Pre-Synaptic Nerve

A

Post Synaptic Nerve

B

The particular type of receptor sites I'd like to talk about are called "opiate receptor sites" on post-synaptic nerve B. The body has its own innate ability to generate chemicals called endorphins, which reach out for acceptance/docking on the post-synaptic receptor sites.

We intervene and attempt to control or block pain by choosing a substance that would take up residence on the receptor's site, blocking the body's natural endorphins from doing their job. Marijuana, morphine, or nicotine are such substances, short-circuiting/blocking the pain pathway to the brain. Coffee appears to play the same role.[17] Laboratory studies have reported that coffee competes for opiate receptors. There was no significant difference between regular coffee and decaffeinated coffee.

Pursuant to this conclusion, a second study reported in *Pub-Med* noted that in spite of caffeine's apparent role in reducing pain perception, it seems to do so in regard to acute pain only. The study found that dietary caffeine consumption, and symptoms reported by patients with chronic back pain, show that caffeine has little to no effect regardless of the quantities consumed.

Therefore, considering that coffee only mildly affects acute pain and is short-lived, its use is counterproductive. Remember, it will take up residence on receptor sites and block other substances as mentioned above, disallowing the body's own (endogenous) painkillers—endorphins, to be exact. Endorphins are not only our own natural painkillers, but they uplift mood, energy, and mental acuity. This is doubly important because when utilizing more natural and longer-lasting efforts to stimulate endorphins and subsequently block pain (such as acupuncture, meditation, exercise, and chiropractic) if you are consuming coffee or other substances, there may be a reduction in receptor sites for endorphins. So we have a situation where coffee consumption could lead one to misjudge the therapeutic effects of natural/drugless therapy.

Osteoporosis and Coffee

Osteoporosis is an additional concern. As aforementioned, coffee has the ability to shift the body chemistry to be more acidic. Acid is a contributory factor to the demineralizing of bones, and bone loss.

The University of Omaha reported that five mg of calcium are lost for every six ounces of regular coffee consumed, due to the acidity.

Arthritis Today reports that caffeine can cause the body to absorb less calcium. But they're not convinced that the studies support osteoporosis as a result of drinking coffee. My opinion is that all we have to know is that increased acidity challenges bone mineralization; calcium will be leached out of bones and used as a buffer to neutralize the acidity. I'm convinced that diets high in acidic residue have contributed to the epidemic proportion of osteoporosis we see, as have diets high in simple carbohydrates, chemical preservatives, processed foods, alcohol, toxins, and coffee.

Rheumatoid Arthritis and Coffee

The American College of Rheumatology reported that women who drink four or more cups of decaffeinated coffee a day are more than twice as likely to develop rheumatoid arthritis, compared to drinking regular coffee. That's not to say that rheumatoid arthritis is caused by drinking coffee; there are many other factors to be considered, such as lifestyle, diet, and emotional factors, as well as genetics. Considering the acid/coffee connection, it makes sense that more acid creates more susceptibility to systemic inflammation, which challenges our nerves, joints, muscles, tendons, ligaments, organs, and digestive system. While we read time and time again that fibromyalgia is not an inflammatory condition, increasing our systemic inflammatory baseline just asks for trouble.

Arthritis Today

I don't mean this section to confuse you, but I do want to make you aware that there is some controversy and more research to be done. In another article in *Arthritis Today,* Sharon Wilder defended coffee against the myriad of attacks it has faced as an alleged contributing factor for heart disease and cancer. She stated that coffee may lower the risk of developing diabetes, gallstones, Parkinson's disease, and Alzheimer's. She claimed that the American College of Rheumatology's study was flawed, as it did not consider other factors such as smoking, diet, or alcohol consumption. In her report, she did note a 2002 study conducted at the University of Alabama that showed no link between regular coffee and the onset of rheumatoid arthritis. The study did determine, however, that women who drank four or more cups a day of decaf had an increased risk for rheumatoid arthritis as they aged. A study conducted by the National Public Health Institute in Helsinki, Finland, backed this up. Dr. Ted Mikuls of Harvard Medical School in Boston claims that there is no relationship between coffee, whether it is regular or decaf, and rheumatoid arthritis.

You can make your own decision as to how to proceed. I would recommend switching to green tea or considering a coffee alternative... or if that doesn't work for you, consider at least organic fair trade coffees and/or low acidic coffees.

Coffee Alternative

Years ago I was introduced to a type of mushroom from the Orient, "Ganoderma Lucidum." At that time the literature and publicity about the mushroom proclaimed its attributes of increasing energy, decreasing stress, aiding in healing, decreasing toxicity, and stimulating the immune system. When we could get our hands on this mushroom we would soak it for days to draw out the beneficial substances, and then drink it as a tea. It actually seemed to work, and we felt we were getting all the benefits that we read about. Patients reported similar results. The extracting of the beneficial substances from the mushroom was a long drawn-out process, plus the mushrooms were hard to find. Fast-forward to today. I have discovered a coffee called "Organo Gold" that's being produced and commercially marketed. This coffee incorporates healthy components of the mushroom Ganoderma Lucidum. It's decaffeinated, but has a natural ability to increase energy without the jitters or the crash (effect on adrenals and insulin aka "rush and crash effect"). Further, it's infused with beneficial herbs. I have to admit I was a skeptic at first. I researched the product on *Pub-Med* and found that the research substantiated their claims of a healthier coffee.

You can order online by going to www.shop.com to find different options and distributors. You may find these coffee substitutes under the name of Organo Gold, Gano Ecel USA, and Royal Reishi.

> Tending to nutrition and general body chemistry takes a lot of commitment, concentration, and preparation. This section was meant to share fundamental perspectives that can be taken into consideration regardless of the specifics of the diet or supplementation regimen you commit to.

CHAPTER 23

Tomorrow:

Real Science, Real Hope—The Future

Chapter Topics:

> Antioxidants
> Glial Cells
> Placebo Effect
> 5th Vital Sign

> Glutathione
> N-Acetyl Cysteine

Antioxidants

Recall the importance of glial cells and the fact that they wear many hats as communicators, modulators, and directors of operation, especially within the brain and spinal cord. One of their most important duties is to detoxify the brain and the neurons, protecting against damage from free radicals.

We've all become very aware of free radicals. Everybody seems to understand that free radicals cause damage and inflammation, and ultimately disease. Free radicals are the byproduct of all physiological and cellular activity in the body. These toxins can damage proteins, lipids, and DNA. When this takes place in the brain, it can cause neurological damage and create disease such as sickle cell anemia, atherosclerosis, Parkinson's disease, and Alzheimer's disease. They have been linked to chronic fatigue syndrome and fibromyalgia.

As discussed previously, there are many antioxidants, aka free-radical scavengers, that reduce the detrimental effects of free radicals. The most common ones are vitamin C, vitamin E, vitamin A, and green tea. Others, such as Oligomertric Proantho-Cyanidins (OPC), are derived from plants; you may know them as polyphenols or flavonoids from grape seed, red wine, bilberry, and pine bark, to name a few. These are exogenous antioxidants, meaning from outside the body. However the most powerful antioxidant is produced by the body, termed an endogenous antioxidant; specifically, I'm referring to glutathione. Glutathione is found in its highest concentration in glial cells.[31] This is of particular interest in the brain's ability to detoxify itself, sparing nerves from free-radical damage. Consider this: the cells of the human brain consume about 20 percent of the oxygen that our bodies use. But the brain equates to only 2 percent of total body weight.[17] This means that the brain is capable of consuming, and in fact does consume, more oxygen and is more metabolically active than any other tissues in the body. Consequently, it has the tendency to create more free radicals and toxins simply due to its high level of activity. Remember, we said some researchers note that glial cells account for about 85 percent of brain matter, and only about 15 percent is accounted for by nerves in the brain.

Considering glial cells' high concentration and responsibility for proper neurological function, it's no surprise that the body dedicates such high levels of glutathione to glial cells so that they can continue their fine work.

When neurodegenerative diseases such as Alzheimer's, Parkinson's and ALS occur, we're able to point a finger at the involvement and compromise of glial cells and their role in generating and utilizing glutathione effectively. This means an increase of oxidative stress, aka toxicity and free radicals. This is sure to cause damage if not mitigated.

Any compromise in glutathione production or effectiveness will reduce the ability of nerve cells not only to function properly, but to protect themselves against further toxins—leading to, as mentioned, neurodegenerative diseases. Again, this emphasizes the importance of antioxidants in the brain.

This of course raises the question: How do we increase antioxidants in the brain--and, more specifically, how do we increase glutathione? It has been demonstrated that glutathione can be synthesized by the enzymes of glutamate and cysteine. While there are other enzymes and amino acids involved in glutathione production, cysteine appears to be the only one that is irreplaceable (the limiting factor) and crucial in glutathione's production.[60]

As an example, in many other systems and other physiological functions, the body is able to recycle substances and chemicals to maintain itself. Glutathione in the brain is no different. The body has the ability to maintain glutathione predominantly by recycling its constituent parts within the brain itself. However, like any other system, it can use as much help as we can give it, especially considering that environmental and lifestyle decisions are so toxic. As we've mentioned, the good news is that cysteine, in particular, will be helpful. And for those who would ask if cysteine can get across the blood-brain barrier, the answer is yes. Amino acids, such as glutamate and cysteine can pass the blood-brain barrier to help replenish and enhance glial cells' production of glutathione.[61] In times of stress (physical and/or emotional), decreased blood circulation in the brain, or decreased glucose, glial cells are able to release more glutathione, recognizing that the brain needs more protection. Not only does glutathione have a detoxifying responsibility, but it also has communication/signaling responsibilities to integrate and coordinate information throughout the brain, including helping to balance hormones.

Glial Cells

Gray matter is the part of the central nervous system that holds glial cells, in contrast to white matter, which primarily consists of tracts of nerves. *The Journal of Neuroscience* reported in 2004 that Dr. Vania Apkarian conducted MRI brain studies of people with chronic pain and compared them to people with no pain. The results were that people with chronic pain had 5-11 percent less gray matter compared to the people with no pain. Further, Dr. Apkarian concluded that more gray matter would be lost the longer that the pain persisted.

As we see from our understanding of glial cells and their evolving importance as likely being more in control of our brain functions than the actual nerves themselves, it's not hard to understand how toxic gray matter along with chronic pain could cause everything from memory and concentration problems (fibro fog) to digestive problems, and problems with energy, fatigue, and sleep—even difficulty with language and expressing oneself.

In an article by Dr. Maha Alattar, April 2011, entitled "Chronic Pain Can Hurt Your Brain," it was reported that different areas of the brain actually work together to maintain balance, similar to the way that the bicep muscle cooperates with the tricep muscle for proper arm function. Contraction of the bicep muscle calls for the tricep muscle to simultaneously relax. By the same token, Dr. Alattar reports that if one region of the brain is active, other areas of the brain will basically deactivate in an attempt to bring a resting state or equilibrium to brain function. We see this function at work when we consider that listening to music activates one area and deactivates others to reduce pain. This is not terribly surprising considering that we all have experienced being able to concentrate on a television show, an article that we're reading, or figuring out some type of a puzzle, which does the same thing by shifting awareness within brain circuits.

Remember someone yelling, "I'm talking to you. Why aren't you paying attention?" And that's the point—your brain was not paying attention, having deactivated one kind of awareness to focus on another. This ability of the brain is very natural; some of it takes place automatically and some by intention. In either case, we refer to it as "selective attention." The brain is so good at this that Trafton Drew, from Harvard Medical School, conducted a study showing that 83 percent of radiologists selectively intent on finding tumors in X-rays and MRIs failed to notice a picture of a gorilla clearly placed within the X-ray films. This is termed "unintentional blindness," aka "perceptual blindness."

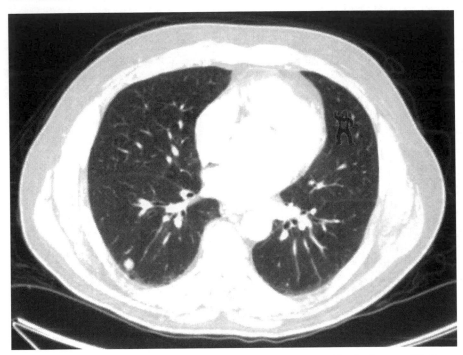

Can you find the tumor in this MRI? Can you find the gorilla?

Dr. Alattar goes on to explain that when people with pain and those with no pain were asked to perform tasks, they seemed to perform equally well. However, studies show that the people with pain had to activate other areas of the brain in order to accomplish the same task—whereas for people with no pain, the activation and deactivation of areas of the brain was much clearer and was more simply compartmentalized. In other words, the balance between selective activation and unintentional blindness became deregulated. I suspect this accounts for some aspects of fibro fog.

His findings suggested that people with chronic pain will not only lose gray matter, but the brain must find a way to make up for that loss by morphing or reorganizing itself. Recall the brain's ability to be "plastic," or basically to recreate itself.

Possible Control

Earlier, we noted that Dr. Christopher deCharms is working in an area of expectation that people can consciously control areas of the brain and activate or deactivate them at will with the assistance of MRI. In reference to pain, the effort would be to reduce or deactivate the area that causes the experienced pain. Theoretically, if a person could control the pain, he could control and preserve the health of gray matter, sparing brain function.

This raises the question: If it's possible to do this in a controlled manner, with intention, is it already happening unintentionally, simply due to fluctuation of emotions or attention? The answer is: Yes; that's the whole point of many of our discussions. This is going on all the time, subconsciously, but we can decide to do it deliberately. Further, it has been shown that the more active a person's mind is—sometimes because that's just the way the person is, other times because a person has a higher level of education or responsibility—higher centers of the brain are more active, causing a natural deactivation of pain centers. I'm sure you've had the experience of pain--a headache, for example--and then you became busy or distracted and went about your daily business, forgetting about the pain--or at least it became more tolerable. Once cognitive gymnastics and activities calm down, you realize the pain is there again, and it becomes more painful and obvious and harder to deal with. In the sufferer's mind this is often perceived as "the pain has gotten worse." This concept then turns out to be quite a conundrum academically, very close to the question of "If a tree falls in the forest and no one hears it, does it make a sound?" Has the pain really gotten worse? What do you think, based on what we've discussed?

The Placebo Effect

A placebo is another way of manipulating focus and altering our experience. A placebo would be like a sugar pill that has no pharmacological value, yet produces an effect mimicking the assumed pharmacological value. I have not seen Dr. deCharms' research in reference to the placebo effect; however, there was a study in 2004 reported by *Journal of Science* that used MRI scans to prove that using a placebo decreased the activity in the areas of the brain that registered pain. So we're clear that the placebo effect is not a spiritual or esoteric concept, but a real neurological influence, no different from taking a medication, receiving a chiropractic adjustment, or employing selective attention, as discussed above—all of which can change the neurology of the brain and hence the experience of pain.

These findings are encouraging, to say the least. This is real science and brings real hope. If a person can be trained to modulate and control her own pain, she can change her life. Keep in mind that once trained, and with the addition of a non-drug treatment such as chiropractic, a real reduction in pain will be evident and possibly the end to medication forever. However, an anti-inflammatory diet and regular exercise will still be necessary for long-term success.

5th Vital Sign: Pain

Traditionally, when speaking of vital signs, we all know them to be blood pressure, respiratory rate, pulse rate, and temperature. In many clinical circles, particularly in nursing and neuromuscular-skeletal venues, we're beginning to accept that the judgment of pain is a fifth vital sign, in spite of the fact that it is subjective and a contradiction to the objectivity of the term "sign." While it's frequently labeled as such, pain is an acceptable standard of health status and a valued clinical perspective.

Unfortunately, to date, its objectivity is still being questioned, particularly when it comes to third parties who may have to foot the bill for that finding. It is conveniently profitable for insurance companies to deny claims. With the fast pace of research studying active pain centers in the brain—as in Dr. deCharms' research—the objectivity of pain will soon become mainstream and will substantiate a reimbursable diagnosis. This is bad news for insurance companies.

However, as of this writing, the objectivity for clinical purposes comes by the use of the visual analog scale whereby a patient simply writes down or circles a numerical designation on a scale of 1 to 10 signifying her pain level, either in a particular region of her body or upon a particular movement or activity. There are various presentations that a patient may see in a doctor's office or hospital. As noted below, they all boil down to the same relative value of judgment: by the patient.

Your doctor may ask you to rate your pain on a scale from zero (no pain) to ten (unbearable pain). This pain scale is called a Visual Analog Scale, or VAS. We like it because it's a combination of words, pictures, and numbers. Most people can comfortably and quite accurately relate to this style.

Wong-Baker FACES® Pain Rating Scale

From Hockenberry MJ, Wilson D, Winkelstein ML: "Wong's Essentials of Pediatric Nursing", cd.7, St.Louis,2005p,. 1259.U;ed with Permission. Copyright, Msbly.

While at first glance it appears to be purely subjective, its ability to track progress as well as integrate the score/opinion of the patient with clinically objective findings by the doctor raises its level of validity and reproducibility, keeping in mind that there are common tests and judgments that doctors make to determine whether or not a patient is malingering.

There are caveats and considerations in judging the VAS when a person is taking medication. Some medications, like opiates or social drugs, could greatly reduce the validity of the score. After taking this into account, the score giving the benefit of the doubt to the patient's reported response is appropriate.

Objective Validity

This discussion puts us on the threshold of scientifically, medically, and legally accepting an objective method of judging pain, thanks to the research of Dr. Jean MacKay, John Gabrielie, and Dr. Christopher deCharms. These research studies, as we've mentioned, revolve around the utilization of MRIs to document the areas of the brain that are active during pain. Presently these tests are impractical and not reimbursable. The analog visual scales will continue to prevail, for now. Nevertheless, there is real science and real hope for fibromyalgia sufferers.

Glutathione

Dr. Gutman, MD, author of *Glutathione: Your Body's Most Powerful Protector*, has shown that glutathione is our body's most powerful antioxidant, and for our purposes, as we've discussed, it is a function of glial cells. Dr. Gutman goes on to say that glutathione is a superb support for health, stress, athletic performance, skin disorders, detoxification, fatigue, digestion, pregnancy and lactation, sleep, psycho-neurobiology, trauma and burns, seizures, stomach and bowel conditions, kidney issues, arthritis, eyesight, hearing loss, sinusitis, lung problems, lung disease, hepatitis, diabetes, heart disease, ear infections, stroke, cholesterol issues, high blood pressure, and, most important to us and our conversation about the brain, Parkinson's and Alzheimer's, and MS as well as ALS. It affects PSA levels, balding and hair loss, infertility, and many other conditions.

This all sounds quite amazing; however, what is more amazing is that we don't have more health problems in the US than we do, particularly considering the prevalence of obesity, the overconsumption of carbohydrates, and poor protein sources. Direct supplementation of glutathione is not very effective due to its vulnerability in the digestive tract. However, many nutrients, in particular cysteine, which is an amino acid (if you recall, amino acids are the biological components of proteins) that when supplied in effective quantities and quality will help increase glutathione production. Most of the research, as we've discussed previously, boils down to cysteine being the primary building block of glutathione. Supplementation with straight cysteine is sometimes not well-tolerated; however, a variation, N-acetyl cysteine, is tolerated well, as it's more efficient and absorbable.[27]

Just like any other substance, cysteine can be toxic if it's not absorbed into the cell efficiently. Again, that's why N-acetyl cysteine is used. When patients suffer from Tylenol (acetaminophen) poisoning, the fastest and best-known way to raise glutathione levels is to administer N-acetyl cysteine.[2] The glutathione then binds to the toxic byproducts of Tylenol poisoning and prevents tissue damage. Tylenol poisoning affects the liver's ability to remove toxic byproducts. When this happens, cellular damage can take place and possibly lead to death.

Of late there have been promising results with transdermal/patch supplementation of glutathione as well as oral sprays, both of which avoid the perils of the digestive system. These are great options; your doctor may have a strong recommendation for one or the other in your case. Supplementation to provide what the body needs to produce glutathione will work for most people.

N-acetyl Cysteine Supplementation
I recommend doing the best you can to bring your food intake up to a healthy and sometimes a needed therapeutic level of antioxidants through natural foods as described above. However, it's a difficult mark to hit. Personally, I supplement my diet by taking antioxidant formulas to enhance and insure glutathione levels.

There are two avenues that I am most fond of: the first through Vicki at the Enfield Pain Clinic and the second through Dr. Jeff Moss of Moss Nutrition.

1. Through the Enfield Pain Clinic order Complete *Detoxification Kit* and *Prime AGE Defense Formula.* Combine these two by the directions.
2. Through Moss you will find Vital Nutrients, *Detox Formula* and Designs for Health *N-Acetyl-Cysteine.* Combine these two by the direction.

(See Appendix for more information and ordering)

> The future is bright for chronic pain sufferers who make an effort to understand evolving neurology and physiology. Becoming a doctor or PhD is not necessary, but at least gain enough savvy to help steer conversations and ask resourceful questions of yourself and your health team.

CHAPTER 24

New Science, Real Hope

Chapter Topics:
   Erasing Pain
   Laser Therapy

Erasing Pain

We've talked about pain that becomes a disease in itself that the body/brain cannot turn off. For the purpose of this section, let's think of pain as a neurological memory that we can't let go of, as opposed to the sensitization and irritation of nerves that keep them firing. So imagine you experience pain, let's say in reference to having been in a fender bender and suffering whiplash. Now let's imagine that you continue to feel pain like a recurring dream, emotion, or fear; the pain is unforgettable by your nervous system and it just keeps showing up. Your body (your brain) remembers/believes (or should I say believes/remembers) that when you move your head, or when your neck/shoulders are touched, that there should be pain. It not only remembers, but it can actually anticipate the pain when you first think about turning your head or anticipate being touched. The memory itself begins to trigger pain. This is the same programming that makes your mouth water and your pancreas start to secrete insulin just from the thought or smell of hot buttered bread.

Research by Karim Nader and Joseph LeDoux showed that the memory of pain in the brain or in the spine is not stagnant and is not as simple as neurological mapping or an inert hardwired circuit, the way electrical wiring in your house is thought of, or that of a child's electric trains as they just keep rotating, following the same track around and around. Rather, it is a living, learning (aka plastic) intelligence, recreating itself into present context each time the memory is brought up. This takes place with all brain functions, but with fibro we are focusing on the marriage of emotions and pain. So what does this mean? It means that each time you feel the pain it literally confirms, resets, and updates itself. This also means that over time it changes, and not only locally in the spine where the pain neurons live, but in self-perpetuating neurological circuits and regions in the brain that change interpretation and the experience of pain. With each memory realized, there is a tendency to change the way you experience and evaluate what it means, what it feels like, how you should move and respond, how threatening it is to you, and how sensitive and protective you should be in the future. This whole process of reinforcement, with its little tweak, is unlikely to be obvious to you. The fact that you don't seem to be getting any better, or possibly getting worse, is confirmation that your "main memory" ability is very efficient.

Whether in the brain or in nerve synapses in the spinal region, the neurological memory is perpetuated by a special protein that just hangs around in nerve synapses waiting to be called to duty. This mechanism has been called consolidation. So when looked at in this respect, the problem seems rather simple. If we can create a drug or a substance that blocks the synthesis of the protein that perpetuates the memory, we can block the efficiency of pain. Keep in mind that we are talking about pain that is inappropriate, meaning there is nothing causing pain happening to you (allodynia). But the body believes that there is still reason to have the pain/memory signal sent when in reality it is untrue; it is just a memory.

Nader and LeDoux's investigation started trying to solve this phenomenon by studying post-traumatic stress disorder. When the stress had passed and people were no longer in the war zone and no longer experiencing the horrors and the stresses, the emotional dramas in their brains persisted. If they could find a way to block/mitigate the perpetuation of the memory, it would be the first time in history that a psychiatric problem could be cured. And although the person could still remember the event, the emotional component stored and reinforced over and over in the brain would no longer trigger emotional suffering. The same principle is being proposed for chronic pain.

The complicating factor with fibromyalgia is that there are two memories involved most of the time. One is the neurological memory outside the brain that perpetuates the stimulation of pain nerves at the spinal level. The most natural and effective way to alleviate this is through diagnosing and correcting spinal subluxations by chiropractic treatment. The second component is the emotional memory and interpretation of the pain that lives in the brain just as post-traumatic stress syndrome does. Nevertheless, the principle is the same. Block/mitigate the proteins that perpetuate the firing of the signals, and you can stop the pain nerves from firing, plus stop the suffering. This is of great importance to fibromyalgia patients.

For those of you who have an interest in post-traumatic stress disorder and would like to know more about the concepts in this section, consider reading Jonah Lehrer's article in *Wired Magazine*, March 2012. You could also contact your local chiropractor, re-read "Spinal Subluxation" in our chapter on History, or contact me at fibro.epc@comcast.net. Many sufferers unable to make progress have not been evaluated correctly for spinal subluxation.

Low-Level Laser Therapy

The National Institute of Health, in 2011 reported on the role that low-level laser therapy plays in neuro-rehabilitation. Low-level laser therapy (LLLT) is effective in treating stroke and traumatic brain injuries as well as central nervous system diseases such as multiple sclerosis, Parkinson's, fibromyalgia, Alzheimer's, and peripheral nerve involvement of neuritis, neuralgia, and idiopathic pain like fibromyalgia. Much of the research came out of Massachusetts General Hospital, Boston, Massachusetts. They concluded;

"Low-level laser therapy is steadily moving into the mainstream of medical practice. As the Western population continue to age, the incidence of degenerative diseases of old age will only continue to increase and produce and ever more severe financial and social burdens. Moreover, despite the best efforts of 'Big Pharma,' distrust of pharmaceuticals is growing in general because of uncertain efficacy and troublesome adverse effects."

Low-Level Lasers

Low-level lasers are different from the more publicized heat lasers that are used in many surgical procedures to cut and cauterize tissue. The Erchonia laser, which is used in therapy at the Enfield Pain Clinic, Enfield, CT, has made history as being the first low-level laser in the world to gain FDA market clearance for the treatment of pain.

The Effects of Laser Light on Tissue and Accelerated Tissue Repair

We are all familiar with plant photosynthesis, a process that converts photons of sunlight energy into chemical energy. The action of laser light on human cells/tissue is quite similar. Photons of light from a laser cascade into tissue and stimulate cells to synthesize adenosine triphosphate (ATP), aka energy.

ATP is a molecule that is a major carrier of energy from one reaction site to another in all living cells. Increases in ATP, as a result of laser light, augment the energy available to cells so that a cell can absorb nutrients faster and expel waste products to bring healing. However, the integrity of the cell membrane is crucial to this process, as well as the effectiveness of the laser. The light photons from the laser must act on and through the cell membrane.

For the sake of general health and effectiveness of the laser, cell membranes must have adequate amounts of fats. For the average fibro patient, the most efficient way to accomplish this is to supplement the diet with fish oil. Refer back to Chapter 22 where we discussed fats, and tests available to find out if your body has a healthy balance. When you are low on Omega-3s, or simply want to support your levels, increase the daily intake of oily Omega-3-rich fish like salmon, tuna, sardines, and anchovies. Other sources such as flax and chia seeds and Omega-3 rich eggs will help also. For most convenience and assurance, fish and flax supplements are available also.

As a review: the healthier the cell membrane, the healthier and more efficient mitochondria will be, hence there will be more ATP available to the cells of tendons, ligaments, muscles, and nerves. Healing/repair and general energy will improve. Healing time can be reduced up to two-thirds with laser therapy compared to normal healing, all other factors remaining equal.

Nerve Pain Response

Laser therapy helps to block pain transmission by decreasing nerve-ending sensitivity. Laser light stimulation also produces high levels of pain-killing chemicals such as endorphins from the brain, adrenal glands, and other areas. It is utilized in the treatment of all pain conditions such as fibromyalgia, low back pain, knee pain, headaches, carpel tunnel, trigeminal neuralgia, muscle and joint pain, etc. To find a doctor trained in laser therapy near you, go to http://www.erchonia.com/physician-search. You'll just need to type in your zip code.

CHAPTER 25

Confident Self-advocacy

Closing Thoughts

Wayne Dwyer tells the story of a man who drops his car keys at the same time that there's a power failure and the lights go out in his house. He reaches down in the dark, shuffling his hands around the floor trying to find his keys. After a few frustrating minutes, he looks up and sees that the streetlight is still on at the end of his driveway. He thinks to himself, *it's too dark in the house to find the keys. I'll go outside where there is light.* He's now outside under the streetlight looking around on the ground for his keys when a neighbor comes along and says, "What are you doing?" "I'm looking for my car keys," he explains. The neighbor says, "Well, I'll help you look for them." So now they're both looking around on the ground under the streetlight. After a few minutes the neighbor says, "Where did you lose them?" The man replies, "Well, I lost them in the house." "You mean to tell me you lost them in the house but you're looking for them out here?" "Well, yeah, I had to have some light. I'll never find them in the house; it's too dark."

Sounds silly, doesn't it? But this is exactly the type of logic we frequently see in the health care community, steadfastly holding on to beliefs, perception, and non-cohesive facts that are relied upon as truth and certainty. This leads doctors, researchers, and patients to look in the wrong places for answers. Consequently, medical and non-medical physicians alike hold themselves and their patients hostage to antiquated paradigms where diagnosis and treatment frequently fail the fibromyalgia, chronic fatigue, and chronic pain patient. How did we get to this point in spite of evolving science, cutting-edge technological advances, and the diverse interdisciplinary opportunities that exist today?

What went wrong? How do so many well-intended doctors perpetuate the unintentional lies, inconsistencies, and misunderstandings that have comfortably settled into a Western paradigm of health care?

We could start with looking at medical education, whereby mentorship of out-of- touch predecessors passes a baton of restricted paradigm to students. This statement considers that there are really two paradigms homogenized into one "health care" paradigm: one is the paradigm of science; the other is the paradigm of the practice of medicine.

Medical people are convinced that their paradigm is the only path to health. This is not dissimilar to the battle between religions, each believing that their God/beliefs will save them. In reference to health care, I'm reminded of the book written by John C. Boyle, *The Battle for the Soul of Capitalism.* He uses the world of health care/doctors as an analogy to prove a point in the world of finance. He describes the difference between *circumstantial ethics* and *absolute ethics,* asking his readers to consider that doctors treat their patients based on circumstantial and contrived ethics created through pressures from insurance companies, corporations, *predecessors, mentors, education,* economics, restriction of time, managed-care demands, and defensive medicine, versus good doctoring that adheres to the *absolute ethics* of their oath as physicians.

In any society, a certain degree of circumstantial ethics seems to be necessary; yet they blur the lines, begging to compromise absolute ethics and contemporary thought leaders.

Let's add one other impediment: patients as well as doctors are swamped with information, literature, and disarticulated research. For most, it's not comfortable to believe that many doctors get their postgraduate information from the same sources as patients, but it's true. Doctors become overwhelmed with ineffective information from articles, drug salespersons, journals, the media, friends and the likes of Dr. Oz; consequently they are confused, if not conflicted, just as patients are. Ultimately, they default to the paradigm of their education and mentors, whether or not it's working.

We are brought up to respect the authority of white coats and stethoscopes. With naïve desperation, many follow a Western paradigm that neither patient nor their doctors realize has passed its prime. On a roller coaster of pain and pills, too many sufferers are frustrated and their families strained. I hope that I can contribute to a new opportunity for sufferers as well as the health care community to re-evaluate their role in fulfilling their hopes, oaths, and promises.

Opportunity
Patients are forced to become students of the sciences, or at the very least take it upon themselves to understand the disciplines and unique opportunities that may exist outside of their medical doctor's

office. Congratulations to you for meeting this challenge with this book in your hands.

I'm guessing that many of these chapters have covered issues and concepts that may have surprised you and challenged lifelong beliefs as well as the conventional wisdom of today.

Whether you're the sufferer, a friend, family member, physician, or caregiver, the most meaningful understandings are frequently contrary to presently held beliefs, the likes of which may rub your doctor the wrong way when you begin to question his or her thoughts. But just to say it one more time: This book may have gotten uncomfortable for you too, raising more questions than supplying answers at times, hoping to help you ask better questions. From the beginning, it was all about you and what could be gathered/learned about science as "usable meaningful knowledge" and pure hope and optimism to change course—an opportunity to rewrite a dead-end future that was almost certain if one stayed on the same old path.

Real Science

Real science inspires real hope. The word "science" comes from the Latin word for "usable knowledge." Usable knowledge is accumulated by observation, natural phenomena, and experimentation. Another component of science is that it strives to minimize objective bias.

Western medicine's paradigm requires science to conform to what's termed "the scientific method." This is a method of investigating and acquiring knowledge that fits scientific principles of reason. The dilemma is that all science is, at best, empirical, regardless of the commitment to the methodology.

Gary Taubes, in his book *Good Calories, Bad Calories*, questions whether real science exists, particularly in the world of nutrition. I have interpolated his thoughts into our concerns about fibromyalgia and neurology. He seems to be troubled, and questions the validity of using the word "science," considering it to be generally debatable in that many of the individuals delivering their beliefs to the general public think of themselves as scientists, but are simply borrowing the authority of the scientific community. And regardless of the tenor of their assertions, they fail to conform to science as most working scientists and philosophers of science would characterize it.

Unfortunately, as we have touched on throughout the book, even the best of our most respected thought leaders in health care have egos and special interests. With the best intentions, they assert their authority and persuasive skills to advance and endorse their own paradigm to the exclusion of other disciplines. This applies even to the most ethical of us, as Richard Feynman in in his commencement address at CalTech in 1974 suggested: *The first principle is that you must not fool yourself...yet you are the easiest person to fool.*

What's true science today may not be considered true science tomorrow. There was a time when science dictated that the world was flat, the sedative qualities of thalidomide were safe and all dietary fats were bad. As insightful learned thinking and evidence evolve, so does science. Hence, a scientific fact does not mean certainty. It's certain only while it's certain. What is certain is that certainty frequently leads to doubt.

"If a man will begin with certainty, he shall end with doubt. But if he will be content to begin with doubt, he shall end in certainty."

Francis Bacon (1605) The Advancement of Learning: Book 1.

Methodology

Methodology and philosophy are important to how we perceive science, especially when diversity exists. Western medicine encompasses a dichotomy between a traditional medical paradigm frequently referred to as allopathic medicine, and a so-called non-medical paradigm. The non-medical paradigm strives to understand and treat maladies without the use of drugs or surgery. Understanding the distinctions could make all the difference in the world in how you relate to fibromyalgia.

Law professor Edmund Gray argues: *Because various sciences maintain different approaches, theories, criteria, and canons of practice, metaphysics and levels of relevance, as well as levels of abstractions, it would be highly naive to suggest that we could expect some basic or universal criteria which could apply consistently to determine "reliability."*[1]

Reliability, in the context of this writing, means "effectiveness in reducing suffering." Professor Gray is suggesting that in law there is science that not everyone will agree on as being "science." Nonetheless, it may be relied upon as scientific information. However, reliability does not mean truth or certainty. And so it is in health care.

Most people along their journey will be involved with some type of medication, treatment, or approach which by the definition of Western science is considered "reliable" and "scientific." Yet the sufferer knows that something is missing—the sufferer still suffers.

In other words, regardless of the reliability, certainty, and confidence professed by any one doctor, pharmaceutical company, or conventional wisdom, you are likely to still need help. You, on the other hand, have broken away from the pack or you wouldn't have read this book and gotten to this page, so congratulations once again. You might now feel motivated to pass this book, or particular chapters, on to others whom you care about.

First Do No Harm

All the information in this book acknowledges that the first calling of any doctor, or caregiver would be "do no harm." The problem is that many patients are discouraged from seeking or are denied access to all therapeutic solutions. This is often due to ignorance and dogma handed down through medical education and mentorship of predecessors who suggest that any path or approach they do not approve may actually cause harm, meaning that anything other than allopathic medicine (primarily drugs and surgery) will cause harm. This attitude is put forth by the same medical community that reported in the *Journal of the American Medical Association* (*JAMA*) that in an average year, 1.6 million people are hospitalized due to the side effects of prescription drugs and up to 160,000 will die from their reactions (Dangerous Drugs, 1992).

You

It's all about you! By now the reader will be better-equipped to sort through the myths, prejudices, ignorance, and arrogance of a Western medical system that has possibly held you back. When you're able to ask questions that help steer your doctors' thoughts, you will be a self-advocating dynamo.

I hope you'll see this writing as a friend, a support, an inspiration, and a doorway to greater possibilities for you and your family. You are called upon to take responsibility and action, as well as to be educated and arrogant enough to educate the doctors whom you want to work with to be better "fibro-docs" for you. I'm sure you've already noticed that you have to be patient and understanding with your doctor. I know that doesn't seem fair. After all you're the sufferer, the patient; why should you have to be the one who is patient and understanding?

The real question is: "What knowledge, perspective, attitude, and action can you adopt as you move forward to get better results?" Dr. Bob Hoffman, DC, suggests, "If you want to improve your life 100 percent, simply improve each area of your life one percent." Chunking it down like this takes out some of the feeling of being overwhelmed and makes it feel more possible, doesn't it? Simply work toward improving your knowledge and understanding, but just one percent. Shoot for just one percent improvement in communication skills, relationships, and your energy; just one percent improvement in your nutrition, exercise, and attitude. Strive to put one percent more effort into preparing for each doctor's appointment so you can ask better questions. Take a minute to make a personal list of areas you could/need to improve, but just one percent. Let the past go, and don't be distracted by those with differing opinions and agendas.

Hopefully, you have read this book from cover to cover. If there are areas where you felt confused and/or you have questions about, don't hesitate to email me at fibro-doc@comcast.net, or go to www.DrRobLangone.com for blogs, research articles, workshops, webinars, Skype coaching, and reference material.

Hope

As Dr. Barbara Fredricksen explained: *"Hope opens us up and removes the blinders of fear and despair. It allows us to see the bigger picture, become creative, and have a belief in a better future."*[4]

Anything we encounter in life that we would consider negative or that will encourage suffering, confusion, and a feeling of being out of control will diminish hope

False Hope

We will define false hope as "hope based on fantasy or any unconfirmed perception." However, the power of hope, any hope, defies reason in that even false hope has the power to bring optimism and change behavior. In the past, the concept of hope changing us in any way was categorized as a psychosomatic or a placebo effect. When based on false hope, the placebo effect must continue to be reinforced more and more diligently than is necessary when based on true hope-- but nevertheless, it is valuable. If nothing else, even false hope helps to keep one on track and open to greater possibilities, frequently evolving into real hope.

Pseudoscience

False hope is in a way related to pseudoscience. They both can carve a path for future discoveries.

When do you feel the least amount of hope and optimism? I don't know about you, but for me it's when I feel a lack of control. So where does the sense of control and optimism come from for Fibros?

Control and Optimism Come From:
- Understanding that fibromyalgia is not your fault.
- Knowing that there are real possibilities to improve your future, not just taking another pill.
- Believing that real science is at hand and evolving at a healthy pace.
- Understanding the cause of fibromyalgia and that you're not going to die from it, yet the term "Stat !" should apply to how you pursue answers.
- Knowing that your doctors' knowledge is limited, and you can and deserve to know what those limits are.
- Being mindful of your values, beliefs, and priorities so as to give yourself the opportunity to strengthen or change them.
- Believing that today does not have to equal tomorrow, and your future is up to you.
- Having a sense of control and knowing you can reset your mind/brain and attitude every day; it's crucial and easy.
- Possessing knowledge and understanding treatment strategies that will help guide you so as to reduce confusion and frustration.
- Having the support of family, caring friends, and caregivers who will provide daily fibro-triage for your success.
- Avoiding being overwhelmed, by using exercises taught in Chapter 19.

Hope Comes From:
- Believing that all things are possible when anchored in reality.
- Knowing that thinking in terms of possibilities is far more powerful than trying to fix, change, or improve things.

Hopefully, you initially completed the "optimism quiz" to uncover emotional roadblocks. If you didn't, that's okay; you can do it now. Go to www.fibro-doc.com and click on the *Members* tab.

Calculate your score and enter it on the back cover of the book. I hope that your results will be inspiring. In any case, as mentioned in the introduction, we would love to hear from you: what happened to your score, what the book meant to you, your thoughts, criticisms, suggestions, and questions. Tell us if you feel more empowered or not. Share with us what it was like trying to put your doctoring team together and what kinds of attitudes and roadblocks came up in the process. Further, we'd love to hear your fibro story right from the beginning. You can do this on our website as well by clicking on "My Fibro Story."

Thank you!

APPENDIX

Cleaning Products:
    *SNAP green cleaning products contact: Vicki G. @ 413 575-3230 or
    Visit: www.shop.com/urbestlife.com   Search SNAP

Nutrition:

Note to Physicians:

Physicians interested in expanding nutritional knowledge and/or
incorporating nutrition into their practice, contact me personally
Dr Rob @ 413-575-7702 or Visit: Nutrametrix.com/DrRobLangone
Click on "Health Professionals", password "Health"

*Detoxification Kit and Prime AGE Defense Formula
  Contact the Enfield Pain Clinic at 860-745-7600 or
  Email: fibro.epc@comcast.net Note "Detox" in the subject

*Detox Formula and N-Acetyl-Cysteine:
  Contact Moss Nutrition; Website: www.mossnutrition.com
  Email: info@mossnutrition.com
  Phone: 800-851-5444

*OPC-3 (Oligomeric Proantho-Cyanidin) Anti-oxidants/Resveratrol:
  Contact My office manager Vicki @ 860 745-7600 or email
  Phil Martin @ pcmgold1@gmail.com (note "Fibromyalgia" in subject)

*ACTS (Adrenal Cortisol Thyroid Support):
  Contact Valerie Martin at Transitions Life Style, (TLS)
  Email; Valeriejeanmartin@gmail.com, Phone: 860-982-2950
  Explain to Valerie that you read; *Fibromyalgia, New Science, Real Hope*

*Fish Oil Omega-3 fats: Heart Health, Essential Omeg-3
  Contact our office: Enfield Integrative Health 860 745-7600
        Email: fibro.epc@comcast.net

*Growth Hormone HGH (secretagogue); Anti-Aging, *Ultra Prime.*
  Contact Dr. Rob Langone at fibro.epc@comcast.net

*Wild-caught young fish (canned): Vital Choice at @
       www.vitalchoice.com

Resources:

*Fats and natural food sources information: Weston A.
  Price Foundation (www.westonaprice.org).

*Fatty Acid Testing: Contact: Lipid Technologies, LLC
  info@LipidLab.com, Toll Free #: (888) 630-6634

*Mitochondria/ATP Testing: Genova Diagnostics; Asheville,
  North Carolina, # (800) 522-4762

BIBLIOGRAPHY

1. "Adrenal Fatigue vs. Hypothyroidism." Dr. Michael Lam. www.drlam, com/articles/adrenalfatiguevshypothrodism.asp (accessed July 25, 2013).

2. Aoyama, Koji, Sang Won Suh, Aaron M. Hamby, Jialing Liu, and Wai Yee Chan. "Neuronal Glutathione Defiency and Aging Dependent Neurodegeration in the EAAC1 Defienct Mouse." *Nature Neuroscience* 9 (2006): 119-126.

3. Badsha, Humeira, *European League Against Rheumatism*, http://www.drbadshamedical.com/our-doctors/humeira-badsha/ (accessed March 16, 2014)

4. Barbara, PhD, Frederickson. *Positivity: Groundbreaking Research Reveals How to Embrace the Hidden Strength of the Postive Emotions, Overcome Negativity, and Thrive.*. New York: Crown Publishing Group, 2009.

5. Bennett, Robert, MD, FRCP, FACP, Professor *of Medicine, Department of Medicine (OP09), Oregon Health and Science University, Portland, OR 97329, USA.*

6. *E-mail: bennetrob1@comcast.net, Clin Exp Rheumatol 2005; 23 (Suppl. 39): S154-S162. © Copyright CLINICAL AND EXPERIMENTAL RHEUMATOLOGY 2005.*

7. Banic, Borut, Steen Petersen-Felix, Ole K. Andersen, Bogdan P. Radanov, P.M. Villiger, Lars Arendt-Nielsen, Michele Curatolo. *The Journal for the international Association for the study of pain, Elsevier, 107 (2004) 7-15*

8. Blaylock, Russell. *"Exotoxins; the Taste That Kills"* Albuquerque, NM, Health Press, 1996

9. Branco, MD, Bernard Bannwarth, MD, Inmaculada Failde, MD, Jordi Abello Carbonell, MD, Francis Blotman, MD, Michael Spaeth, MD, Fernando Saraiva, MD, Francesca Nacci, MD, Eric Thomas, MD, Jean-Paul Caubère, MD, Katell Le Lay, MD, Charles Taieb, MD, Marco Matucci-Cerinic, MD,. *Prevalence of Fibromyalgia: A Survey in Five European Countries,* Elsevier, Article in Press, 2009

10. Browning LM, Hsieh SD, Ashwell M. "A systematic review of waist-to-height ratio as a screening tool for the prediction of cardiovascular disease and diabetes: 0·5 could be a suitable global boundary value." Nutr Res Rev. 2010 Dec;23(2):247-69. Epub 2010 Sep 7.

11. Boublik, JH. "Coffee Contains Potent Opiate Receptor Binding Activity." *Nature* 301 (1983): 246-248.

12. Browning LM, Hsieh SD, Ashwell M. "A systematic review of waist-to-height ratio as a screening tool for the prediction of cardiovascular disease and diabetes: 0·5 could be a suitable global boundary value." Nutr Res Rev. 2010 Dec;23(2):247-69. Epub 2010 Sep

13. Buskila, Dan, and Piercarlo Sarzi-Puttini. "Biology and therapy of fibromyalgia. Genetic aspects of fibromyalgia syndrome." *Arthritis research & therapy* 8.5 (2006): 218.

14. Caudill, David S. "Expert Scientific Testimony in Courts, The Ideal and Illusion of Value Free Science. Villanova University School of Law *The Pantaneto Forum*, Issue 39, July 2010.

15. Camacho, A: Massieu, L. "Role of glutamate transporters in the clearance and release of glutamate during ischemia its relationship to neuronal death". Archives of medical research 37, 2006.

16. Chaitow, Leon. *Fibromyalgia Syndrome, A Practioner's Guide.* New York: Churchill Livingstone/Elsevier, 2010.

17. Clark and Sokoloff, "Coffee contains potent opiate receptor binding activity" Pub med 1983 January (1999

18. Clarke, Donald, and Louis Sokoloff. *Circulation and Energy Metabolism of the Brain: Basic Neurochemistry in Molecular, Cellular, Medical Aspects.* 6th ed. Philidelphia: Lippincott-Raven, 1999.

19. Cohen, Phd., Suzy. *Drug Muggers: Which Medications are Robbing Your Body of Essential Nutrients-And Natural Ways to Restore Them.* New York: Rodale, 2011.

20. Cordain, Loren, Ph.D. *The Paleo Diet.* Hoboken, New Jersey, John Wiley & Sons Incorporated, 2002

21. Curtis, Kathryn, Anna Osadchuk, and Joel Katz. "An Eight-Week Yoga Intervention is Associated with Improvements in Pain, Psychological Functioning, and Mindfulness, and Changes in Cortisol Levels in Women with Fibromyalgia." *Journal of Pain Research* 4 (2011): 189-201.

22. Davis, Glenda H., and Patricia Stephens. "ADD/ADHD and Fibromyalgia:Where Is The a Connection." *Advance Magazine,* Jan. - Feb. 2000.

23. Defense Mechanism." *Diabetes and Obesity Program* 101 (2009): 17787-92.

24. De Rosa SC, Zaretsky MD, Dubs JG, Roederer M, Anderson M, Green A, Mitra D, Watanabe N, Nakamura H, Tjioe I, Deresinski SC, Moore WA, Ela SW, Parks D, Herzenberg LA, Herzenberg LA. N-acetylcysteine replenishes glutathione in HIV infection. Eur J Clin Invest. 2000 Oct;30(10):915-29

25. *Dorland's Illustrated Medical Dictionary.* 32 ed. New York: Elsevier, 2013.
26. Drigen, R. "Metabolism and Functions of Glutathoine in the Brain." *Progress in Neurology* 62, no. 6 (2000): 649-671.
27. Dröge W. "Is aging a cystine deficiency syndrome?" *Oxidative Stress and Ageing philos trans r soc lond B biol sci. 2005*
28. Engleman, David, *Incognito:The Secret Lives of the Brain.* New York: Pantheon, 2011
29. Fallon BA, Lipkin RB, Corbera KM, Yu S, Nobler MS, Keilp JG, Petkova E, Lisanby SH, Moeller JR, Slavov I, Van Heertum R, Mensh BD, Sackeim HA. : Regional Cerebral Blood Flow and Metabolic Rate in Persistent Lyme Encephalopathy.. Archives of General Psychiatry 2009;66: 554-563
30. Fallon BA, Keilp JG, Corbera KM, Petkova E, Britton CB, Dwyer E, Slavov I, Cheng J, Dobkin J, Nelson DR, Sackeim HA. : A Randomized, Placebo-Controlled Trial of Repeated IV Antibiotic Therapy for Lyme Encephalopathy. 2008; 70 (13); 992-1003) (Epub 10/2007). Neurology 2008;70: 992-1003
31. Fields, Douglas, R., Phd. *The Other Brain.* New York: Simon&Schuster, 2009.
32. Field, Tiffany, et al. "Fibromyalgia pain and Substance P decrease and sleep improves after massage therapy." *JCR: Journal of Clinical Rheumatology* 8.2 (2002): 72-76.
33. Fujikawa, DG. "Prolonged seizures and cellular injury: understanding the connection.". Epilepsy and behavior. (//www.ncbi.nlm.nih.gov/pub med/16278099). (accessed 2007)
34. Gerwin, Robert, S Shannon, C-Z Hong, and DR Hubbard. " Myofascial trigger point examination: interrater reliability." *Pain* 69 (1997): 65-73.
35. Häuser, Winfried, et al. "Treatment of fibromyalgia syndrome with antidepressants." JAMA: the journal of the American Medical Association301.2 (2009): 198.
36. Hoehn, KL, AB Salmon, C. Behrens-Hohnen, N., Turner, AJ Hoy, GJ Maghzai, R. Stocker,
37. H.Van Remmen, E.W. Kraegen, and G.J. Cooney. "Insulin Resistance is a Cellular Antioxidant
38. "Is 500 Mg of Niacin Too Much? | LIVESTRONG.COM." LIVESTRONG.COM - Lose Weight & Get Fit with Diet, Nutrition & Fitness Tools | LIVESTRONG.COM. http://www.livestrong.com/article/226390-does-niacin-raise-hdl-levels/#ixzz2QG5JQA82 (accessed July 25, 2013).

39. Jaffe, Russell. "Xenobiotics: managing Toxic Metals, Biocides, Hormone Mimics, Solvents and Chemical Disruptors."www. drrusselljaffe.com/#/publisheddcience, accessed Jan 24, 2014.

40. Janda MD, DS, Vladimir, and CE Morris. "Tribute to a Master of Rehabilitation." *Spine* 31 (2006): 1060-1064

41. Knuston. DC, Gary A. "Dysafferentation:A Novel Term to Describe the Neuro-Pathologic Effects of Joint Complex Dysfunction. A Look at Likely Mechanisms of Symptom Generation." *Journal of Manipulative and Physiological Therapies* 22 (1999): 491-494.

42. Korr, D, KJ Barwell, C Sjuken, CD Gajewski, G Manefredi, and S Ackerman. "MTG1 Codes Required For Mitochondrial Translation." *Molecular Bioligical Sciences* 14 (2003): 292-302.

43. Kurzweil, Terry Grossman, MD. "Transcend: Nine Steps To Living Well Forever," New York, NY, Rodale Press, 2009.

44. Landmark Education, "The Forum", Headquarters 353 Sacramento St., Ste. 200 San Francisco, CA 94111. Cromwell, Connecticut, March, 2006.

45. Lee CM, Huxley RR, Wildman RP, Woodward M., "Indices of abdominal obesity are better discriminators of cardiovascular risk factors than BMI: a meta-analysis". J Clin Epidemiol. 2008 Jul;61(7):646-53. Epub 2008 Mar 21.

46. Le Goff, Paul. "Is fibromyalgia a muscle disorder?." *Joint Bone Spine* 73.3 (2006): 239-242.

47. Marek, Claudia Craig. *The First Year; Fibromyalgia.* Cambridge Massachusetts, Da Capo Press, 2003.

48. Martínez-Jauand M, Sitges C, Femenia J, Cifre I, González S, Chialvo D, Montoya P. "Age-of- onset of menopause is associated with enhanced painful and non-painful sensitivity in fibromyalgia". Research Institute on Health Sciences (IUNICS), University of the Balearic Islands, Cra. de Valldemossa km 7.5, 07122, Palma de Mallorca, Spain.)

49. McEwen, B. S. "Protective and damaging effects of stress mediators". New England Journal of Medicine, 338:171 – 179, 1998

50. Mavros Y[1], Kay S, Simpson KA, Baker MK, Wang Y, Zhao RR, Meiklejohn J, Climstein M, O'Sullivan AJ, de Vos N, Baune BT, Blair SN, Simar D, Rooney K, Singh NA, Fiatarone Singh MA. "Reductions in C-reactive protein in older adults with Type II diabetes are related to improvements in body composition following a randomized controlled trial of resistance training."

J Cachexia Sarcopenia Muscle. 2014 Feb 12. [Epub ahead of print]

51. Northrup, Christiane, MD *The Wisdom of Menopause.* New York: Bantam. 2006.

52. Nuttall S., Martin U., Sinclair A, Kendall M. 1998. Glutathione: in sickness and in health. The *Lancet* 351(9103):645-646

53. Oschman, James, L. *Energy Medicine, The Scientific Basis.* London: Churchill Livingstone, 2000

54. "Oxidative Stress and Aging: Is Aging a Cyeteine Defiency Syndrome?" *Philisophical Transactions of Royal Society B: Biological Sciences* 360, no. 1464 (2005): 2355-2372.

55. Rolf, Ida P. *Rolfing: Integration of the Human Structures.* Santa Monica: Dennis-Landman, 1977.

56. Russell IJ, et al. "Treatment of fibromyalgia syndrome with Super Malic: a randomized, double blind, placebo controlled, crossover pilot study." PubMed.gov, *Journal of Rheumatology.* 1995 May; 22(5):953-8.

57. Russell, Gibbons. "As Seeing the Oracle Through the Fountainhead:BJ Palmer and his Times, 1902-1961." *Chiropratic History* 7 (1981): 9-14.

58. Roizen, Mehmet C. Oz, MD, *You Staying Young,* New York, NY, Free Press, Simon & Schuster, Inc. 2007.

59. Romano, T. J. "Clinical experiences with post-traumatic fibromyalgia syndrome." *The West Virginia medical journal* 86.5 (1990): 198.

60. Seaman, David. *Clinical Tradition, or pain, inflammation and tissue healing,* Hendersonville, NC, *1998.*

61. Schuh-Hofer S¹, Wodarski R, Pfau DB, Caspani O, Magerl W, Kennedy JD, Treede RD. *"One night of total sleep deprivation promotes a state of generalized hyperalgesia: a surrogate pain model to study the relationship of insomnia and pain."* Pain. 2013 Sep;154(9):1613-21. doi: 10.1016/j.pain.2013.04.046. Epub 2013 May 11.

62. Shomon, Mary J. *Living Well With Chronic Fatigue Syndrome and Fibromyalgia,* New York, NY, Harper Collins, 2004.

63. Vasquez, Alex*, Fibromyalgia in a Nutshell: A Safe and Effective Functional Medicine Strategy,* Portland, Oregon; integrative and biological medicine research and consulting, LLC.

64. Sacerdote, Paola; Suzanne Denis-Donini; Paola Paglia; Francesca Granucci; Alberto E. Panerai; and P Castagnoli-Riccardi. "Cloned Microglial Cells but not Macrophages Synethesize Beta-Endorphine in Response to CRH Activation." *Glia* 9 (1993): 1305-1310.

65. "Self-Tests by Psychology Today." Psychology Today. http://
psychologytoday.tests.psychtests.com/bin/transfer?req=
MTF8MTMyMHw0NDUIOTUIfDF8MQ==&refempt=)
arrangethisaddressthroughourwebsite. (accessed July 25, 2013).
66. St. Amand, Paul, MD, Claudia Craig Marek. *What Your Dr. May Not
Tell You About Fibromyalgia.* New York, NY: Grand Central Life &
Style, 2012.
67. Staud, Roland, MD, Christine Adamec. *Fibromyalgia for Dummies.*
Indianapolis, Indiana, Wiley, 2002.
68. "Tick Disease Plea to Moor Users." BBC NEWS. http://news.bbc.
co.uk/2/hi/uk_news/england/south/_yorkshire/8070935.stm
(accessed July 25, 2013).
69. Travell, Janet, David G. Simmons, and Lios S. Simmons. *Myofacial
Pain and Dsyfunction: The Trigger Point Manual.* New York:
Lippincott, Williams&Wilkins, 1999.
70. Turk, V., J. Kos, and B. Turk. "Cyestine Cathepsins (Proteases)-On
the Main Stage of Cancer." *Cancer Cell.* 4 (2004): 409-411.
71. Van West, Dirk, and Michael Maes. "Lower Baseline Plasma
Cortisol and Prolactin together with Increased Body Temperature
and Higher mCPP-Induced Cortisol Responses in Men with
Pedophilia." *Neuropsychopharmacology* 24 (2001): 37-46.
72. Wang, MD, Chenchen, and Schmid, PhD. "Prevalence of
Fibromyalgia: A Survey in Five European Countries." *Seminar in
Arthritis and Rheumatism* 39 (2010): 448-453.
73. Wood PB, Schweinhardt P, Jaeger E, Dagher A, Hakyemez H,
Rabiner EA, Bushnell MC, Chizh BA. "Fibromyalgia patients show
an abnormal dopamine response to pain". Eur J Neurosci. 2007
Jun; 25(12):3576-82.
74. Yellin, Jackie, and John C. Lowe, MA. "Triiodothyronine (T3)
Treatment of Euthyroid Fibromyalgia." *Clinical Bulletin if Myofacial
Therapy* 2 (1997): 71-88.
75. Yunus, Muhammed B. "Suffering, Sciene, and Sabotage." *Journal
Of Musculoskeletal Pain* 12 2004: 3-18
76. Myhill, Norman E Booth2, John McLaren-Howard3 "Targeting
mitochondrial dysfunction in the treatment of Myalgic
Encephalomyelitis/Chronic Fatigue Syndrome (ME/CFS)" – a
clinical audit Int J Clin Exp Med 2013;6(1):1-15 www.ijcem.com /
ISSN:1940-5901/IJCEM1207003

INDEX

Abbreviations "FM" and "fibro" stand for the term "fibromyalgia."

A
acid reflux, 362–63
acid-alkaline balance (pH/body chemistry)
    breathing/blood oxygenation, 89
    cellular functions and, 348
    defined/described, 343–45
    diabetes and, 349
    effect of diet and food choices, 90, 317, 345–47
    high pH (alkalosis), 348–49
    linkage to FM, 349–50
active trigger points, 151
acupuncturists. See non medical professionals
addictions, 101, 107, 362
adenosine triphosphate (ATP). See cells/cellular functions
adrenal glands
    catecholamine production, 222
    coffee as stimulant, 362–63
    cortisol production, 64–67, 94, 234, 236–37, 312–16, 320
    DHEA production, 312–13, 320
    exhaustion/fatigue, 23, 31, 312–17
    hypothyroidism interactions, 322–24
    laser light stimulation, 379
    location and functions, 311–12
    stress effects, 309–10
    See also endocrine system

advanced practice registered nurse (APRN)/nurse practitioner, 138, 254
The Advancement of Learning: Book I (Bacon), 383
aerobic vs. anaerobic exercise, 338–40
affirmations and self-talk, 114, 304–08
Agency for Toxic Substances and Disease Registry (ATSDR), 174
aging/anti-aging properties
    adrenal exhaustion, 314, 324
    alcohol and, 209–10
    allostatic load (stress), 158
    exercise, 337, 340–42
    genetics and, 218
    glutamate and, 161
    heavy metals and plastics, 170
    linkage to FM, 11
    pain and, 109
    vitamin D, 233
    wellness care, 86–87
Alattar, Maha (Dr.), 369–71
alcohol/alcohol consumption
    benefits vs. side effects, 209–10
    chronic fatigue syndrome and, 33
    diet and, 344–45, 365
    dopamine effects, 222–23
    fetal alcohol syndrome, 215, 216
    linkage to FM, 215–16
    reduction in cravings, 203
    sleep issues, 237

high fructose corn syrup and, 172–73

hypoglycemia and, 75–80, 85

pH/body chemistry and, 349

Type I (diabetes mellitus), 82–83

Type II (adult onset), 77, 79, 82–83, 211, 331

See also insulin

diagnostic testing

about Western medicine and, 270–74

blood test for FM, 219–20

cellular mitochondrial/ATP, 360–61, 390

DNA gene-snip test for FM, 67

fatty acids, 354, 390

finding the right doctor, 277–78

heavy metals, 177, 185

Lyme disease, 43

making a FM diagnosis, 274–81

plasma thiol test, 158, 187–88

results and retesting, 110–11

diarrhea, 22, 33, 61, 321. *See also* gut

diet and nutrition

advice for a healthy life, 206–07, 343

body chemistry and pH, 343–49

chemical stress, 81, 83–85

comprehensive nutrition, 101–02

concept of "treat the body, not the disease," 17–18

controlling stress with, 66–67

diabetes, 210–11, 331, 349, 353

dietary protein, 90–91, 206–08, 312, 316–17, 332

foods as a source of toxins, 165–68

functional medicine and, 41

linkage to FM, 349–50

overeating/emotional eating, 90–91

phosphorus/phosphate levels, 27–29, 219–20, 334

weight loss myth, 205

wheat-free diet, 14

See also carbohydrates; essential fatty acids; gluten/gluten sensitivity; sugar and sugar substitutes

diet soda, artificial sweeteners and, 160, 200–201

diffusion-weighted magnetic resonance imaging, 51

digestive system. *See* gut

digital palpation, 8–10, 34, 220

Dintyala, Kiran (Dr.), 261

disclaimer, iii

Dobbin, Michael (Dr.), 355

doctors - medical

choosing a rheumatologist vs. neurologist?, 11–12

defined/described, 248

education and training, 236

finding the right doctor, 126, 241–43, 265–69, 384

integration with non-medical services, 261–62

osteopaths, 21, 41, 72, 84–85, 100–101, 108, 128–29, 146–47, 254, 256

physician's assistant/nurse practitioner, 138

primary care physician (PCP)

finding the right doctor, 14

as part of a healthcare team, 227–28, 267–68

X
X-ray, 15, 51, 129, 370

Y
yerba dulce. *See* stevia
yoga, 71, 101, 132, 135–36, 138, 244, 264, 300–302, 335, 338

Z
The Zone: The Dietary Roadmap (Sears), 163
ZRT Laboratory, 314

Made in the USA
Charleston, SC
02 December 2015